# Community
# Health
# Nursing
## Second Edition

**KATHLEEN M. LEAHY, M.S., R.N.**
Professor Emeritus of Nursing
University of Washington, Seattle

**M. MARGUERITE COBB, M.N., R.N.**
Associate Professor of Nursing
University of Washington, Seattle

**MARY C. JONES, M.S., R.N.**
Assistant Professor of Nursing
University of Washington, Seattle

**McGRAW-HILL BOOK COMPANY**
A BLAKISTON PUBLICATION
New York     San Francisco     St. Louis     Düsseldorf
Johannesburg     Kuala Lumpur     London     Mexico
Montreal     New Delhi     Panama
Rio de Janeiro     Singapore     Sydney     Toronto

This book was set in Eterna Medium by Datagraphics, Inc., and printed and bound by R. R. Donnelley & Sons Company. The designer was Janet Bollow; the drawings were done by Judith McCarty. The editors were Cathy L. Dilworth and Eva Marie Strock. Charles A. Goehring supervised production.

**Community
Health
Nursing**

Printed in the United States of America.

Library of Congress catalog card number: 72-179080

7890  DODO  798765

07-036830-9

# Contents

Foreword by Madeleine Leininger    ix

Preface to Second Edition    xi

Preface to First Edition    xiii


## PART ONE

**1** Community Health and Community Health Nursing    3

**2** Relationship Skills    38

**3** Community Characteristics and Health Practices    74

**4** The Family    89

**5** The Home Visit    118

**6** The Community Health Nurse and Communication    168

**7** Family Nutrition    194

**8** Selected Concerns for Community Health Nurses    214

**9** The Community Health Nurse and Statistics    235

**10** History, Trends, and Philosophy of Community Health Nursing    258


## PART TWO

Introduction    279

### Case Situations

**1** A Failure in Communication    280

**2** Family Stress    281

**3** Planning the Teaching for a Mild Diabetic    282

**4** A Hospital Extension Program Patient    284

**5** Need—A Factor in Learning    286

**6** Recognition of a Nonverbal Communication    287

**7** Syphilis in an Itinerant Family    289

**8** A Family with an Alcoholic Member    290

**9** A Family's Reaction to Death    292

**10** A Family with a Mentally Ill Member    294

**11** A Marijuana Smoker    296

**Case Records**

**1** Stroke    298

**2** Rehabilitation    302

**3** Married Expectant Mother    306

**4** Single Expectant Mother    314

**5** Communicable Disease—Typhoid Fever    318

**6** Tuberculosis    323

**7** Terminal Cancer    327

**8** Venereal Disease    334

**9** Alcoholism    336

**10** Cuban Refugee Family    342

**11** Rediscovery of a Tuberculous Patient    346

**12** Infant Health Supervision    349

Index    354

# Foreword

In recent years we have been experiencing a world of unprecedented rapid changes, a world of hope for peace, a world of scientific knowledge explosion, and a world of diverse people with many different ideas and ways of living. We have not only felt the need to respond to these compelling cultural changes in our society, but we also have been trying to shape our future in light of these developments.

These American cultural trends well characterize some of the developments in the field of nursing, in which persistent efforts seek to make nursing a visible scientific and humanistic field sensitive to the needs of others. With the growing body of nursing knowledge and innovative nursing practices, nursing is rapidly becoming a specialized professional field. There are, however, a wealth of concepts and processes that remain relevant to the generalized health needs of people. These generalized needs are still the active concern of community health nurses in the profession.

Among the many changes in nursing is the central focus upon people who live in designated communities with health needs, interests, and cultural styles that challenge nurses to think anew in ways to understand and work effectively with people. The community concept and community groups with both special and general health needs must become a more integral part of *all* nursing theory and practice. It is logical that community health nurses are in a natural position to take the active leadership in spearheading the development of new and broad conceptualizations of nursing that need to be distinctly community-based and community-implemented. In the past, community health nurses have made some significant strides toward this goal; however, they have been handicapped by several educational, normative, and professional practices. The impact of institutional practices upon community health nursing has limited broad and new conceptualizations of community health for the future.

It is, indeed, an exciting and promising period in nursing and one in which nurses with strong community orientation can give leadership to new kinds of health care delivery practices, new roles in nursing practice, and new guidelines for undergraduate and graduate nursing programs. Nursing students of today are interested in becoming an active part of the new community focus and participating in the general changes in nursing.

The authors of this book are experienced leaders,

educators, and practitioners in community-based nursing. Through many years of experience they have worked closely with students, faculty, and community staff to help students use concepts and practices that support dynamic community nursing endeavors. They have been sensitive and amenable to changes occurring in the field of nursing and have integrated many concepts into community health nursing from the four major subfields of nursing and from the social sciences, natural sciences, and humanities, as well as from other health science fields.

This new edition identifies and clarifies content of and approaches to the practice of community health nursing. New content areas have been introduced, such as interpersonal relationship skills, working with groups, cultural concepts, the family, family nutrition, and communication factors in relating to people with different social and cultural backgrounds. These new areas greatly enhance the usefulness of the book. In addition, the authors have written the book with a focus on the nurse's understanding herself and others in order to be an effective health worker under diverse cultural, social, and economic conditions. The extremely rich student accounts of patient-nurse encounters and the analysis of these situations make this book especially valuable in helping the reader understand the many earthy kinds of problems that the nurse encounters in the helping process.

Another noteworthy feature of the book is its emphasis on the problem solving approach as an important means of identifying and examining nursing problems in light of multiple factors and circumstances. This book has a warm and sensitive approach to the needs and proclivities of nursing students as they work with people under varying kinds of stress. The reader can cast herself into common community-based problems and explore the problems of common life situations. The authors are to be highly commended for making the above additions to enrich the book. This new material should help the student realistically face today's world of community health nursing.

**Madeleine Leininger, Ph.D., R.N.**
Professor of Nursing
Lecturer in Anthropology
Dean, School of Nursing
University of Washington, Seattle

x

Many years ago, Winston Churchill warned the world that scientists were at the point of having "the keys to all the chambers hitherto forbidden to mankind." Churchill believed that without an equal development of such attributes as mercy, pity, peace, and love, science could not only destroy itself, but all that makes life "majestic and tolerable."

The many momentous changes that have occurred in recent years may substantiate Churchill's foreboding (see Preface to first edition). The attendant problems of recent change highlight the new responsibilities for the community health nurse who, by means of her knowledge, skills, understanding, and appreciation, can help to avoid that destruction of all that makes human life "majestic and tolerable."

Changes in society's social attitudes and patterns of living, such as political philosophy, social mores, industrialization, transportation (even to the moon), housing, food, and dress all have an impact on community health nursing today.

For example, many individuals feel that they are unable to cope with either change or the *lack* of change; this has brought about an increase in suicide attempts at all levels of society. The use of drugs to escape life's situations has become a habit for some people. The apparent efforts of some drug users to "kick" the habit and return to society provide a challenge to health workers to meet those efforts with understanding, knowledge, and objectivity and to assist the individual to find and establish new life values in his return to both mental and physical health.

Recognizing the changes that have taken place and, at the same time, some of the old problems that remain as before, the authors have tried in their revision of *Community Health Nursing* to help the student see some of the evolving phases of the work. The term *public health nursing* has been changed to *community health nursing* as being more applicable to the field of health nursing today. The terms *nurse* and *community health nurse* are used interchangeably throughout the book; usually *community health nurse* is used for emphasis and clarity. As in the previous edition, the authors have presented a discussion of the field, and by means of case situations and case records have attempted to show what the nurse can do for patients, families, and community.

The aim of the book is to present community health nursing for all nursing students desiring to become acquainted with its practice. Since it is anticipated that health services will be focused increasingly in the community setting rather than the institutional setting, the content of this book is intended to stimulate comprehensive nursing practices that will effectively meet the existing health needs of all citizens. Although the book recognizes new developments in the health care field, it does not present a complete discussion of the community health nursing field and must be implemented by the instructor's own philosophy, experience, and knowledge of community health nursing.

Miss Mary C. Jones, Assistant Professor of Nursing, University of Washington, who has wide experience in community health agencies, has become a coauthor of this book.

We are grateful for the interest and assistance of many of our friends and coworkers in community health fields. We appreciate particularly the helpful suggestions of Miss Gladys H. Mathewson, Nutrition Consultant, Community Health Services, U.S.P.H.S., Mrs. Margaret Willhoit James, Nursing Consultant, Community Health Services, U.S.P.H.S. (ret.), and the written contributions of former nursing students, who, by sharing their feelings and experiences with their nurse instructors, have added the extra dimension of humanistic appeal to the book.

**Kathleen M. Leahy**
**M. Marguerite Cobb**
**Mary C. Jones**

Writing in *The Lancet* some time ago, Sir Francis Fraser pointed out that a "fundamental difficulty for universities is how to develop the specialization needed to train their graduates for careers in technical callings" [referring to medical students] "and at the same time insist on the broad education which it is their traditional aim to provide."[1]

For many years collegiate schools of nursing have contended with this problem, which becomes more pronounced with the steadily increasing body of scientific knowledge that must be included in today's curriculum for the nurse. In curriculum committees, faculties ponder how to ensure that nursing students will secure the necessary preparation in science and at the same time acquire a sound background in the humanities.

Foreseeing the future, Winston Churchill wrote in 1932, "The busy hands of the scientists are already fumbling with the keys of all the chambers hitherto forbidden to mankind. Without the equal growth of Mercy, Pity, Peace and Love, science herself may destroy all that makes human life majestic and tolerable."[2]

With this in mind, the writers have tried not only to present the fundamentals of public health nursing but also, by means of case situations and case records, to illustrate what public health nurses do and to show that more than a knowledge of the natural, physical, and behavioral sciences, valuable as they are, is essential for today's nurse.

This book, then, presents some fundamentals of public health nursing for basic-degree students in collegiate programs of nursing. It is not a complete discussion of the field, for the writers recognize that instructors will wish to develop their teaching in the light of their own public health nursing experiences and the philosophy of the individual schools of nursing in each college or university. The writers suggest that this book be used as a basis for classroom discussion and for student reading, implemented by current professional literature, not only in nursing and in the public health sciences, but also in the supporting disciplines such as sociology, psychology, cultural anthropology, and the humanities. Some instructors may wish to use this book as supplemental reading to help the student, early in her pro-

[1]Sir Francis Fraser, "Power and Responsibility," *The Lancet.* 262:61–64, 1952.
[2]*Ibid.*

gram, gain insight into the work of the public health nurse and into the community approach to all nursing.

Since students in collegiate schools of nursing learn to use the problem-solving approach in all their work, it seemed appropriate to present some basic principles of public health nursing that the writers, through their experiences in working with families and in their classroom and field teaching, believe to be essential to the safe, effective practice of public health nursing. For the purposes of this presentation, Lambertsen's statement that a principle might be considered "an accepted truth, the evidence of which might be empirical or scientific" was accepted.[3] It is recognized that many of these principles, discussed in Chap. 2, are inherent in all nursing, but attention is called to their application in public health nursing practice.

The case situations and case records in Part Two have been selected from agency records in many parts of the country. Names and other identifying material have been changed. Some of the cases were carried by senior students in collegiate schools of nursing during their field experiences, and others were selected from the files of both rural and urban agencies. In some instances certain principles were violated; but the case material was not selected for the perfection of the work done. Rather, it was chosen for its value in illustrating some of the needs of patient, family, and community that were encountered by the public health nurse and how she met them.

In some situations, the nurse is inadequate to meet the needs of the family. This may be not only because of her own deficiencies but also because of lacks in the agency program and the community resources, as well as the inability of the patient and family to accept and utilize the help offered by the nurse. What knowledge and skills is it essential for the nurse to have in order to meet these needs? This was the central thought in preparing this book. The discussion topics at the end of each case situation and case record were designed to bring this question to the attention of the student.

The terms *nurse* and *public health nurse* are used interchangeably throughout the book. For the most part public health nurse is used for clarity or emphasis.

[3]Eleanor C. Lambertsen, *Education for Nursing Leadership*, J. B. Lippincott Company, Philadelphia, 1958, p. vi.

We are grateful for the interest of our many friends and colleagues, and for their encouragement and support. We appreciate particularly the helpful comments and suggestions of Miss Ann Hill, Associate Professor of Public Health Nursing, School of Nursing, University of California Medical Center, San Francisco; Miss Edna J. Brandt, Chief, Bureau of Nursing, California State Department of Health; Dr. Ole Sand, National Education Association, Washington, D.C.; and Dr. Blair M. Bennett, Associate Professor of Preventive Medicine, School of Medicine, University of Washington, Seattle, all of whom read parts of the manuscript; and the cooperation of Miss Josephine Hawes, Assistant Professor, School of Nursing, Stanford University, and the instructors in schools of nursing and supervisors in public health agencies who so generously shared illustrative case material from their files.

**Kathleen M. Leahy**
**M. Marguerite Cobb**

# PART ONE

**1**
Community
Health
and
Community
Health
Nursing

## COMMUNITY HEALTH

The promotion and improvement of man's total health has a significant bearing on the social revolution now in progress throughout the world (see *The Family of Man*). New thinking and approaches to better health care become mandatory in solving such long-term problems as lack of sanitation, insufficient food and clothing, inadequate housing, and control of communicable diseases and such noncommunicable disease conditions as heart disease, accidents, or disaster. Emerging problems of family pathology, drug abuse and addiction, air and water pollution, polarization of the races, and overpopulation require new methods of solution. Increased scientific knowledge and more imaginative skills and techniques in teaching health care are in order for all community health work.

Community health or public health as a profession had its beginnings about a hundred years ago. Its early responsibility was the control of communicable disease, which was attempted by such measures as control of environment, better sanitation, and strict isolation procedures, particularly for typhoid fever and tuberculosis. As laboratory techniques were developed from increased knowledge of microbiology earlier diagnoses became possible and medical care became more effective. Other control measures also were developed, such as immunization and the provision of safe water supplies and waste disposal.

Gradually the six basic functions of public health evolved—communicable disease control, environmental sanitation, laboratory services, vital statistics, maternal and child health care, and health education. Public health agencies began to base their programs on these six functions, the emphasis being on people. To carry out these functions effectively school and industrial health programs

3

were developed, since large segments of the population could be reached in this way.

Community health programs built on the six basic functions, including school and industrial health programs, continue to be important, but nearly every nation is experiencing *new* health hazards that demand fresh approaches to their solutions. Problems stemming from the population explosion include environmental problems of overcrowding, air and water pollution, accidents, and, frequently, drug abuse and alcoholism. Current pollution of the environment affects not only human beings and domestic animals, but also fish and wildlife in many parts of the world. This presents a pressing need for concerted community action as well as action on an international basis. Finally, there is the urgent need of many people for more care from the medical and paramedical professions—care that is better organized and equally available to all segments of society.

Public health appears to be shifting its emphasis to both people and environment, accentuating the relationship of the *total* man to his *total* environment. Underlying this ecologic approach to public health is the vast amount of knowledge that has been accumulated within the past fifty years in the biologic, physical, and social sciences that must be adapted and utilized by the several professions, e.g., medicine, nursing, dentistry, and engineering in the public health field. The field of public and community health becomes "the meeting ground of all areas of knowledge and professional activity relevant to the health of the public."[1]

## Community Health Nursing

A description or definition of community health nursing should be based on an understanding and appreciation of the entire spectrum of nursing. Virginia Henderson considers the function of the present-day nurse to be unique. It is, she writes, "to assist the individual, sick or well, in the performance of those activities contributing to health or its recovery (or to peaceful death) that he would perform if he had the necessary strength, will or knowledge. And to do this in such a way as to help him gain independence as rapidly as possible."[2]

Health teaching and counseling and the skilled care of the sick in their homes by community health nurses from official or voluntary health agencies is recognized as an essential service in the community's total health program. The nurse functions within the framework of both the nursing and the public health professions, utilizing effectively her knowledge of the

[1]Hilary G. Fry, in collaboration with William P. Shepard and Ray H. Elling, *Education for Manpower and Community Health*, The University of Pittsburgh Press, Pittsburgh, 1967, p. 8.
[2]Virginia Henderson, "The Nature of Nursing," *The American Journal of Nursing*, 64:64–68 (August) 1964.

content and methods of both professions in her service to the individual patient, his family, and the community.

## Community Health Nursing Practice Defined
In 1969 the following definition was established:

> Community health nursing practice is a synthesis of nursing practice and public health practice applied to promoting and preserving the health of populations. The nature of this practice is general and comprehensive; not limited to a particular age or diagnostic group; it is continuing not episodic. The dominant responsibility is to the population as a whole. Therefore, nursing directed to individuals, families or groups becomes a valid component of the practice as it intrinsically relates to and contributes to the health of the total population.[3]

## Concepts of Community Health Nursing Practice
Based on the above definition, six concepts of community health nursing practice were stated to be:

1.  The primary focus of community health nursing practice is on health promotion. The community health nurse has a greater contact with people who are seeking health care—to "reach" the community—and has more opportunity and responsibility for evaluating the health status of such persons and groups and relating them to practice.

2.  Although the primary concern and initial contact with a family may be with or in relation to an individual, community health nursing practice is extended to benefit the whole family and community.

3.  The community health nurse is a generalist in terms of her practice throughout life's continuum—its full range of health problems and needs.

4.  Contact with patient and/or family may continue over a long period of time—include all ages and all types of health care.

5.  The nature of community health nursing practice requires that current knowledge derived from the biological and social sciences, ecology, clinical nursing and community organization be utilized.

6.  The dynamic nursing process of assessing, planning, implementing and intervening, periodic measurements of progress, evaluation and a continuum of the cycle until termination of nursing is implicit in the practice of community health nursing.[4]

---

[3]The Executive Committee, Division on Community Health Nursing Practice, American Nurses' Association, New York, 1969.
[4]*Ibid.*

## FUNCTIONS AND SETTING

The community health nurse encounters problems and conditions never imagined by her predecessors. In addition to conditions previously mentioned, the nurse meets such situations as poverty amid affluence, urban sprawl and decay, social injustices, racial strife and tensions, and in many areas, a decline in the quality and integrity of community life and efforts to improve it. Facing these situations requires marked objectivity on the part of the nursing and public health professions, coupled with the realization that specific knowledge and skills are essential in contributing to the solution.

The family (see Chap. 2) is usually the unit of service for the nurse; therefore the major part of community health nursing is carried on in the home, where health care is needed for patients of all ages. In many communities there is an increasing demand for skilled geriatric nursing, largely for the following reasons:

**1.** The increasing number of elderly people in the population, with many living alone rather than as part of a family group, as in former generations

**2.** The growing incidence of chronic diseases usually found in older age groups, e.g., cancer and cardiac vascular conditions

**3.** The emphasis placed today by the medical and nursing professions on commencing rehabilitation of the patient at the onset of the disease or disabling condition or as early as possible

In her contact with the patient and family, the nurse needs to develop opportunities and plans for teaching health concepts and practices to all members involved. Many parents need help in understanding and appreciating the growth and development—physical, mental, and emotional—of their children at different age levels, including infancy (the terrible twos and the trusting threes), school age, adolescence, and early maturity. Parents sometimes need assistance in guiding their children to learn to accept the demands for living, not only within their own group, but to learn to understand, respect, accept, live, and work with people of other races, cultures, mores, religions, and backgrounds.

When entering the home, the nurse is responsible for teaching the patient or the family member or other person available for his daily care. This requires a sound knowledge of underlying principles of the physical, biologic, and social sciences, as well as the ability to teach, demonstrate, and use nursing skills, such as the application of sterile dressings to an open, draining wound to minimize the spread of infection and to teach the safe disposal of dressings that have been saturated with drainage. Although a comparatively simple procedure, it requires, if done safely, that the nurse have a knowledge of microbiology, anatomy and physiology, sanitation, and psychology, as well as a deft, sure nursing skill.

The nurse is concerned with the health of the entire family including those in school, industrial plants, and other places of work, as well as those in the home when she visits. She must be aware of extraneous community health hazards, such as poor housing conditions, insufficient and unsafe water supply and waste disposal facilities, faulty fire protection and traffic safety. She must be cognizant of possible sources of disease in the community and the routes of spread and methods of their control.

The scope of the nurse's activities in the school setting is changing. In 1902, when the first school nursing program was initiated in the New York City schools through the efforts of Lillian Wald, the nurse's work consisted mainly of first aid and communicable disease control. Now the nurse's work is more that of a health counselor and adviser for general health and nutrition matters and in mental and emotional health, with such problems as drug abuse and teen-age pregnancies. The nurse works closely with teachers, students, and parents in helping to meet and work through these problems.

Nurses participating in health programs in industry and other places of employment find the emphasis there changing also. Although first aid and health and safety supervision continue to be important activities, there is an increasing need for health education and health counseling for adults in general health practices such as physical activities, rest, nutrition, mental and emotional health, and mild chronic diseases.

A new dimension being added in community health nursing is the mental and emotional health services and their integration into the other services the nurse can offer in the home, the school, and places of employment. This integration has been triggered by a wider knowledge and awareness of the behavioral sciences, a developing recognition by communities of their responsibilities toward their emotionally disturbed citizens, and a growing understanding of the value of the nurse-patient and nurse-family relationships. Possibly, by the end of the twentieth century, these and other services will have made an impact on the health aspects of people and communities similar to those results brought about by the control of diphtheria, smallpox, poliomyelitis, and insectborne diseases in the past century. These changing social and health patterns have been the impetus for new and experimental programs and activities in community health services, including nursing.

The need is growing for more nursing services in the home that will provide bedside care and health supervision to patients of all ages and social and economic backgrounds. There is some increase in nursing services through the provisions for nursing care and supervision in the various health insurance plans, both private and governmental, in programs for rehabilitation nursing in the home, and programs for continuity of medical and nursing care between hospital and home in urban and rural areas. This increase in service to patients and families in their homes widens opportunities for teaching principles and practice of positive health, as well as for nursing care of the ill. Group teaching is increasing wherever the nurse can bring like-interest groups together for such classes as prenatal care, child care, nutrition, and home nursing. The nurse should be on the alert for opportunities to develop such classes in housing projects, health centers, or prenatal clinics.

## AGENCIES
In a community health nursing program, the nurse works within the framework of an organization set up to carry out certain health-related functions in the community. These organizations may be "official" or "nonofficial" (voluntary) agencies. Official agencies are tax-supported; nonofficial agencies have various sources of support, such as gifts, patient fees, United Fund or United Crusade, and contracts with insurance companies and with Medicare and Medicaid.

Examples of official agencies are the Public Health Service, state health departments, and county, district, or city health departments. Examples of voluntary or nonofficial agencies include visiting nurse services which provide bedside care in the home or the agency having private sources of income whose function is to assist in meeting certain community health problems. The American Heart Association and its components is such an agency. Official and voluntary health agencies are generally referred to as "public health agencies" or "community health agencies." They are concerned with the health of the entire community and serve all citizens.

## THE UNITED STATES CONSTITUTION AND PUBLIC HEALTH
The United States Constitution, adopted in 1787, provided in article I, section 8, that the Federal government shall have the power to provide for the general welfare of the United States, and to regulate commerce with foreign powers and among the several states. On this basis and within the limitations of this authority, the newly established Federal government became the responsible agent for

1.  Those health matters in the new country that involved interstate and international relations
2.  Scientific research for the general welfare[5]

---

[5]Harry S. Mustard, *Rural Health Practice,* The Commonwealth Fund, New York, 1936, p. 3.

The Tenth Amendment to the Constitution, as quoted by Mustard, provided that "powers not delegated to the United States by the Constitution, nor prohibited to it by the States, are reserved to the states respectively, or to the people."[6] Therefore the ordinary day-to-day health problems within the confines of a given state and their solutions became the responsibilities of that state.

The American colonies had had individual experiences in caring for sick merchant seamen. Influenced by the British system of collecting "hospital money" from sailors' wages for their care while ill, the seaports of New York, Boston, and Norfolk, Virginia, had undertaken similar programs prior to 1780. At its beginning session in 1789, the First Congress of the United States recognized an obligation to care for sick and disabled seamen by appointing a committee to prepare a bill or bills which would provide for the establishment of hospitals for sick and disabled seamen, both American and foreign.


## THE PUBLIC HEALTH SERVICE

The agency now known as the Public Health Service of the Department of Health, Education and Welfare was established in 1798. Its main work then was to protect the young nation from disease from without by providing hospitals for ill and injured American and foreign seamen, and to protect the country as a whole from diseases that might spread from one state to another.

Although these original functions are still important, other functions have developed to meet increasing health needs. These include: (1) to carry on research and training in medical and related sciences and community health administration; (2) to aid communities in their planning and development of hospitals, health centers, and related facilities; and (3) to assist states and possessions with finances and trained personnel to apply new knowledge in prevention and control of diseases, maintenance of healthful environments, and development of appropriate community health services.

Medicine, nursing, dentistry, epidemiology, engineering, veterinary science, health education, nutrition, and biostatistics are among the disciplines making specific contributions to the carrying out of these functions. Effective use also is being made of the social sciences. Anthropology, psychology, sociology, political science, and public administration have enabled health workers to gain increased knowledge and understanding of people, aiding them in their work with patients, families, neighborhoods, and the wider community.

[6] *Ibid.*

## STATE HEALTH DEPARTMENTS

Massachusetts established the first state board of health in 1869. Today, all fifty states have health departments functioning as a recognized part of state government. These departments are charged with the responsibility for assisting local health departments—city, county, district—to promote health in all its phases and provide the safest possible environment for all members of the community.

State health departments are administered in most states by qualified health officers assisted by staff drawn from the many public health disciplines mentioned previously. Other specialists are added depending on the types of industries, health problems, and hazards peculiar to any one state. Each state develops individual programs according to its own needs and resources. Health programs appropriate to Alaska might not meet the needs or be feasible in Kansas or Connecticut.

In the early part of this century programs were developed to meet pressing community health needs. These programs were built on the "six basic functions" mentioned before. Programs were developed around these functions, with nursing participating to some degree in all of them. While it is still important to carry out *these* functions, other functions and programs have become necessary if current community problems are to be attacked. In addition to those previously mentioned, these problems include an increase in recognized mental illness, the need to provide and extend medical care, the toll of accidents with resultant deaths or severe disabling injuries, the increase in drug addiction, alcoholism, and venereal diseases, and the need for family planning and, in some states, abortion counseling.

Some state health departments provide direct services, including community health nursing service to local communities. This may be done for demonstration purposes or, especially in remote areas, from necessity because of a lack of local facilities or scarcity of nursing personnel.

A trend apparent in some states is combination of state departments of welfare and health into one organization. There is insufficient experience at present to determine the feasibility of this move. Students should watch for developments of this and similar trends in their own states.

## LOCAL HEALTH DEPARTMENTS

Many counties in the fifty states have county, bicounty or tricounty health departments or health districts. The idea of a county health department originated in 1911. The first such departments were in Yakima County, Washington, and Guilford County, North Carolina, and they were set up almost simultaneously. In Yakima County an organization was needed to control a typhoid fever epidemic, and in Guilford County health promotion of school children was the immediate objective. All large cities and many smaller ones have municipal health departments, some having functioned since the beginning of the nineteenth century, when their main interest was the control of communicable diseases.

The legal basis for the authority of municipal, county, or district health departments lies in the laws of the several states and in the rules and regulations that define the mandatory activities of local government units relating to health matters. Local ordinances may define additional activities.

Historically, local health departments have come to be charged with responsibilities for (1) developing programs based on the health needs of the community; (2) providing necessary facilities and qualified staff to carry out these programs; and (3) making surveys of community needs and evaluating existing programs as necessary to ensure that these responsibilities are being met. Most local health departments developed their programs around the basic six functions, placing emphasis on the most pressing current problems; for instance, at one time tuberculosis, with its high incidence and death rates, was the most pressing problem in many communities. Health departments in those communities devoted much medical and nursing time to the prevention and control of this disease.

The nucleus of any local health department staff continues to be the health officer (usually a physician), the nurse, the environmental specialist, and the secretary, who is responsible for keeping records and vital statistics. Local programs were and still are instituted and maintained depending on community interest, health needs, budgets, the vision and leadership of the professional staff, and staff availability. As communities come to recognize their health needs and to demand additional professional services, they are more willing to support increased budgets for programs and staff.

With the shift of emphasis from concern for environment to greater concern for people, health departments are changing their roles. This results in part from laws recently enacted in the 1960s by the United States Congress in relation to Social Security. Some states followed the Federal government and passed similar legislation to meet emerging health problems in their jurisdiction.

This period of transition from the old, accepted "prevention" programs to the wider, more comprehensive, and direct approach to the solutions of health problems with emphasis on the individual and his family, raises questions regarding the adequacy of health departments as now organized and administered to meet current problems. Many shifts of practice and emphasis in the health organizations and their administration will become necessary in the near future. There is need also for a careful appraisal and the spending of available financial resources so that the greatest benefit for all people in the community may be obtained, for air pollution and other environmental hazards directly or indirectly affect the health of people in every part of a community.

This changing concept of community health needs should be implemented by constant study and evaluation of health problems of the individual—such as physical and mental diseases, physical defects, and maternal and child health needs—and of environmental dangers—such as traffic accidents, poor housing, and unsafe dairies and other sources of foods. Following such studies, programs for community protection and safety can be established. The social and economic components of illness must be considered in any assessment and program planning.

Within the metropolitan areas, population shifts have modified the needs for certain health programs and services, and intensified the needs for others. For example, the child population tends to be centered in the suburbs today, thus increasing the needs there for more maternal and child health services; an older age group tends to become centered in cities, necessitating such programs as nursing homes and long-term home nursing services. Furthermore, it is becoming obvious that the child population remaining in the metropolitan areas is to be found, for the most part, in the dependent and low-income groups, who have many health needs.

Many urban, suburban, and rural communities in the past two decades have been experimenting with methods of merging local health departments. The weight of their experiences has shown that essential health services can be maintained with greater efficiency and economy and more effective use of staffs by a combined agency of some type. Various patterns of merged health agencies have been developed by communities, depending on local needs, resources, customs, government, and the interest and participation of the citizens.

Mergers range from a permanent consolidation of two or more agencies into a "combined health district" to the "contract-for-services" type, which allows for an annual contract between two or more health agencies or health departments, stating the specific services to be rendered by one agency to another and the financial obligations and administrative responsibilities involved.

The experiences of agencies that serve wide geographic areas show that communities can be served more efficiently if there is a decentralization to several health districts but with all of them functioning under the same health department policies and practices. Community planning for health programs will continue, but in order to meet new needs and to provide better and more efficient health services, other approaches to health agency reorganization must be developed and tested.

## INTERNATIONAL HEALTH ORGANIZATIONS

Agencies with public health programs function on an international level also. Two whose programs are particularly related to health are the World Health Organization and the Food and Agricultural Organization, member agencies of the United Nations.

## World Health Organization

After World War II many nations became aware of the need for global cooperation in health matters. This concern led to the founding of the World Health Organization (WHO) in 1948. In setting up its constitution, the WHO defined health to be "a state of complete physical, mental and social well being, and not merely the absence of disease or infirmity."[7] Article I of the constitution states that the objective of the WHO "shall be the attainment by all peoples of the highest possible level of health."[8]

This organization is a coordinating and cooperating body. Representatives from each member nation comprise the WHO assembly, which meets annually, usually in the spring, to vote the budget, hear reports, and confirm programs. Supervision of the various programs is the responsibility of the Executive Committee. The Secretariat Headquarters are in Geneva, Switzerland, and there are six Regional Offices located in Copenhagen, for the European area; Alexandria, for the Mediterranean area; Brazzaville, for the remainder of Africa; New Delhi, for Southeast Asia; Manila, for the Western area; and Washington, D.C., for the Americas.

The major part of the financial support of the WHO comes from its 127 (1969) member nations. Requests for financial assistance and trained personnel for desired programs are usually presented by governments through their ministries of health to the Regional Office for consideration and study. For example, a request for assistance with a maternal-child health program in Taiwan would be sent to the Regional Office in Manila. If deemed feasible and in order, it would be approved and forwarded to the General Headquarters in Geneva for further approval and implementation.

By means of its annual spring meetings and the work of its regional conferences and Expert Committees, which consider the many health problems facing countries around the globe, WHO provides valuable exchange of ideas and of expert knowledge. Much of this has been published in several languages and distributed worldwide.

The WHO has nearly twenty-five years of international health experience. Although striking advances have been made in meeting many health problems, they are not all solved by far, and work must continue. The health potential of nations handicapped by centuries of economic difficulties, social restrictions, and lack of technical skills and knowledge has not been realized. In many countries health services are yet to be developed, well-trained personnel continue to be in short supply, and some countries report little progress in health planning. Some countries also have grave problems of overpopulation. Qualified manpower is an increasing problem in many nations.

[7]Neville M. Goodman, *International Health Organizations*, J. and A. Churchill, Ltd., London, 1952, p. 187.
[8]*Ibid.*, p. 188.

## Food and Agricultural Organization

The Food and Agricultural Organization (FAO) is another widely known specialized agency of the United Nations concerned with health at the international level. It was founded in 1945. The need for this agency was evident when it was recognized at the end of World War II that two-thirds of the world's population was undernourished and that its health would be greatly improved by adequate nutrition. FAO's organization is somewhat similar to that of WHO but is not so extensive. The headquarters of its Secretariat are in Rome.

The FAO has six major programs: (1) Agriculture; (2) Economics, Marketing and Statistics; (3) Forestry; (4) Fisheries; (5) Nutrition; and (6) Rural Welfare. It has carried out special studies in nutrition and agriculture in many parts of the world, especially in the developing countries.

The FAO works closely with the WHO in their common interests in human welfare, nutrition, and improved sanitation in rural areas. This was dramatically emphasized in the 1950s, when expansion of food production in a potentially fertile area in Southeast Asia became possible owing to a successful WHO program of malaria control in that region.

## COMMUNITY HEALTH NURSING AGENCIES

Many members of different social and economic groups in society have a growing awareness of the intrinsic value of health to each individual. There is an increasing recognition that health is no longer a *privilege* of the few who can pay for it, but a *right* to which every citizen is entitled. There is a definite trend on the part of many communities to accept this belief and to regard adequate health services as one of the responsibilities of government. Communities are realizing, more and more, that not only is a healthful environment essential but that health services and health supervision are basic to the maintenance of the health of the entire community. This has led to an increase in the number of agencies organized to provide nursing service in homes, health centers, schools, and places of employment.

### Support, Responsibilities, and Programs

An agency conducting programs in community health nursing of some type or other may be classified as a public, official, or governmental agency,[9] or as a private, nonofficial, or voluntary agency.[10]

A community health nursing agency formed by the merging of two or more agencies may receive support from both public and private sources.

[9]The terms *public, official,* and *governmental* are used here interchangeably in referring to a health agency administered by a department of health.
[10]The terms *private, voluntary,* and *nonofficial* are used here interchangeably in referring to a community health nursing agency not administered by a health department.

Such an agency is referred to in a number of ways, depending on its organization pattern. Some are known as "combination services." Health agencies with either public or private support have existed in this country in some form or other for about one hundred fifty years. Agencies described as public, official, or governmental are usually tax-supported. Those described as private, voluntary, or nonofficial receive most of their support from private sources, such as united funds, health-insurance groups, gifts, contributions, endowments, and patient payment for services. Medicare and Medicaid funds may be used to pay these agencies for nursing services rendered. Previously, one clear difference between the two general types of organization was that tax-supported agencies had certain obligations and restrictions imposed on them by law or by rules and regulations, while private agencies, less restricted, were freer to carry on experimentation and demonstration in new fields of community health service. This distinction is disappearing and currently many agencies with public support are able to budget for some experimentation and research. Another type of community nursing service is appearing in some large cities, a proprietary agency. Usually it is an extension of private proprietary hospitals or nursing homes into the community. Sources of support are private patient fees and such funds as Medicare or Medicaid. In general these agencies are required to meet the rules and regulations of the state department of health in the state where they function.

Tax-supported health agencies are to be found on the various governmental levels—Federal, state, county, or municipal and township. Agencies on any one of these levels usually function with the advice of boards of health comprised of professional and lay members. Under the law in some states, the county boards of supervisors or commissioners form the county boards of health. In other states, the county boards of health are appointed in various ways. These boards of health may act as interpreters of the community to the agencies' professional staffs, and also as interpreters of the agency staff to the community. Their contribution can be on a two-way basis.

Privately supported agencies carry on health programs on a national, state, county, or municipal and township basis. An example is the National Tuberculosis Association with its component state and county associations. A visiting nurse association is an example of a private agency on the local level. There is no national organization of visiting nurse associations in the United States such as exists in some countries, e.g., Canada.

The responsibility for the health of the community rests not only with the official health department but also with the medical, dental, nursing, and allied professions, with voluntary health agencies, hospitals, schools, and, most of all, with the general public or the community itself. Each community develops its own health patterns at its own rate of speed. It must have freedom of choice in the type and scope of its health programs. Through its members, the community should participate responsibly in the overall planning of the work, to its interpretation, and to its implementation. The final responsibility for the health of the community lies with the appointed health officer (usually a physician), for he has the necessary legal authority. The community has delegated this authority to him in his appointment, and he is considered to be the community's health expert. Hanlon says that he [the health officer], "by virtue of his position, is ultimately responsible for all phases of the health program of the department, and for that matter, of the community as a whole."[11]

A well-prepared staff is essential to an agency's program if the services are to meet the health needs of the community. These needs are not static but change with the developing social, economic, industrial, and health conditions in the community. For example, an industry moving into a new community might create certain health hazards, such as the need for safe waste disposal or for air pollution control. It might create also an urgent need for additional housing for its employees. For some communities this would cause such problems as an increased need for health services, additional school facilities, playfields, and shopping centers. On the other hand, the construction of a new expressway might necessitate destruction of many homes, apartment buildings, and other living facilities, resulting in families and individuals having to move to other parts of the community, thus increasing the needs for health and other services elsewhere.

Health programs should be flexible, designed in terms of both the needs and resources of the community, and capable of modification to meet new problems pertaining to health as they arise. Certain health programs, so important to the community in the past, have served their purpose.

Planning for health programs in neighborhoods or communities should involve the expression of needs, thinking, and participation of the local inhabitants, as the local area is their home and they are aware of many facets of community living that professional workers would have no way of knowing. If the residents of these communities make mistakes in their planning and decisions, it's their community and their mistake, and they will soon recognize it and work out other solutions. They may need a new health center that could be utilized by all community members, and they could suggest certain locations where few opposing forces would be evident. For example, in a low-socioeconomic neighborhood, the location of a health center near a police station may act as a deterrent for some citizens. The suggestions of the local citizens regarding the best location should be

[11]John J. Hanlon, *Principles of Public Health Administration,* 4th ed., The C. V. Mosby Company, St. Louis, 1964, p. 458.

heeded. When they participate as planners, leadership qualities appear, on which professional workers can build (see *9226 Kercheval,* by Nancy Milio).

The professional workers have certain responsibilities for the safety aspects for programs such as traffic hazards, sanitation and environmental health, control of population density, and satisfactory layouts for sewage systems and control of surface drainage. Even in these programs, local residents should be kept informed and their advice sought and heeded. They should have the responsibility for decisions for locations of health centers, schools, and recreational facilities such as playgrounds, parks, and libraries in their area.

This shift in the philosophy of community health work has occurred for several reasons, some old and some new. When health programs were being developed years ago, many people were new arrivals from European countries or were from rural areas seeking industrial employment and unaware of city ways. They accepted what was available to them in health services but had no thought of participation. Their descendents are products of the American schools and they are eager, for the most part, to participate in their own neighborhood and community development, where they have become property owners, earn their living, and raise their families.

Today's public health programs must provide for continuous comprehensive services to the community, prevention as well as care, including nursing service to patients in their homes as needed, with rehabilitation as an integral part of all phases of the work. The age shifts in population, and the increase in degenerative diseases in all ages, today demand health programs with a different focus from those of the past. These new programs should meet the need for control and care of cancer, the prevention and care of cardiac diseases, the prevention and care of mental diseases, and the necessary rehabilitative measures. Public health agencies must plan to meet these new and different problems and to revise their programs with the help of their citizens' committees as they review community needs each year.

### Visiting Nurse Agencies

Beginning in the early 1880s in this country, a growing sense of community responsibility on the part of many citizens led to the establishment, under private auspices, of visiting nurse associations, particularly in such large Eastern cities as Buffalo, Philadelphia, Boston, and Baltimore. These agencies differed from the existing official health agencies as they were founded for the sole purpose of sending graduate nurses into homes—usually the homes of the poor—for the care of new mothers and their babies and for the care of the sick. From their inception the visiting nurse organizations in this country emphasized the teaching function of the public health nurse,

and frequently the word "instructive" appeared in the name of the organization, as the "Instructive District Nursing Association of Baltimore."

These organizations drew inspiration from similar organizations commenced five to ten years earlier in some of the big industrial cities of England. The British set up a national organization for the development of
visiting nursing in the home, with definite standards for staff qualifications,
agency records, procedures, and uniforms. Local organizations were responsible to the national organization for maintaining these standards.
However, in this country, each visiting nurse association developed independently, with little interagency contact until the National Organization for
Public Health Nursing, one of the forerunners of the present National
League for Nursing, was founded in 1912. The National Organization for
Public Health Nursing provided for membership of nurses, of laity, and of
agencies. It gave board members and directors of nursing services an opportunity to discuss and attack their problems with those who were carrying
on similar programs in other communities.

The visiting nurse organizations were governed by boards of directors
of interested citizens, usually women, who gave freely of their time and
effort to the development of these agencies. In recent years, men have
shown an increasing interest in the administration and development of this
type of community service, and today many agencies have men serving on
their boards. Many boards found it advantageous to incorporate under state
laws. Through experience, boards of directors learned to see their responsibilities as determining policies, setting up rules and regulations governing
agency services, selecting the director of nursing services, and raising most
of the necessary funds to finance the work.

As communities came to recognize the contribution these agencies
made to the health and social betterment of its citizens, financing became
less of a problem. In many cities, agencies were able to secure some assistance from united fund drives. Contracts with insurance companies to provide nursing services to their policy holders for a stated fee, as well as
similar contracts with certain industries for home nursing services to their
employees, became sources of further financial aid. Furthermore, a growing
concept that community health nursing was not a charity but should be
available to all in the community, families paying for the nursing service
according to their financial abilities, increased the scope and financial resources of many agencies. Relief from some of the financial pressures for
agency support enabled boards of directors to give more time to the study
of community needs in relation to public health nursing services and, with
the director of the nursing service, to make long-range plans for meeting
them.

A letter by Miss Nightingale to the *London Times* in 1876 regarding
the London district nurses gives an interesting sidelight on the matter of

families paying for community health nursing services according to their abilities. She wrote:

> The present Association wants to foster the spirit of work (not relief) in the district nurse, and for her to foster the same in her sick poor.
>
> Nor are these District Nurses without hearing and receiving evidence that this spirit is now becoming really understood among the sick.
>
> One poor old woman was heard saying to her younger neighbor: "Them nurses is real blessings: now husbands and fathers did ought to pay a penny a week as 'ud give us a right to call upon they nurses when we wants they."

"This," comments Miss Nightingale, "is the real spirit of the thing."[12]

## Health Department Nursing Services

While the development of visiting nursing under private auspices and support was in progress in many of the Eastern cities, Los Angeles, California, initiated a public health nursing service supported by public funds. In 1898, a nurse employed by the College Settlement, a private organization, received her salary from city funds. In 1910, it was reported that the nursing staff at the Settlement had seven nurses, all on the city payroll but receiving supervision from the nursing committee of the College Settlement. Their responsibilities included especially the control of tuberculosis and other communicable diseases and the care of mothers and children. In 1913, a city ordinance created a bureau of municipal nursing, and the program became a part of the city health department.[13]

The value of a community health nurse, visiting the sick poor in their homes to teach care and control of tuberculosis and mother and child care, slowly became apparent. Cities and counties throughout the country began to add community health nurses to their health department staffs. After 1911, many counties in rural areas, particularly in the West, set up health departments as a service of county government. Frequently the nurse was the only full-time employee of the department. In some instances her salary was underwritten by the American Red Cross or by state and local tuberculosis associations on a demonstration basis and later assumed by the county government.

In addition to accepted programs of care and control of tuberculosis and other communicable diseases and maternal and child care, the health of school children became part of the rural nurse's responsibility. Follow-up

---

[12]Lucy Ridgely Seymer, compiler, *Selected Writings of Florence Nightingale,* The Macmillan Company, New York, 1954, pp. 315–316.
[13]Annie M. Brainard, *Evolution of Public Health Nursing,* W. B. Saunders Company, Philadelphia, 1922, p. 258.

home visits for school children gave the nurse valuable opportunities for health teaching, such as the importance of immunizations and nutrition and for finding antenatal mothers with newborn infants.

## Specialized Services

Specialization as a field of public health nursing began in 1895 with the employment of the first occupational health nurse by the Vermont Marble Works for the care of its employees. The program spread to department stores, factories, and other industrial plants, reaching peaks of development during World War I and World War II.

In 1902, Lillian Wald, the founder of the Henry Street Nursing Service in New York City, and at that time its director, convinced the city health department of the value of health services for the school child to implement the control of communicable diseases, especially such diseases as scabies, impetigo, scarlet fever, and diphtheria. The immediate success of this program was evident, and schools in other communities soon adopted it. Specialized school nursing continues to function in some urban areas, but in most rural areas it has become part of the program of county health departments.

Other specialties in public health nursing developed, such as tuberculosis control nursing. However, because of the increased costs of services, and with more and better-prepared public health nurses available, specialization in most fields of public health nursing is not feasible. Currently, most specialists in public health nursing function as consultants to staff nurses in generalized programs. These consultants are public health nurses with experience and advanced preparation in their specialty. Although specialized programs of school nursing and occupational health nursing are to be found, many communities now include school nursing in the generalized public health nursing program, and some are experimenting with the inclusion of occupational health nursing.

## Combination Public Health Nursing Agencies

This type of nursing service has been defined as an agency that is "administered jointly by a voluntary and an official agency, and supported by tax funds, community chests and united funds, earnings and contributions, in which the combined field of service offered by the participating agency is rendered by a single staff of nurses."[14]

---

[14]U.S. Department of Health, Education and Welfare, *Nurses in Public Health,* publication 785, 1964, p. 52.

During and immediately following World War II, many communities began searching for more effective utilization of the services of the public health nurse. Professional and lay leaders recognized that the duplication of travel and services of both staffs was costly in time and money. Studies relating to the situation revealed that staff nurses from both official and voluntary agencies were visiting the same families, often on the same day.

Combined public health nursing agencies function in approximately one hundred communities in the United States, as a part of both health departments and visiting nurse organizations, and in some instances of the schools. The degree to which a combination or merging of nursing services takes place varies with the community. Experimentation with this form of nursing service continues, and new patterns in organization will emerge with study, research, and experience.

## COMMUNITY HEALTH NURSING PRACTICE

The practice of nursing with the community being the field of action is based on the foundations of general nursing. The community health nurse draws on her knowledge of nursing theory and skills gained in the care of patients in hospital and clinic settings, and supplemented with studies in the humanities and the social and natural sciences. She works with healthy families and with nonhospitalized ill persons and their families, with special groups, such as school children, and with problems involving the health of the community as a whole, e.g., epidemiology.

The knowledge gained from theory and practice in the clinical setting becomes such a part of the nurse's thinking that she can react readily and intelligently to a situation. The very nature of public health nursing often places the nurse in circumstances where she must make judgments without the resources of immediate help and supervision from medical and nursing staffs that were available to her in the hospital environment.

In addition to a knowledge of the theory and practice of nursing, other competencies required in public health nursing in order to meet the needs of patients, family, and community include:

1. Abilities and skills in communications: interviewing, listening, teaching, and also the sharing of pertinent information as necessary with professional colleagues

2. Observation skills: the ability to note signs and symptoms of *health,* as well as those of disease, in relation to the physical, mental, and emotional health of the patient and his family

3. A knowledge of the community resources that can be utilized to meet the individual needs of the patient and of the family

4. As complete an understanding of human behavior as possible

**Services of the Community Health Nurse**
The concept of the community health nurse as teacher, though long recognized, is increasing in importance. The demand for direct nursing care in the home is also increasing, but with a different emphasis from that of the past, when the greatest need in home nursing was for the care of patients with communicable disease, e.g., scarlet fever or typhoid. Today's greatest need is home nursing care for patients of all ages, but especially for older persons, because of the increased emphasis on rehabilitation at the onset of patient illness or disability.

Community health nursing services are becoming available to more families than formerly because of (1) provision of nursing care in health insurance plans, both private and governmental; (2) development and extension of rehabilitation care in the home; and (3) expanding programs for continuity in care of patients from home to hospital to home in rural as well as urban areas. This makes possible many challenging opportunities for both teaching and nursing service in the home.

The significant social legislation passed by Congress during the 1960s provided for increased health services and their funding. Examples of this legislation of interest to health workers include:

1. Heart Disease, Cancer and Stroke Amendments of 1965 (Public Law 89–239)

2. Health Professions Education Assistance Amendment of 1965 (Public Law 89–290)

3. The Social Security Amendments Act of 1965 (Public Law 89–97)

4. The Housing and Urban Development Act of 1965 (Public Law 89–117)

5. The Comprehensive Health Planning and Public Health Services Amendments of 1966 (Public Law 89–749) and 1967 (Public Law 90–174)

**PRECEPTS**
Community health nursing as an organized community service has functioned in one form or another for over 300 years. From the experience of several countries under varying situations and conditions certain basic ideas of conduct, or precepts, have evolved that assist the nurse and her agency in carrying out work in the home and the community. Some of the earlier precepts are no longer pertinent because of social and economic changes in our society, while others have been added as need arose. This process will continue.

A *precept* has been defined as a rule for action or conduct. Another source says a precept is a command or a principle for a general rule of action. In order to assist the nurse in achieving the goals she and her agency have for work with patient, family, and community, certain precepts have to be recognized and observed. By following precepts of community health nursing the nurse is able to maintain a continuity and balance in her work. Adherence to these precepts, and to others as they develop, is a protection to the patient, his family, the nurse, and the agency.

## HISTORICAL BACKGROUND

St. Vincent de Paul, in the seventeenth century, founded and directed the work of the Sisters of Charity as visiting nurses to the sick poor in their region of France. He recognized that certain basic precepts would have to be observed if the Sisters were to be successful. These included:

**1.** Recognition of the family as the unit of service

**2.** The responsibility not only of the rich and influential but also of the poor and the humble to contribute within their means to the relief of distress

**3.** Appraisal from time to time of the family situation in order to determine the causes of need and the possible remedies

More than 200 years later, William Rathbone of Liverpool, England, founded the first modern visiting nurse organization on a secular basis, as a memorial to his wife. He recognized also that adherence to certain precepts would facilitate the work of the nurses and the agency to the benefit of patient and family. He recognized the following three precepts as essential to safe functioning of the nursing program:

**1.** The public health nurse should not give financial assistance; "even sick relief should not be given indiscriminately."

**2.** The nurse should not interfere with the religious convictions of her patient.

**3.** The nurse should be educationally prepared for her work as a district nurse.

Florence Nightingale, vitally interested at that time in home care of the sick, added another precept widely accepted today, that the nurse is responsible for teaching basic health principles and practices to the patient and his family.

## PRECEPTS PRACTICED IN COMMUNITY HEALTH NURSING

In the United States, as community health nursing developed in the large cities and rural areas, changing socioeconomic conditions pinpointed other precepts that should be observed to enable the nurse to practice with safety and meet the needs of patient, family, and community. These changing conditions include new findings and practices relating to health, economic, social, and industrial changes, and changes in attitudes of patients, families, and neighborhoods toward health values.

**Precept 1**   Community health nursing is an established activity, based on recognized needs and functioning within the total health program.

As an activity to meet recognized community health needs, nursing provides supervision and counseling for health promotion, health appraisal, rehabilitation, and prevention of disease and provides care for the sick, toward cure or a peaceful death, in their homes. In addition to the home, nursing services may be carried out in the health center, clinics, schools, and places of employment. Community health nursing is an integral part of the total public health program, coordinating its plans and activities with those of other social and health agencies, and does not function or stand alone in the community.

Nursing services are supported by public and private funds to the degree that the community understands and appreciates its own health needs. The community has the obligation to study and evaluate continuously the nursing services it receives to determine trends of changing family and community needs, to develop new programs as necessary, and to discontinue those no longer pertinent. The decrease in communicable disease incidence resulting from education, immunization, and other control programs, and the increasing need to provide nursing service and rehabilitation for persons in their homes are examples.

**Precept 2**   The community health nursing agency has clearly defined objectives and purposes for its services.

The multiplicity of social and health agencies in any given community demands that each agency have clearly defined and stated objectives and purposes in order to prevent duplication of certain community services and omission of others. Objectives and purposes vary with the type of agency and the community but should be related to the goals of the agency for nursing service so that every citizen may be helped to achieve and maintain optimal health.

The philosophy, now in evidence, of the consumer of nursing service having a voice in the development of the objectives and purposes of community nursing is important to implementation of this precept. Such constructive participation by the consumer can result in a more effective nursing service.

The community health nurse works within the administrative framework of her agency, being fully aware of its objectives, purposes, and policies and adhering to them carefully. For the most part, the nurse works alone in the district and frequently is faced with decisions that relate to her work with families and coworkers, such as social workers, school, and industrial personnel. Her complete knowledge and understanding of the agency's objectives, purposes, and policies will help prevent errors that might involve the agency and even community health nursing itself.

**Precept 3**   An active, organized citizens' group, representative of the community, is an integral part of the community health nursing program.

Community health nursing agencies, public and private, need to share their problems with and seek advice from representative community groups. Nearly every community includes among its citizens men and women who have been a part of its past and who will continue to be a part of its future. Their knowledge and experience, shared with the professional workers, can be of inestimable value to the community as a whole and can provide the professional workers with an understanding and awareness of the elements of the complex backgrounds of the community's life, development, and experiences.

An active, organized citizens' group, representing the public, should be invited to participate in the planning and development of health programs that will meet community needs and interests. Such a group can provide continuity for the planning and service of the agency and contribute to the interpretation of community health nursing. It can serve also as a valuable liaison between the agency and the community.

The composition of this group varies according to whether the community is urban, suburban, or rural. Since consideration of community needs is an important function of the group, members should be selected for the contribution they are able to make. Their period of service should be limited, e.g., to three or six years, depending on the needs of the community and its resources. Members may be drawn from such organizations as parent-teacher associations, men's civic and service clubs, women's organizations, church councils, professional groups such as lawyers or physicians, schools, labor and management, and industrial and agricultural groups. Representatives of diverse religious and ethnic groups will aid in the general understanding of community problems, e.g., housing and unemployment.

A citizens' group functions in various ways. Its members may make selected home calls with the nurse so that they can interpret her work with more understanding to other community groups. They can point out to the agency needs for nursing services as they see them in their neighborhoods, districts, or parishes. They can discuss and offer solutions to problem cases presented by the agency. They can assist in the extension and development of nursing services, either geographically or in depth. They can keep the agency informed of trends relating to the economic and social conditions in the community; this is especially valuable when a trend is just beginning. The interest and assistance of this group can also be of great value at budget planning time.

The precept that a citizens' group should be an integral part of the community health nursing program points up that just as the public health nurse should work *with* patient and family, rather than *for* them, community health nursing should plan health programs *with* community members, rather than *for* them.

An advisory committee should meet at regular intervals to be kept informed of the agency's program and to contribute from their personal and community experiences to the solution of problems. They are entitled to share in the successes of the program as well as the failures. Recognition and implementation of this precept is important, as many citizens spend practically their entire life in the community and have much invested in it, and the valuable contributions they can make to the work and success of the public health agency should not be lost.

On occasion, the nurse will find small, informal groups of residents in her district who can be of great help to her in her work, for they can interpret the local needs, cultures, and mores of their neighborhood. Many of these men and women have a potential for leadership and might be considered for membership on communitywide health committees, where their experience and understanding of such neighborhood problems as lack of health centers, child-care centers, and hospital facilities, can contribute to the entire community. Recognition and utilization of this resource can add stability and continuity to the agency's program.

**Precept 4**  Community health nursing services are available to the entire community regardless of origin, culture, or social and economic resources.

Community health nursing is a field of specialization within the broad spectrum of organized public health practice. Its services should be available to all persons according to their health needs, physical and emotional, and regardless of ethnic origin, cultural background, or social and economic resources. Deviation from health of any one member of a family or of the community may affect the health of the entire family or community. The background of the individual or family should not interfere with their receiving the needed services the nurse can provide, e.g., skilled nursing care and health teaching relating to maternal and child care, nutrition, immunizations, and mental and emotional problems. Although community health nursing had its inception in the work of the early church, it is not necessarily a charity and has adapted itself to changes in the social order.

Nonofficial agencies, such as visiting nurse associations, charge for nursing care if the family can arrange to pay. Fees should be within the range of the family's financial resources and should reflect the value placed on the service by the community, the family, and the agency. Fees for visits are charged on a full- or part-pay basis, depending on the ability of the family or patient to pay, especially when the patient is the family's breadwinner. The nurse needs to estimate the period of time care will be needed, as it will be a factor in establishing the fee. Many families who might be able to pay full fees for the nurse's visits for a short-term illness might be unable to do so if faced with a long-term illness, such as cancer. When the family can arrange to pay at least part of the fee, they should be encouraged to do so. Necessary nursing care should not be discontinued because of an inability to pay for it. Part of the nurse's plan is to assist the patient and family in their rehabilitation to attain optimal health so that they may function independently and assume, as soon as possible, their responsibilities for their own health problems. But when for economic reasons a patient has to forego essential nursing care, the goals of the nurse and her agency are lost. In some agencies after the nurse has assessed the situation, arrangements for fee collection are made by the clerical help.

Current policies in most official nursing agencies do not provide bedside nursing care except on a demonstration basis. In some areas this practice is changing; the present trend is for local health department staffs to provide bedside nursing when the community lacks other home nursing facilities. Some states have passed legislation that makes it possible for local official agencies to charge for these nursing visits when feasible.

The precept that community health nursing services are available to everyone is broad in its concept. It permeates all nurse-patient and nurse-family relationships. It contributes to the goals of the overall community health nursing program.

**Precept 5**   In community health nursing the *family,* rather than the *individual patient,* is recognized as the unit of service.

The community health nurse's work is family-centered, rather than patient-centered, with the home being the usual setting. This is a different approach from that of patient-centered care in the hospital environment. It recognizes the patient or family as the hostess and the nurse as the guest in the situation. The effect of health or illness (physical or emotional) of any one member on the lives of other family members is more obvious in the home than in the hospital, and the nurse is able to observe more closely in the home than in the hospital the effect of suffering, fear, and death on the family (see Case Record 7).

In studying and trying to understand the home situation, the nurse draws widely on her knowledge and background of the social and behavioral sciences. On the basis of her knowledge of the family composition, its history, resources, and current problems, she employs the epidemiologic approach in meeting family needs. She makes frequent appraisals of the health progress of the family and patient. She recognizes that the family is a segment of the community and of society, and she utilizes the available community resources in her planning. Frequently she functions as a liaison person with other community agencies in securing health and social resources for the family.

The nurse's ultimate goal is to make the entire family independent and knowledgeable regarding health principles and practices. Achieving her goal is facilitated when she plans *with* them rather than *for* them. Her emphasis is primarily on health promotion for all the family through health counseling, emotional support and understanding, teaching, demonstrating, and nursing care; at the same time she provides for the patient's needs.

**Precept 6**   Health education and counseling for patient, family, and community are integral parts of community health nursing.

Teaching health concepts and practices to the community, family, and patient is interwoven throughout the work of the community health nurse. On a community level she participates with other members of the health team in planning and carrying out community health education concerning mass x-ray surveys, immunization programs, safety programs, dependable food and water supplies, reliable waste disposal, or development of mental health programs. Media used to provide community health education include news stories, films, posters, radio and television programs, and talks to individuals and groups. County and state fairs offer excellent opportunities for educating the general public about the control of tuberculosis and other diseases, and for programs on vision conservation, better nutrition, and accident prevention, among other topics.

In the home the nurse works closely with patient and family in health counseling, focusing on individual needs. She plans with them to meet their goals in health promotion, rehabilitation, and independence in health matters. Teaching the family the importance of immunization and environmental sanitation and teaching prospective parents the care of mothers and babies are examples. As far as possible, the nurse should coordinate her teaching in the home with that of the family physician.

In the schools, the nurse cooperates with principals and teachers in health matters. She acts as a resource for health education, and is available for conferences on health matters with children, parents, teachers, and administrative personnel. In industrial plants, she assists supervisory personnel and others in instituting health and safety programs, and she coordinates her work with other health education activities in the plant and in the community.

The general public is interested in many health matters and fairly well informed regarding them. However, since much of the layman's information is received from current lay periodicals, the nurse needs to be aware of this source of "health" literature, as it sometimes contains half-truths and needs interpretation. On the other hand, she also needs to keep herself well informed regarding knowledge currently presented in the literature of the medical, nursing, and allied fields.

The nurse's goal in all health teaching and health counseling is to help the individual, the family, and the community to be so well informed regarding sound health principles and practices that they achieve and maintain optimal health by means of their own knowledge and efforts.

**Precept 7**   The patient and family participate fully in all decision making relating to goals for the attainment of health.

The community health nurse recognizes and respects the right of patient and family to participate in all decision making relating to their health goals. The nurse's function is to help the patient and/or family to recognize the existence of a health need, to assess all aspects of the situation, to consider appropriate activities that will improve the situation, and to arrive at the decision which is deemed most suitable by the patient and family. Implicit in the decision-making process is that the patient and family comprehend fully the meaning of the decision and accept the responsibility for consequential events. An example is the parents' decision to have a rubella immunization for their child after weighing the pros and cons of immunization versus voluntary exposure to a "childhood disease," rubella.

A more involved situation would be the decision a patient and his family would have to make regarding open-heart surgery. Although this surgical technique has reached a fairly high degree of safety, there are certain elements of danger in individual cases. The nurse needs to be objective in her teaching, helping the patient and family to make their own decision, and at the same time help them to make a free and responsible choice on their own and to gain independence for future decision making through the experience.

The nurse also observes this precept when working with community groups. Her aim is to involve community members in the planning and provision of health care to the highest possible degree and to help create independent thinking and action on the part of consumers, as well as the ability to live with their decisions. If a community fails to pass a bond issue for necessary money to ensure safe water supplies or a well-equipped fire department, they may have to accept the results of a water-borne epidemic or a heavy loss of life and property following a disastrous fire, but the decision should lie with the community.

**Precept 8**   Periodic and continuing appraisal and evaluation of the health situation of the community, family, and patient are basic to community health nursing.

Although this precept has been recognized for a long time, its importance has been accentuated in recent years by the rapidly changing patterns in community and family life and by the new discoveries in medicine that shorten recovery and convalescent periods. In some situations, changes in the circumstances of the community, family, or patient may be so subtle that they pass unnoticed unless the nurse and the agency maintain continuous appraisal and are fully aware of their implications. The term "periodic" is a fluid one, and its meaning depends on many factors. In a family, community, or neighborhood experiencing rapid changes, it may mean every month or oftener; in other situations a review or appraisal might not be necessary more than once every six months.

The family health appraisal is a tool for the nurse in helping the family to achieve health independence. Family situations can be dynamic, a birth or death may cause a complete family reorganization, and a severe illness or change in the health status of any one member may have repercussions for every member. Also a change of residence or a change of occupation with resultant change in income may have marked effects on the physical and emotional health situation. At intervals, these changes need to be assessed by family and nurse in the interests of planning for the family health program. By consultation with family and patient and by careful observation and case recording, the nurse can evaluate the family health progress, determine the priorities, and adjust her nursing plans.

An awareness of the progress that is being made and of the degree of independence that the family seems to be achieving helps the nurse to establish her priorities in planning for her daily work in the district and the home calls to be made.

Communities, too, are dynamic and changing constantly for better or worse, some at a quicker rate than others. Periodic study of the neighborhoods in her district enables the nurse to be informed of changes that will affect the lives of the families there. What changes are taking place in relation to population shifts, age groups, business areas, recreational facilities, and housing? Changing transportation facilities, such as an increase or decrease in bus routes, parking lots, arterials, and highways, affect a neighborhood. The need for additional buildings for schools and hospitals, or their abandonment, points up community changes involving growth or decay.

From these periodic appraisals of patient, family, and community, the nurse gains a basis for evaluating the effectiveness of her work and of her own growth and development.

**Precept 9**  The nurse is prepared professionally to function as a health worker in the community.

A hundred years of experience with community health nursing has proved to society that the nurse must be prepared professionally to serve as health worker in the community and that this preparation should be based on a firm foundation of nursing knowledge and skills, including theory and practice in community health procedures. She needs special competence in adapting learned nursing procedures to the home care and rehabilitation of the patient. Since community health nursing is a family-centered activity rather than a patient-centered one as in the hospital, the nurse also needs a broad background in such social and behavioral sciences as anthropology, sociology, and psychology to meet effectively problems that involve interpersonal relationships, community organization, and social pathology.

The community health nurse brings not only broad preparation and technical skills to her work, but she also must continue to grow and to improve her performance skills in interviewing, teaching, problem solving, group work, and leadership. She needs to keep up with recent knowledge in nutrition, social work, epidemiology, and behavioral sciences as well as in nursing and medical care.

This precept that the nurse be prepared professionally for her work is the cornerstone in the foundation of community nursing, for without previous professional preparation and an awareness of current knowledge in nursing and medical care, as well as in the allied fields, her work could not measure up to the community's needs.

**Precept 10**  The community health nurse functions as a member of the health team in serving community, family, and patient.

All successful teamwork is based on a common interest of the team members and there should be no division of concern among them. The community health nurse often finds herself functioning on various teams at one time or another. One such team would include members from her own agency or nursing division such as other staff nurses, paranursing personnel, students, the district supervisor, the nursing director, clerks, volunteers, and other nonprofessional personnel, all of whom work together to provide the best possible community nursing service.

The nurse also participates on a community team composed of workers from the allied health fields and interested community members. Although the ultimate goals of this team are the same as those of the nursing team, the emphases may vary. This interdisciplinary team usually includes, besides the nurse, a health officer, family physician, social worker, nutritionist, and environmental specialist. Members of other health disciplines can be added as needed, as well as such interested community members as school personnel, clergymen, volunteer community workers, and in most situations, the patient or his family.

The nurse has several roles on the interdisciplinary team. She acts as an interpreter of nursing in the team's assessment of the patient's physical, mental, and social needs and in planning means to meet these needs, and in turn keeps the nursing team aware of the thinking and action of the community team. She also participates in the team action regarding improvement of environmental resources. The nurse also functions as a leader by influencing the quality of health and nursing care that can be provided to the community by helping it to become aware of the need for health programs.

With the recognition of the value of continuity of nursing care, it is possible that a third team is emerging composed of hospital personnel as the head nurse, staff nurse, resident, intern and/or family physician, and the community health nurse, all of whom would know the patient. This team can coordinate plans for continuity of nursing care, thus providing for fewer interruptions in the care of the patient during his transition from home to hospital to home. The patient and family frequently participate on this team and assist with the making of plans and their implementation.

In making the team effective, each member must recognize the contribution of all other team members in achieving the planned goals and objectives, which are the health, safety, and comfort of patient and community.

**Precept 11**  The community health nurse provides nursing care for the individual patient as ordered by his physician.

The provision of nursing care for the individual patient as ordered by his physician is basic to all nursing. Every nurse, in her care of the sick, works under the direction of the physician in charge of the patient. Violation of this precept jeopardizes the entire community health nursing program. The nurse receives orders for care from the physician responsible for the medical care and supervision of the patient. In most instances this is the family physician, but it might be a physician from a hospital clinic, a school system, or an industrial plant.

When a family or patient refuses medical care, although it appears necessary to the nurse, she has no recourse but to withdraw from the situation. This has occurred on occasion. It is a difficult step for the nurse to take, especially if the patient is an infant or a child, but this precept must be held inviolate. Before taking such a radical step, however, the nurse should report the situation to her nursing supervisor or her health officer. Except in great emergency, a nurse does not care for a sick patient without medical orders.

Most community health nursing agencies have a policy, approved by the local medical society, that the nurse may make, without medical supervision, two nursing visits to a family with illness for the purpose of providing nursing care. If during the first visit, the nurse believes that the patient should be under medical supervision—and he is not—she must advise the family that a physician should be called. Depending on her judgment, she may give nursing care during the visit according to the agency's standing orders, which have been approved by the medical advisory committee of the agency, the county medical society, or the local health officer. At this time also she may counsel the family on health matters such as general nutrition, rest, comfort, and safety of the patient. The next day, the nurse may visit the family to see whether a physician was called and to ascertain his orders for nursing care. If the family has not called a physician and does not plan to do so, the nurse should determine their reasons. If it is a matter of finances she can explain the community resources for free medical care. If the family does not wish to have medical care for other reasons, the nurse cannot continue to provide nursing care.

As in the hospital, the nurse in the public health field reports regularly to the physician in charge, regarding his patient's condition, and secures additional orders from him as necessary. When the nurse visits the home for health teaching and counseling, she keeps the family physician informed, in writing or by telephone, so that they may work together in assisting the family to achieve independence and self-sufficiency in health matters.

**Precept 12**  The community health nursing agency makes full use of family and other service records.

The maintenance of accurate records and their use are important to both family and agency. The family record is indispensable to the nurse in her daily work and is an important element in making continuity of nursing care possible. Good recording covers all nurse-family, as well as all nurse-patient contacts and interaction. The nurse uses patient and family records in planning for home visits and for other means of serving the patient. Her visit plans will be based on the accomplishments of previous visits that she and other nurses, if any, have made to the family or patient and on the current situation of the patient or family. Records are invaluable to the nurse assuming care of the patient for the first time. A review of the records prior to her first visit will save both her time and that of the family. The nurse's knowledge and understanding of situations will reduce family stress at the time of a first visit by a new nurse.

The quality of the agency's services to the community is reflected in its records. A periodic critical study of them helps the agency to evaluate its program in relation to its current objectives, and assists in determining its long-term objectives. The records are a source of statistical information and are valuable in determining costs, in ascertaining needs for additional staff members, and in planning budgets. They provide a guide in making staff assignments to the different nursing districts.

Community health nursing agencies have legal authorization to operate, their records are legal documents and as such are subject to subpoena by the courts, but in all other situations they are strictly confidential. Within the policies of the agency, a report of the contents of the record is shared with the family physician or with a professional staff member of another agency, such as a social worker, when requested.

The staff nurse is responsible for maintaining her records so that they are current, accurate, complete, and legible. The information should be recorded objectively, the nurse being aware at all times of the many uses the agency will make of the record.

**Precept 13** The community health nurse does not provide material relief but directs the patient or family to appropriate community resources for necessary financial and social assistance.

The community health nurse does not provide material relief, since there are community agencies organized for this purpose. The nurse's concern is for the patient's immediate health needs and for the promotion of health, physical and emotional, and prevention of disease. By providing material relief, even transportation to the clinic or health center, except on the request and approval of the cooperating agency, the nurse might be jeopardizing the long-range planning of other community workers. The nurse is responsible for knowing the programs and functions available from social agencies and for cooperating with them, utilizing their services, and referring patients and families to them as necessary.

The timing for the referral and the family's readiness to accept it needs careful consideration. The family should participate in the planning for the referral, which should never be made against their will but only with their understanding and acceptance.

It is basic to this precept that when a nurse provides material relief, no matter how little, she tends to nullify her teaching. Unconsciously she is buying patient and family cooperation in health matters, for instead of incorporating her teaching into their thinking and making it their own practice and action, they are waiting to be paid for it (see Case Situation 1).

In the early days of district nursing in London and Liverpool, Miss Nightingale recognized the importance of this precept and its implications to the nurse. She wrote: "So nothing is *given* but the nursing and some day, let us hope that the old woman's sensible plan will be carried out. In the meantime the nurses are nurses—not cooks, nor yet almoners (social workers) nor relieving officers. But, if needed, things are procured from the proper agencies and sick comforts made as well as given by these agencies."[15]

**Precept 14** Nursing supervision of the staff nurse is provided by qualified nursing personnel.

[15]Seymer, *op. cit.,* p. 316.

Supervision is an educational and advisory relationship between supervisor and staff nurse. Its aim is to develop the abilities and skills of the nurse so that she can meet her professional responsibilities with an increasing productivity and effectiveness.

Supervision in community health agencies by qualified nurses is essential for continuous improvement of the nursing service to patient and family, for the overall planning of the staff nurses' work, and for coordination of their activities within the agency. It is also a stimulus and guide for the individual staff nurse in her health teaching, family counseling, and nursing service, and for her own growth and development.

Methods of supervision vary with agencies, but the methods most frequently employed include planned and continuing staff orientation, joint study and review of family case records by supervisor and nurse, supervised home calls or clinic experiences, and individual and group conferences relating to the nurse's work and to the continuing development of the agency's program. Staff members need to be aware at all times of the agency's planning and work if a balanced development is to be maintained. An adequate and satisfactory program of supervision will assist not only in the growth and development of each staff member but also in the continued improvement of the quality of nursing service that the agency provides the community.

**Precept 15**   The community health nursing agency provides a continuing staff education program.

Such a staff education program is essential to maintain sound nursing practice in hospitals and community health agencies. Planning for in-service education takes into account the professional needs and interests of the staff nurses. Consideration is given also to the special skills and knowledge required by the agency. The staff must be kept informed of new situations and conditions arising in the community, such as a sudden increase in the incidence of a communicable disease, a change in the health and welfare resources in the community, e.g., the formation of a local council for alcoholism, and new Federal, state, and local regulations relating to health matters.

Periodic, planned staff meetings for sharing experiences and information with other members of the health team in the community also provide an opportunity for widening professional knowledge and skills, not only in nursing, but in other phases of the community health program as well. Many agencies send one or more staff members to conferences, institutes, summer schools, or professional meetings in other parts of the state or country on the premise that the entire staff will share in the reports of these educational experiences.

A sound in-service program is based on the dynamics of medical and nursing care and an appreciation of the ever-increasing body of knowledge with which the nurse must be familiar and the additional skills she must acquire for use in her daily practice with patients and families and in her contacts with coworkers.

**Precept 16** The nurse assumes responsibility for her own continuing professional development.

The responsibility of the nurse for her own continuing professional development is a precept basic to all nursing; it is the other side of the coin of the precept just stated relating to the agency's recognized responsibility and obligation for providing in-service and staff development programs. The staff nurse is equally responsible for her own continuing professional growth and education. It has been said that the ultimate goal of an education program is to shift to the student the burden of pursuing his own education. Continuing education is considered by many leaders in all fields to be the greatest single challenge to professional personnel.

Each nurse needs to establish her own immediate and long-term goals in order to continue building and developing her education, both professional and general. She can do this by various methods, such as reading professional journals and periodicals on nursing and allied subjects, by attending and participating in the meetings of her professional organizations, and by not neglecting books, journals, and lectures in the humanities and the arts. For the most part, the nurse will find libraries, art galleries, concert and lecture series available in either her own community or an adjacent one. As a professional person, the nurse should plan to invest some of her own time and money in her growth and development through attendance at summer sessions in colleges and universities, and by working toward higher degrees whenever possible.

## SUMMARY

The precepts of community health nursing relate to the *organization* of community health nursing, to the *work* of the individual nurse, and to the *nurse* herself. They are guidelines only and are to be followed in any situation with sound judgment and common sense. The majority of these precepts pertain to nursing in general, not to community health nursing alone. Their implications for all nursing will tend to increase as the philosophy and practice of continuous care of the patient from home to hospital to home becomes accepted by patient, family, and community, as well as by the nursing, medical, and allied professions. Students of nursing have become aware of many of these precepts from their experience in clinical situations in the hospitals. They are stated here, however, within the framework of community nursing.

The responsibilities of today's community health nurses are succinctly summarized by Cline and Howell as "to help individuals, families and communities to develop and utilize their potential for healthful living through cultivation and use of their own and external resources, and to provide nursing care for the sick and disabled in their homes. . . ."[16]

The means by which the nurse carries out these responsibilities include home visits to patient and family, work with neighborhood groups, such as parents' classes and prenatal classes, by health supervision in places of employment, and by assisting teachers of children of all age groups. Community health nursing must be based on an understanding and appreciation of the needs, social relationships, and cultural mores of the patient, family, or group.

[16]Nora Cline and Roger W. Howell, "Public Health Nursing and Mental Health," in Stephen E. Goldston (ed.), *Mental Health Considerations in Public Health,* U.S. Department of Health, Education and Welfare, Public Health Service, Health Services and Mental Health Administration, National Institute of Mental Health, Maryland, 1969, p. 146.

## SUGGESTED READING

Abelson, Philip M., et al.: "Manmade Environmental Hazards," *American Journal of Public Health,* 58:20–43 (November) 1968.

Adam, Martha: "This I Believe about Public Health Nursing," *Nursing Outlook,* 17: 44–46 (August) 1969.

Brown, Esther Lucile: *Newer Dimensions of Patient Care,* Part 3, Russell Sage Foundation, New York, 1965.

Byrne, Mary Woods: "This I Believe About the Baccalaureate Graduate in a VNA," *Nursing Outlook,* 18:28–31 (July) 1970.

Caskey, Kathryn K., Enid V. Blaylock, and Beryl M. Wauson: "The School Nurse and Drug Abusers," *Nursing Outlook* 18:27–30 (December) 1970.

Colt, Avery M.: "Elements of Comprehensive Health Planning," *American Journal of Public Health,* 60:1194–1204 (July) 1970.

Doster, Daphine D.: "Utilization of Available Nurse Power in Public Health," *American Journal of Public Health,* 60:25–37 (January) 1970.

Freeman, Ruth B.: *Community Health Nursing Practice,* W. B. Saunders Company, Philadelphia, 1970, Chapter 1.

Goerke, Lenor S., and Ernest L. Stebbins: *Mustard's Introduction to Public Health,* 5th ed., The Macmillan Company, New York, 1969, Chapter 3.

Hanlon, John J.: "An Ecologic Viewpoint of Public Health," *American Journal of Public Health,* 59:4 (January) 1969.

Ingraham, Norman R., and Walter J. Lear: "A Big City Strives for Relevance in its Community Health Services," *American Journal of Public Health,* 60:804–809 (May) 1970.

Milio, Nancy: *9226 Kercheval: The Storefront That Did Not Burn,* The University of Michigan Press, Ann Arbor, 1970.

Remillet, June, and Sadie Reading: "Adapting to Changing Community Health Needs," *Nursing Outlook,* 18:47–49 (October) 1970.

Shannon, Iris R.: "Nursing Service at the Mile Square Health Center of Presbyterean-St. Luke's Hospital," *American Journal of Public Health,* 60:1726–1732 (September) 1970.

Steichen, Edward: *The Family of Man,* published for the Museum of Modern Art, New York, by the MaCO Magazine Corporation, New York, 1955.

# 2

# Relationship Skills

For the nurse beginning to practice community health nursing, the necessity for relating effectively and productively with others is known to be a crucial determinant for her subsequent practice. Because of inner awareness of this knowledge, many nurses often approach the first families with high anxiety and attempt to practice the role of the community health nurse according to accurate or inaccurate preconceived ideas, past experiences with community health nurses, and expectations of proper professional nurse behavior. What happens thereafter is dependent upon the innate skills of the nurse and the behavior of the family receiving the visit.

The nurse must know *why* she is knocking on the door and meeting the family, and she must be able to convey the purpose for her visit in words that the family can understand and accept and with behavior that is congruent with her words. She must be open, honest, and genuine. With an approach like this, the family is inclined to reciprocate with similar behavior. Because it is important to work *with* families, understand reciprocal verbal and nonverbal communications, and work toward goals which are agreed upon together, it is vital that the nurse initiate the relationship process in a way that the family member can accept and support.

## USE OF SELF WITH OTHERS

Many books have described the advisability of knowing oneself and have explored ways of increasing self-knowledge, but few have interpreted the difficulty of knowing oneself both as a person and as a nurse. Nurses frequently ask themselves, "Can I be me and a nurse too?" In encouraging a senior nursing student to be genuine with the family she was visiting, an instructor was told, "For three years I have been told how to behave professionally. I don't know if I know how to be me!"

In a book written for the purpose of getting better acquainted with oneself, the author pointed out that we all make two wishes in life. One is for success in our relationship to other people and the second is for success in our undertakings. If we were to make a third wish, it should be to understand ourselves, since if that wish can be made to come true, the first is certain to be fulfilled and the second is likely to be. The initial step in understanding the self is observation of how we act in the world.[1]

In all the fields of nursing, understanding the self is important; however, in the setting of the community, the observation and cognizance of the behavior of self is often thrust upon one like an unexpected stiletto. The action and reaction of the consumer of health services has to be taken into account and given careful consideration, and subsequent behavior of the nurse intervener must be modified in accordance with the purpose of the encounter. The nurse frequently represents the middle-class setting and culture and consequently interacts with people from a middle-class point of view, which involves an expectation of others to have values and beliefs similar to her own. Meeting consumers from settings and cultures different from her own requires acute observation skills, sensitivity to verbal and nonverbal cues, ability to be adaptable and flexible, and an intuitive sixth sense, which is sometimes needed to guide her toward appropriate behavior. An early sufficient grasp of the characteristics of lower-class families in poverty and the cultures of minority families such as blacks, Chicanos, Indians, and Orientals must be known so that the establishment of a beginning relationship can be facilitated.

Consumers who live in poverty tend to distrust helping persons on first acquaintance, particularly if the nurse or health representative epitomizes characteristics that they lack. The distrust is based on several factors, some of which are (1) despondency regarding their own potential for achievement; (2) disbelief that their life and environment can be changed; and (3) negative previous experiences with professional people who tried to help but lacked understanding of vital essentialities inherent in their culture or life style. In preparation for working with consumers who are different, it is imperative for the nurse to be accepting of all differences, no matter how great or small, and to be cognizant of the effect she induces in others.

To start with, the nurse should be aware of her personality style as a *Self-Awareness* person and as a nurse. Is she friendly, charming, talkative, serious, reserved, or quiet? How do others respond to her? What is their verbal and nonverbal feedback? Jourard stated that many nurses acquire a fixed way of behaving in the presence of patients. He called it their bedside manner or character armor. Use of the bedside manner stifles spontaneity in the person using it and protects the nurse from possible hurt coming from the outside. Charac-

---

[1]Jo Coudert, *Advice From a Failure*, Dell Publishing Co., Inc., New York, 1965, p. 245.

ter armor serves effectively to hide a person's real self, both from himself and from others.[2] If a person avoids a bedside manner or a "charming front," how can a nurse "sell" her purpose for visiting the consumer? By being herself and believing deeply that she can assist the consumer toward greater health. An inescapable nurse is one who is open to her own experience, who genuinely cares about people and about herself. She knows it is important to care about herself. She is a person who is always in process of maturing and growing. She can look into her own memory, background, and experience and find that she has suffered, thought, felt, wished, and enjoyed just about everything human beings anywhere under the sun have experienced. This openness to herself makes it possible for her to establish empathic contact with families.[3]

### Talking and Listening

When the nurse is a spontaneously talkative person, she must be aware of the effect of her verbosity on the consumer. If the constant output of words is repelling or elicits few responses from the patient, the purpose of the encounter may be nullified. The gabby nurse needs to be able to control her talk, be sensitive when her words dominate the dialogue, and maintain a discipline of self-articulation. On the other hand, the quiet nurse who finds it difficult to verbalize extensively generally is able to elicit responses from patients fairly easily because she is often a good listener. Her difficulty arises when she meets another quiet person and the conversation is filled with frequent uncomfortable silences. The quiet nurse needs to be particularly prepared before a home visit with specific information to which the consumer may be responsive and be able to force herself to talk when the conversation takes a lull and needs direction. If she practices role-playing or rehearsal of information she wishes to give with another person before making the home visit, this may make her feel more at ease during the actual visit. Learning to talk effectively is facilitated when the nurse is accepting of herself, honest, and spontaneously open to her experiences, and does not hide behind the mask of being a quiet person.

*Listening — key to successful interview*

Intelligent and effective listening takes conscious effort and is the key on which a successful interview is based. Listening to a patient takes skill, which is best accomplished in a competent, professional, and friendly way. It denotes a voluntary effort to comprehend meanings and can be used in several ways. It can mean that (1) the nurse acts as a sounding board against which the patient can ventilate and recognize what he feels; (2) the nurse elaborates and expands the words the patient has used and gives him a sense of prestige and importance as he exerts greater effort to clarify or

---

[2]From *The Transparent Self* by Sidney M. Jourard, Copyright © 1964 by Litton Educational Publishing, Inc., by permission of D. Van Nostrand Company, Inc., New York, p. 112.
[3]*Ibid.*, pp. 136–137.

crystallize his meanings; (3) the nurse provides psychological support by listening to the patient's feelings in relation to the problem, and his burden is lessened because the problem is shared; (4) the nurse creates an environment in which the patient is comfortable in expressing his thoughts; and (5) the nurse is willing to expend energy toward gaining greater understanding and empathy with the patient.

A patient's willingness to verbalize is highly dependent upon the nurse's response to what he says, and if she listens with sensitivity she plays a major role in facilitating her own recognition of the patient's expressed needs. Wilson stated that it is desirable for nurses to do reflective listening and described it as a process that involves the listener's conscious or unconscious assessment and selection of clues from the auditory influx of data, his interweaving and interconnecting of this data with his own existing psychic organization, and his resultant behavioral responses.[4] Reflective listening implies an integral *relation* between verbalization, listening, and response and promotes a creative, progressive relationship between nurse and patient that is dependent on their mutual listening abilities. When both nurse and patient experience feelings of satisfaction about their interactions, this implies cooperation and responsibility regarding the purpose of their exchange and provides impetus to strive toward accomplishment of their mutually set goals.

### Friendliness and Professionalism

Many nurses feel a deep concern about their manifestation of professionalism. They wish to be open, honest, and genuine, but these attributes seem to conflict with their concept of professionalism. Nursing students report that they receive ambivalent messages from experienced nurses about the characteristics of professionalism. Can a professional nurse be a friendly nurse? Can she reveal herself as a personable being?

Not many years ago the professional nurse image purported to be organized, orderly, clean, courteous, and knowledgeable and her manner was one of crisp efficiency. She was called "Miss Doe" and never revealed any personal characteristics that would betray the fact that she had human weaknesses. This imagery tends to persist even though behavioral scientists currently encourage more openness, genuineness, and warmth.

To be involved in a helping relationship, Carl Rogers has set some penetrating questions upon which to reflect. They are:

**1.** Can I *be* in some way which will be perceived by the other person as trustworthy, as dependable or consistent in some deep sense?

[4]Lucille M. Wilson, "Listening," in *Behavioral Concepts and Nursing Intervention,* Carolyn E. Carlson (ed.), J. B. Lippincott Company, Philadelphia, 1970, pp. 153–168.

**2.** Can I be expressive enough as a person that what I am will be communicated unambiguously?

**3.** Can I let myself experience positive attitudes toward this other person —attitudes of warmth, caring, liking, interest, respect?

**4.** Can I be strong enough as a person to be separate from the other?

**5.** Am I secure enough within myself to permit him his separateness?

**6.** Can I let myself enter fully into the world of his feelings and personal meanings and see these as he does?

**7.** Can I receive him as he is? Or can I only receive him conditionally, acceptant of some aspects of his feelings and silently or openly disapproving of other aspects?

**8.** Can I act with sufficient sensitivity in the relationship that my behavior will not be perceived as a threat?

**9.** Can I free him from the threat of external evaluation?

**10.** Can I meet this other individual as a person who is in process of *becoming,* or will I be bound by his past and by my past?[5]

If the nurse internalizes these questions and uses them as a guide for her behavior with the patient, she is less apt to hide behind a mask of "professional" helpfulness and is more inclined to be genuine and honest with the person to whom she is relating. She is comfortable about revealing significant personal thoughts and feelings and sharing past experiences when a disclosure seems purposeful and has potential meaning for the patient.

In a nutshell, the friendly nurse also can be the professional nurse. The friendly nurse is preferred by most consumers. The difference between a purely friendly and a professional relationship is that the professional is purposeful and goal-directed in her behavior with the patient, whereas the friend responds to interactions spontaneously and with no particular intent to change behavior.

**Well and Sick Patients**
Since most nurses are perceived as persons who work mainly with sick patients, an initial difficulty for some beginning community health nurses is to relate with "well" persons as the focus of their attention. They may be accustomed to working with patients who are sick enough to be bedridden or who are in the process of being rehabilitated to activities of daily living.

[5]Carl R. Rogers, *On Becoming a Person,* Houghton Mifflin Company, Boston, 1961, pp. 50–55.

Such patients have the advantage of a diagnosis and a prognosis, and the nurse feels comfortable in her role as caretaker. However, many of the consumers of health services in community nursing are well persons who are coping in their own way with the conditions of their world. The community health nurse is an intervener who becomes acquainted and offers her services in an effort to improve their health status. They may recognize a need for improved health but are not always cognizant of the role that a community health nurse can play in assisting them. This fact requires the nurse to interpret and communicate to the consumer her special ability to relate, to give services purposefully and in a nonthreatening manner, and in so doing, to imply that the coping measures of the consumer will be greatly enhanced by her intervention, and he will be able to adapt more effectively to ever-changing daily tasks.

To elaborate, all human beings experience some degree of tension daily and have individual ways of coping with stress, which they regard as *Maintaining* perfectly normal or as their own idiosyncrasies. In an effort to maintain *Balance* balance or order in their lives, they make use of coping measures which have been satisfying to them in the past, such as chewing gum, cursing, taking a long walk, and other common activities which help to release excess energy. However, when equilibrium is not achieved at a particular time and tensions seem to mount, as evidenced by exaggerated or irritated reactions to minor daily events, coping devices inevitably become more pronounced, are less effective in alleviating stress, and a state of emergency or crisis ensues. It is at this strategic time that the nurse intervener can most effectively initiate a helping relationship. Jones cited the case history of a woman who was pregnant, had marital problems, an alcoholic husband, and little money. The patient was coping with her problems by feeling discouraged, eating quantities of bread and jam, and constantly criticizing her husband. The nurse on early acquaintance was responsive to the patient's concerns, listened to the description of her worries with sensitivity, and by means of discussion, encouraged ideas or activities that the patient could try that she had not considered or attempted previously. As a result of the progressively supportive nature of the relationship between the patient and nurse, changes occurred within the family because the patient voluntarily started to try new methods of coping, such as dieting and attempting to praise her husband instead of nagging him. As the patient noticed subtle, perceptible improvements within her household, her self-confidence gradually returned and her eagerness to try more and more measures to alleviate trying conditions within the home was accentuated. She reported her accomplishments to the nurse with satisfaction and pleasure.[6]

[6]Mary C. Jones, "An Analysis Of a Family Folder," *Nursing Outlook,* 16:48–51 (December) 1968.

### Salesmanship of Self

In community health nursing the nurse sometimes recognizes that she may be mistakenly received as a salesperson at the door. To counteract such an impression she immediately introduces herself, the agency she represents, and her purpose for visiting. At the same time, if the visit is her first one to the family, she presents herself as favorably and convincingly as she is able in order to gain entrance into the home. Because of the initial need to "sell" herself and her services, the nurse must be conscious of her personality style, her approach, her strengths, and her limitations. She must also be aware of her behavior on an initial visit if she is anxious and uncomfortable, so that accurate evaluations of nurse-patient interactions later can be studied by her or with the help of a consultant or supervisor. She can increase awareness of her style by attempting to objectively view herself as a third party by writing process recordings of her interaction, by listening to herself and the patient on a tape recorder, or by use of videotapes if they are available. Preceding a home visit she can role-play an anticipated situation with other nurses or with her supervisor, or following a home visit, a description of an actual situation can be enacted with the nurse playing herself or the role of the patient. New insights are often gained through role-playing or psychodrama because the enactment of a role not only causes words to be spoken but actual physical sensations are felt that are autonomous to the situation. Another effective method of increasing self-understanding is to role-play yourself in a given situation with another person, followed by a reversal of roles. Observing another person playing your role according to their perception of your behavior can be illuminating and clarifying. When the nurse's general style is known, there are times when a conscious attempt has to be made to break a generally successful behavior pattern because the consumer is not responsive to the presenting behavior. Since not all persons react similarly to a given behavior, the nurse must be able to adapt her style to one which may be more appropriate for the patient with whom she is communicating. This requires an accurate and sensitive appraisal of verbal and nonverbal cues forthcoming from the patient. For example, when the interviewing style of the nurse is indirect and makes allowances for the patient to go at his own pace, this may not be at all effective for the person who will respond only to a forceful, prodding style. An adaptable nurse role-plays a part that is unlike her own style when she believes the patient will respond favorably to the changed style. In other words, the effective nurse is flexible, adaptable, and responsive to the cues received from the patient. The necessity to be constantly alert to the behavior of the patient guides the nurse to select the nursing approach she believes will be successful. The fact that she must have several possible roles at her disposal challenges her resourcefulness.

The Effective Nurse

## WORKING WITH INDIVIDUALS

A wide variety of people are encountered in community health nursing, representing the basic fabric of which the community is composed. The nurse must be aware that she interacts with differentiation, dependent upon her degree of comfort, to representative members of the community whether they are members of lower, middle, or upper classes, minority and cultural groups, youth, middle-aged, and geriatric groups, or those with special disease classifications. Her encounter with a specified patient will be based on her experiences, observations, understanding, and acceptance of the different characteristics of which the individual is representative. For example, a young, middle-class nurse who has never entered a poverty-stricken home might initially relate differently to a representative of the lower-economic classes, particularly if the home is filthy according to her standards and the consumer is apathetic and unresponsive to her suggestions, than she would to a representative of the upper class whose home is beautifully furnished and whose manner is pleasantly courteous. The manner in which a nurse responds to a given situation is often dependent upon her expectations, past experiences, values, prejudices, and adaptability to unfamiliar stimuli.

Because she must deal with all types of persons, the nurse is best prepared to function effectively when she feels a deep interest and curiosity about others. By consciously transferring her thoughts to the identified patient or family member, she helps herself to communicate clearly, to be responsive to the other's reactions, and to judge if the encounter has meaning. Her interactional skill also is enhanced by reading references about the characteristics of the group of which the patient is a member because clues and guidelines given in readings aid in observation and verification of existing or nonexisting patterns of behavior. By being attentive to the patient and accepting him as he is, the nurse communicates a respect for his autonomy and a sense of "caring" for him as a distinctive individual. In Chap. 3 characteristics of a variety of representatives of a community are discussed. By delving deeply into additional books and periodicals, the nurse can prepare herself effectively to be cognizant of the many physical, economic, environmental, social, and psychological factors which are affecting the consumer in his life style.

## INTERPERSONAL APPROACHES

Since consumers of health services are individuals and families representative of widely different backgrounds and experiences, the interpersonal approach of the nurse must be sensitive to the responsive patient behavior. Professional books and periodicals representing nursing, social work, medicine, and psychology have described a variety of known approaches that can be implemented. In addition, new methods of interacting with patients and families are reported with increasing frequency. This fact emphasizes the importance of continuing self-education and maintaining familiarity with up-to-date literature and references. The selection of a given approach or mixture of components can be adopted for use and attention given to the responses of the patient to determine if the selected approach is effective in securing the patient's attention and implementing the desired change of behavior. At the same time the nurse must be aware of her interviewing skills and constantly practice to improve her ways of relating so that the patient is helped to feel at ease in talking to a professional person. Some of the known therapeutic and nontherapeutic interpersonal statements or responses have been described in detail by Hays and Larson. They claim that every comment the nurse makes to the patient (or within his hearing) can be evaluated as having therapeutic or nontherapeutic value; i.e., it either contributes to his emotional growth or it reinforces his illness.[7] When a nurse consciously practices the described therapeutic techniques, she finds that they do facilitate commentary from patients, and that with practice her interactional therapeutic skills become more spontaneous and natural.

Some therapeutic questions or statements that are helpful in eliciting information or commentary from the patient are "How have you been managing the past few days?"; "Is there some way I can be of service to you?"; "You appear worried about something"; "How have things been going lately?"; or "It sometimes helps to talk about your concerns with someone who is not a member of the family." At the same time that the nurse verbalizes these questions or statements, her nonverbal behavior should be one of interested concern and intent listening. By making brief comments or asking pertinent, open-ended questions, which are used to encourage the patient to continue talking, the nurse gains an impression of the patient's perspective or the way the patient views his own concerns. By eliciting the patient's perception of his immediate health problems *first,* the nurse then has a base from which to operate. She is made aware of the patient's attitude, and his method of handling current problems, and consequently she is able to devise a plan of implementation that is feasible for the patient's situation.

Some approaches which have been used successfully with consumers and which recognize them as necessary participants in the interactional process include the mutual, strengthening, inquiry, and goal-oriented approaches.

**Mutual Approach**
This approach makes use of the patient and the nurse as equal participants in any interchange that involves determining the purpose for visits, planning

[7]Joyce Samhammer Hays and Kenneth Larson, *Interacting With Patients,* The Macmillan Company, New York, 1964, p. 2.

for implementation of goals, evaluating outcomes, and clarification of feelings and/or behavior. The rationale for this approach is based on precept 7, which was discussed in Chap. 1.

When the purpose for visits on a continuing basis is the focus of attention, a discussion takes place whereby the patient is encouraged to pinpoint a health problem with which he would like assistance or a difficulty in daily life with which he is dissatisfied, and the nurse then interprets skills, resources, and materials to which she has access that may be of assistance to the patient. As a consequence of this interchange of information, a *mutual agreement* or *contract* is made by the patient and nurse to work toward the stated, agreed upon goal, and plans are made for continued contact. At the same time, it is desirable that each participant know what constitutes the work he must do to prepare for the next visit, so that movement toward the stated goal will be achieved in progressive steps and at a pace that is reasonable for both the patient and the nurse.

*The Contract*

For clarification of feelings and/or behavior, the nurse is generally the one who initiates the discussion to take this focus. The following example was recorded in a family record by a student nurse:

> Sue appeared uncomfortable and did not know what to say. I then told her how I felt about our nonexistent relationship and that I too was uncomfortable. Sue then told me a little about herself. It is hard for her to talk with strangers and she doesn't talk much anyway. After this, she talked more freely.

By recognizing the patient's nonverbal behavior and revealing her own feelings, the nurse communicated a discomfort with the one-way conversation, requested the patient to share her feelings, and facilitated a much more satisfactory interchange.

## Strengthening Approach

During the educational period when a student is learning to become a nurse, she is encouraged to look for deviances from the norm. She is alerted to symptoms that are indicative of a pathology and patterns of behavior that are not accepted as healthy behavior. For example, symptoms can be identified that are descriptive or indicative of specific biologic diseases, emotional dysfunctions, or unacceptable social conditions. Because of the identifiable nature of the symptoms, the student learns to look for those signs which represent pathology and often anticipates manifestations of progressive disease. Concurrent with learning to identify and anticipate pathology, the nurse also experiences performance evaluations of her work with ill patients. When her nursing performance is evaluated, she seems to be conditioned to expect critical statements rather than positive reinforcing statements regarding her skills. Otto stated that in our problem-centered culture most people's perception of their own personality strengths and resources is very limited. Research has shown that the average healthy, well-functioning person with one or more years of college training, on being asked to list his strengths, writes down only five or six items. If asked to list his weaknesses, he can usually fill one or two pages.[8]

It is generally accepted that all persons have unrealized potential and frequently live a life within self-imposed boundaries or limitations inflicted by others. One way for assisting that person, including patients and/or nurses, to recognize his strengths and disclose thoughts about potential is to do a personality inventory of strengths. This method is new to many persons, and the results of such an inventory can be strengthening to the individual as his self-image and self-confidence soar to a new level of acceptability. Sometimes a false idea of humbleness blocks his receptivity to the idea of personality strengths. Yet if this person believes in himself and his innate skills, he must recognize those strengths that exist and realize that a deepening and broadening of his positive capabilities can yield results beneficial to himself and to those around him.

Nurses themselves and patients are enriched mentally and emotionally from a personality inventory of strengths. It is a procedure that a person can do alone or one in which two persons can share identification of strengths for each other. Herbert Otto prepared a list of headings under which strengths could be identified.

Sports and outdoor activities
Hobbies and crafts
Expressive arts
Health
Education, training, and related areas
Work, vocation, job, or position
Special aptitudes or resources
Strengths through family and others
Intellectual strengths
Aesthetic strengths
Organizational strengths
Imaginative and creative strengths
Relationship strengths
Spiritual strengths
Emotional strengths
Other strengths such as a sense of humor[9]

In the practice of writing down assets, additional related strengths often come to a person's mind and should be added to the list. When two people

[8]Herbert A. Otto, *Guide to Developing Your Potential,* Charles Scribner's Sons, New York, 1967, pp. 171–172.
[9]*Ibid.,* pp. 236–239.

are using the inventory method, they inspire each other with many additional ideas. It must be remembered that the process of taking inventory of strengths is strengthening in itself to all participants.

Nurses who have used the strengthening approach with patients have received a variety of reactions, mainly positive. Patients are initially surprised to have strengths pointed out to them but respond with pleasure, and if the approach is a consistent one, they increasingly show evidence of an improved self-image and confidence in decision making. One situation in which the strengthening approach was conducive in moving the patient toward an increase in self-respect involved a nurse's weekly visits to a young mother for emotional and practical support; the nurse decided to try the method, explained the process to the patient, and asked her to write down her own strengths in preparation for the next visit. The nurse assured the patient that she too would write down the patient's strengths as she had observed them. On the subsequent visit the patient read her list of strengths first. They were mainly positive statements regarding her relationship with her husband and child. None made a direct reference to herself. When the nurse read the list of strengths that she had observed in the patient's behavior and life style, the young mother perceptibly straightened up in her chair, responded with a radiant glow, and exclaimed, "Do you really see that in me?" In this case, by accepting the positive opinion of the nurse, the young mother was started on the road toward development of greater self-respect, which involved the recognition and internalization of *her* strengths. This she needed, the nurse believed, in order to cope more effectively with her daily life.

## Inquiry or Problem-Solving Approach
The inquiry approach is based on the idea of encouraging the patient or family member to think his way through to new understandings by himself. The nurse serves as a facilitator in introducing this process and making use of questions that stimulate thought, expression, and divulgence of new insights. It is known that thoughts are often fuzzy when the mind is mulling all aspects of a given problem, and the act of verbalizing one's thoughts tends to clarify and crystallize ideas which have been previously vague and disjointed. Language influences thought and the putting together of an idea verbally helps to organize and clarify the problem. When the individual attentively figures out his own problem with the assistance of a facilitator and considers possible methods for solution, he attains greater depth of understanding of the issues involved, is more apt to follow through with his own devised solutions, and feels satisfaction with his conclusions and self-directed learning.

Nurse = a facilitator

*Facilitating Role of Nurse*

The role of the nurse in facilitating an inquiry approach is to elicit those problems that are of concern to the patient. As the concerns of the patient unfold, by being responsive to the patient, the nurse can pose questions that enable the patient to delve investigatively and sometimes with discovery into all aspects of the problem. If there are omissions or patterns of information given, the nurse can assist in looking for the gaps by asking the patient pertinent questions or recognize the patterning by making comparative analogies or checking her perception of the information she has heard from the patient. The nurse's goal in the inquiry approach is to stimulate the patient to think by creating an environment responsive to the patient and enabling him to verbalize his concerns in a self-investigative, creative way. Rather than giving direct suggestions or advice, the nurse elicits the knowledge the patient has about his problems, the possible solutions and resources with which he is acquainted, and the possibility of implementing activities which the patient believes to be feasible. Through this approach the patient is an active participant in his own learning, is enabled to find answers to his own questions, discovers the joys of doing his own problem solving, and consequently feels a boost of self-esteem. The nurse may have known the best answer to the problem and given the needed advice early in the interview, but by engaging the patient into doing his own problem solving, the probability that the patient will carry through with the "discovered" solution is greatly enhanced. At the same time the sharing of information and wrestling with a problem between nurse and patient produces a supportive relationship that is satisfying to both. There are times when the patient is unaware of the role the nurse plays when she facilitates inquiry, and the patient thinks he has done all the problem solving himself. At these times the nurse may express pleasure that the patient is so adept at problem solving or she may recap the sequence of the interview as it progressed.

The following example illustrates the facilitating role of the nurse as she talked to a mother who was concerned about her fourteen-year-old boy, who had been known to steal but on the day of the interview was playing hooky from school. The nurse makes use of the inquiry approach and she also takes advantage of the teachable moment when it occurs.

NURSE: Now, why do you think Mike played hooky today? He hasn't been in any real trouble for quite awhile, although he has been stealing by picking things up.

MOTHER: (then recounted his habit of "lifting things" and told about her husband's sister, who is married and has a habit of "lifting things.") I don't intend to excuse myself, but really, there has been no stealing on my side of the family. I've thought about it very carefully. My husband and his sister and her twin brother do "lift things," but the sister does it more than any of the others.

NURSE: (getting back to Mike) You asked me why Mike stole and why I think he may have played hooky. Shall we look at this together?

MOTHER: Well, I sure would like to understand why he does things like this.

NURSE: There are several theories or ideas why children steal. We can look at these and think about it. One idea is that the child is looking for love and affection and he steals because he is trying to grab on to love. Another idea is that stealing is attention-getting. It is one way to be a "big man" around one's friends, to be important. Another idea is that stealing and behaving badly is a way of getting back at your parents or authority figures. It will get your parents in trouble. Because he has not stolen this time, but played hooky, and you and Mike have been fighting about the dishes this week, I would tend to subscribe to an underlying dynamic that he is hitting back at *you*. Here is one way that will really hurt you, and get you into trouble.

MOTHER: I hadn't thought about that. I really would like to understand him better. (Said with sincerity.)

NURSE: He knows you have been angry with him. Have you said any kind things to him at all this week?

MOTHER: (looked at the table for awhile in thought. Then she raised her head and said) No, I don't think I have.

NURSE: Well, no matter how badly the children have behaved, they need praise. You may have to look hard sometimes to find something to praise them about that is real, but look, and look hard and give praise and appreciation to the children, especially those who misbehave the most. At the same time you need to stand firm—as you are doing—on your expectations for them.

MOTHER: I wonder what I should do to him.

NURSE: What do you plan to do?

MOTHER: I'm really going to lay into him when he comes home. I'm really going to tell him what I think about him and his friend (a pause). But I've done that before and it doesn't work.

NURSE: I offer this as a thought. Why not tell him you know he is angry with you about this past week and you realize he's trying to get back at you and hurt you. Tell him he has succeeded. Let him know he really has hurt you, and ask him how he feels now and if hurting you has done him any good.

MOTHER: I never thought of that. Do you suppose it would help?

NURSE: I really don't know, but it is an honest approach, isn't it?

MOTHER: Yes, it is. I've never approached him in that manner. I suppose I might as well try it. Nothing I have done has worked.

NURSE: There is one thing about discipline; you must fit it into the framework of *your* family and the values *you* hold. Consistency is the key, and teenagers in the rebellion of seeking the independence of adulthood still want the security of limit setting. This is how you tell them you love them, that you care what happens to them.

## Goal-oriented Approach

The goal-oriented approach makes use of the fact that any person will actively strive to attain a goal that he truly desires when he believes that it is within his reach. The optimal time to set a goal or goals is when the individual feels dissatisfied with a specific condition or aspect of his life. Upon reflection and considerable thought, he can be encouraged to decide what he wants, then set definite, desired goals. Goals must be known and desired, must be clearly stated and preferably written, must have a deadline for achievement, and in reality, must have the possibility for attainment.

Life is a continuous process of development and maturation from birth to death. Developmental tasks are dealt with as the person progresses in age. Tasks such as learning to walk and talk, to relate effectively with others, preparing for marriage, adjusting to physical changes of middle age, and adjusting to retirement often are taken for granted and managed as the particular stage of development and age are reached. However, life at any stage also has periods of obstacles and challenges which each individual can view as opportunities if he wishes to realize his potential for growth and make optimal use of any situation. One method of coping with life's problems is to set goals. Goals help to focus attention on coping mechanisms, facilitate movement or progression toward a desired end, help in motivation, give a sense of inner, compelling urge, and often expand the individual's view of existing opportunities. When goals are reached, the reward of achievement develops increased self-esteem and confidence.

The role of the nurse in utilizing the goal-oriented approach is to introduce it as a method for the patient, explain the purpose and desired ends of goal setting, and offer encouragement and support as the patient needs it when obstacles are encountered. When the nurse makes use of goal setting in her own life, she can serve as an excellent model and proponent of the efficacy of the method. She can offer examples of benefits and pitfalls from her own experience. She can stress the importance of *clearly stated goals, written goals,* and *time limits* for achievement. She can discuss the difference between goals and wishes as one of commitment. A wish is a desire that a person may dream about and truly want. It can be changed from a wish and become a goal when one is committed to achieving it by writing the culmination of the desire in clearly stated terms, setting a target date for achievement, and persisting in the belief that the goal can be and will be attained, regardless of the obstacles that may appear.

The nurse can utilize the goal-oriented approach in planning her own work for and with the patient. This is shown in the nursing care plan written specifically for the patient. The nurse can also introduce the patient to goals by advocating the use of the goal-oriented approach. She can assist the patient in writing a clearly stated goal that is conceivably attainable within a specified time limit. Together they can work toward achieving the stated goal. By involving the patient in goal setting and demonstrating success in achievement, the nurse serves as a teacher in opening up new avenues for the use of goal setting. For example, the patient may be encouraged to write his own personal goals which will benefit his life. Personal goals do not necessarily need to be shared with others; sometimes a personal goal is best attained when the individual writes it privately and works toward it alone. At other times the individual needs the reinforcement of a helping person such as a husband, wife, friend, or nurse. This person's role is to give positive encouragement as it is needed to overcome motivational obstacles and periods of discouragement and to reinforce the individual's belief in his ability to attain his goals.

An example of a goal-oriented approach utilized by one nurse with a patient was demonstrated when the nurse visited a young woman who stated the desire to lose weight. A discussion ensued about the variety of crash diets which the patient had utilized in the past, the successes and failures that had been experienced, and the pitfalls that often occurred. The nurse asked the patient what weight she wished to attain and tried to determine if the patient were truly in earnest about wishing to lose weight. When the nurse sensed that the patient's motivation was purposeful, she suggested the goal-oriented approach. Together the nurse and patient wrote down the desired loss in weight and the target date for achievement. In this instance, the patient weighed 135 pounds and wished to lose fifteen pounds. A target date for achievement was set for two months hence. The weekly goal of weight loss was determined to be a minimum of two pounds. A chart for notation of weekly weights and specified target dates was devised. The nurse advised the young woman to set up the chart where it would be seen constantly and remind the patient of her resolve to lose weight. The nurse also encouraged the patient to cut out pictures that would image her goal and put them where she would see them frequently. In this case the patient chose a photograph of herself when she had weighed 120 pounds. She put the chart with blank spaces for weekly weights and target dates and the photograph of herself on the door of her refrigerator. In addition, she pasted a statement in large lettering which read, "I weigh 120 pounds and it looks *good.*" Together the nurse and patient worked out a low-calorie diet that the patient felt she would be able to follow and that would enable her to lose the two pounds needed per week. On every subsequent visit the nurse requested the patient's account of how things were going. When success was achieved in losing the two pounds weekly, the nurse gave praise and reinforced the patient's self-discipline. When pitfalls were encountered, the nurse encouraged the patient to recall the events preceding the period when the diet was forgotten. Together the nurse and patient looked at the stresses which the patient had experienced and talked about ways in which the patient might respond differently if a similar event or temptation occurred. The nurse maintained a constant belief in the patient's ability to lose and communicated this belief to the patient verbally and nonverbally. When the patient attained her goal of fifteen pounds weight loss ahead of her target date of two months, she felt elated and proud of her accomplishment and emanated a new sense of self-confidence in her demeanor.

## THERAPEUTIC RELATIONSHIP SKILLS

"First"
Impressions
Important

When the nurse meets a family for the first time, a relationship is initiated which has the possibility for moving in any number of directions. If the nurse is offering her skills to help the family with a health problem, she desires the relationship to become a therapeutic one. Initially, as two people interact, they work out together what type of communicative behavior will take place in their relationship. From all the possible messages given to each other, they select which messages are acceptable or unacceptable. The cues for acceptability or unacceptability are given verbally or by nonverbal behavior. In this way they reach a mutual definition of the relationship. For example, on making a home visit and meeting a mother with a young baby for the first time, the nurse may enter the living room of the home and say, "That is a beautiful flower arrangement. Did you do it?" The mother may respond with pleasure and the conversation will focus on flowers temporarily. Later in the interview, the family cat may choose to jump on the nurse's lap, whereupon the nurse reacts with horror and pushes the cat away. The look of displeasure on the mother's face will be a cue to the nurse that her behavior was unacceptable. By being observant of all cues and initiating different subjects for discussion, the nurse and patient consciously and indirectly agree on limits within which the relationship can be developed.

Guide to
Success-
ful Relation-
ships.
Characteristics'
① Accurate
Empathy
② Nonposses-
sive Warmth
③ Genuineness

In order for any relationship to be successful, Truax and Carkhuff state that three characteristics are essential for the therapist to possess. These are accurate empathy, nonpossessive warmth, and genuineness.[10] To be facilitative toward another human being requires that the therapist be deeply sensitive to the other's moment-to-moment experience, grasping both the core meaning and significance and the content of his experiences and feelings. To understand empathically means that the therapist must have some warmth and respect for the other person. This is best expressed by being "real" or truly genuine with the other person. To be genuine means to be honest and open, to meet the other person without defensiveness or without playing a role that is "phony." Nonpossessive warmth is of central importance to any trusting relationship. The warm person has a sense of

[10]Charles B. Truax and Robert R. Carkhuff, *Toward Effective Counseling and Psychotherapy,* Aldine Publishing Company, Chicago, 1967, p. 25.

liking people and practices a friendly interest and acceptance of the other, regardless of differences or appearances. The quality of being nonjudgmental is of vital importance and has to be constantly exercised before it becomes a natural aptitude. To have a truly empathic understanding of another person, warmth, respect, trust, and even love for that person must be mutually communicated.[11] It is caring deeply about what is happening and what might happen to that person. It is at this point that a therapeutic relationship is established and the growth of the patient begins to take place. The development of a therapeutic relationship takes time and several contacts. It does not happen immediately.

*Caring*

### Rapport and Therapeutic Relationship

Rapport can happen immediately between two persons, but not necessarily between all persons. Rapport is a process, a happening, an experience undergone simultaneously by the nurse and patient. It is composed of a cluster of interrelated thoughts and feelings which are transmitted and communicated to each other. The nurse and patient remain separate and distinct human beings who share a series of mutually significant experiences together.[12] Both are involved. They perceive each other and relate as human being to human being, instead of as nurse to patient. For example, when two people's eyes meet and something "clicks," it often means a good rapport in which meanings of words are understood, enthusiasm is transmitted, and a mutual warmth of liking for each other occurs. Humor is shared and all behavior is accepted at face value. However, if two people meet, are courteous to each other, listen attentively and politely to all words spoken, but nothing is communicated when the eyes meet, this represents a pleasant acceptance but not necessarily a rapport. Because there are individuals in the community who have had little opportunity to experience moments of relatedness, it is particularly vital for the community health nurse, if possible, to facilitate the vivid awakening of a meaningful human-to-human encounter with specified patients. Rapport is a dynamic process and is developed with consecutive contacts and interactions, which lead eventually to a therapeutic relationship.

*Developing a Rapport*

The therapeutic relationship may be developed slowly or rapidly, depending on the circumstances of the nurse-patient situation. The nurse facilitates the development of trust by being warm, open, honest, genuine, and flexible. She creates an atmosphere in which the patient feels free to express his feelings, whether positive or negative. She actively tries to understand why the patient feels as he does and assists him to understand

---

[11]*Ibid.,* p. 32.

[12]Joyce Travelbee, *Interpersonal Aspects of Nursing,* F. A. Davis Company, Philadelphia, 1966, pp. 155–156.

his own feelings. She listens keenly, sensitively, and with complete attention. She communicates that she genuinely "cares." The patient responds
to the relationship by feeling secure and comfortable. His initial anxiety is
reduced and he feels a reassuring sense of worthiness and respect. He feels
that perhaps he can be helped and becomes ready to change his views or
behavior if it seems expedient. All interactions are directed purposefully
toward a mutually agreed goal of health. During the early stages of the
relationship, there are periods of progression and regression. It is the
nurse's task to be sensitive to the moments of regression and identify possible reasons for the patient's behavior. She may need assistance from special consultants to define the weakened link in the process and to be able
to intervene subsequently in a helpful manner with the patient.

Defn.:
Therapeutic
Relationship

In conclusion, the therapeutic relationship is a connection or bond
between nurse and patient that connotes mutual trust, respect, caring, sharing, and understanding. By its nature, it facilitates the growth of the patient
toward a goal of health which he desires and is made possible through the
purposeful intervention of the assisting nurse.

## WORKING WITH FAMILIES

In the life of the community health nurse the traditional unit for service is
the family and the setting for her interaction is the home. The family unit
generally consists of two or more people; therefore, when a nurse meets
with a family, she is dealing with a more complex situation than interacting
with one individual. She is faced with a group of two or more persons who
are in a particular phase of their life cycle dependent upon their ages, have
particular needs (possibly in health), and are accustomed to dealing with
stresses dependent upon the particular dynamics and patterns of that particular family. Oftentimes the life style of the family is affected by their
particular social class, culture, neighborhood environment, and economy.
Because the family is a more complex unit than the individual, the nurse
must be prepared to observe multiple facets of data and deal with presenting health problems. This entails the ability to assess a family situation
comprehensively, to sift out the factors that need immediate attention, and
to set priorities that have the most meaning to the family members. It involves establishing an effective interpersonal relationship with family members, an activity that necessitates a succession of home visits. In a study by
Highriter, families gave the highest performance ratings to those nurses
who were enthusiastic about their relationship with the family and seemed
to have a special liking of the family. In addition, families who received more
than ten nursing visits showed significantly more progress in the nursing
care areas studied than those who received fewer visits.[13]

[13]Marion E. Highriter, "Nurse Characteristics and Patient Progress," *Nursing Research,* 18:484–
501 (November-December) 1969.

## Patterns of Behavior of Community Health Nurses

Community health nurses working with families were found to differentiate their roles in two ways, according to Zola and Croog. One group was medically oriented and the second was socially oriented. The medically oriented nurse saw her role in terms of more traditional tasks, such as giving technical medical assistance and supervision. She was essentially patient-centered. The socially oriented nurse used the comprehensive health approach and conceived of her "core" role as one that emphasized teaching and counseling. She was more family-centered than patient-centered.[14]

*Medically oriented vs. Social orientation ↓*

In working with health needs of families, the *social orientation* of the community health nurse is imperative, but it *must be balanced* with *medical orientation* because it is generally through association with the physical health of the family that a contact by the nurse is gained and maintained. Sometimes the nurse feels helpless and inadequate when confronted with a complex family situation with multiple problems, but if she focuses on (1) what is happening in the here and now; (2) the family's interactions and interrelationships; and (3) the family's strengths, she can determine where to start. — *Frame of Reference*

*Need for Balance*

On early contact the nurse must become acquainted with all the members in the household. She must learn their ages and be observant of interactional patterns between family members whenever feasible. It is extremely important to meet the father or head of the household, since he often holds an influential role in the family. In the past, many nurses have not made a practice of meeting the man in the family because they do not know how to cope with him for one reason or another.[15] However, when the organizational makeup of any family is studied, the conclusion reached is that the man holds an important position of influence and power and therefore must be involved. Sometimes, in order to meet the man in the family, special arrangements have to be made, such as a visit in the evening or an appointment visit near the father's place of employment. Generally when the nurse expresses a desire to meet the man of the family, the response of family members is favorable. Until all members of the household are met and actively involved, a truly accurate assessment of a complex family health situation cannot be accomplished.

*Meet the Father*

When entering a home, the nurse must consciously greet all the family members present. If she recognizes by verbal or nonverbal means all members of the household, she is making her presence known and is in a position of catching their attention even though the initial response of individual family members may be one of indifference or withdrawal. Even the family's

[14]Irving Kenneth Zola and Sydney H. Croog, "Work Perceptions and Their Implications For Professional Identity: An Exploratory Analysis of Public Health Nurses," *Social Science and Medicine,* 2:15–25, Pergamon Press, New York (March) 1968.
[15]Rosemary Pittman, "The Man In the Family," *Nursing Outlook,* 16:62–64 (April) 1968.

pets should be acknowledged, particularly if they seem to hold a position of esteem. For example, a staff nurse who was visiting a young couple with a new baby recognized early that the friendly Dalmatian held an important position in the affections of the new mother. It was not until several visits had been made that she came to the realization that the dog was treated as a firstborn and the new baby was regarded in attitude very similarly to that of a second-born child. By making this assessment of the dynamics of family life, the nurse was able to give more appropriate, cogent assistance to the young mother.

If the household contains a sick member who is unable to respond verbally or tangibly, the nurse should make a point of speaking directly to the patient, in a manner which indicates her belief that he understands. By recognizing the existence of the patient, the nurse communicates a respect for the patient's dignity and serves as a model to family members regarding the appropriate attitude to assume toward the sick person.

### Beginning Relationship with a Family

By recognizing all the members of the household and being cognizant of the interrelationships and family dynamics, the nurse is in an excellent position of soliciting and gaining cooperation from family members and eliciting health goals which will be beneficial to all. When she wants to meet with the family as a whole, she must purposefully make an appointment with the family, specifically stating that all are to be present. When the appointed time arrives, she should take the initiative for starting the conversation by introducing her reasons for wanting to talk with all the family members. She should consciously create a setting that is relaxed and aimed to put family members at ease. Encouragement of each individual to state his particular view of the health issue should be done by asking direct questions in a nonthreatening manner. She should realize that her presence in the family group is essentially that of an outsider or a third party, and this role will enable her to facilitate conversation between family members which is not usually openly expressed. She should give feedback to individuals within the family about their verbalizations as perceived by her. She should be accepting of positive and negative information and, by listening carefully, should request further information which is clarifying and factual. She should be cognizant of assets and express recognition of individual and family strengths as they become apparent. By engaging the family as a whole, the nurse is able to assess the family situation, enable the family to focus on the issue of the moment, and provide the impetus to move toward stated, desired, unified goals. Because all family members have been brought together and encouraged to discuss a health situation openly, and decisions regarding goals to be achieved have been elicited and perhaps decided upon, the predictability of a favorable outcome for future events is much more assured.

To cite an example, a student nurse who was visiting on a regular basis a family with multiple problems frequently discussed with the mother the current problems of the father's unemployment, finances, transportation, school adjustment of the four children, and discipline in the home. There was no noticeable progress in the family's ability to cope with their daily problems as reported by the mother until the nurse conceived the idea to meet the father and arrange a family conference. An appointment was made to meet the entire family and an open discussion of their situation was aired. No issues were resolved as a consequence of the meeting other than a complete reassessment of the family by the nurse. After three more meetings, during which several health issues were discussed, the family demonstrated much more unity, a happier and more secure attitude, a better insight into some of their behaviors, and an improved ability to cope with daily events. Because of the positive change in the family's functioning, the nurse felt that she benefitted most because she learned that <u>all families are a dynamic whole, made up of individuals who must be met and involved as participating members, and resolution of health needs is facilitated with the least amount of nurse energy.</u>

## WORKING WITH GROUPS

With the changes that are occurring so rapidly in our society, the realization that nurses must work more actively with community health groups in planning and implementing programs is strikingly apparent. Consumers from a variety of community settings are declaring their right to be heard and demanding health services from a number of different resources and for a number of different reasons. However, they are not necessarily remembering that community health nurses are an excellent resource for assistance. Consequently, nurses must initiate their willingness to become actively involved in the particular health sphere in which they are interested. In doing so, they must become knowledgeable about working with groups. Some examples of community groups that would benefit from the participation of the nurse include prenatal, weight-watching, mental health, child discipline, special disease conditions, geriatric, discussion, and many other groups. The opportunity for the nurse to be truly creative is potentially inherent in community group work.

The community health nurse generally has a range of membership in different professional groups such as staff, team, or in-service education meetings in agencies and interdisciplinary meetings with persons from other professions. However, she should become much more involved in community health meetings in which many of the participating members

Working with all Resources

are lay people or nonprofessional representatives. By attending these meetings, she will be exposed to a variety of people with a variety of expectations. She must know *why* she is a member of the group and what is to be her role and purpose. Specifically, a group may be defined as a plurality of individuals who are in contact with one another, who take one another into account, and who are aware of some significant commonality. It is essential that members have something in common and that they believe that what they have in common makes a difference.[16] Olmsted stated that there are two groups, primary and secondary. Primary groups are composed of members who are warm, intimate, and have personal ties with each other. They are usually of a small, face-to-face sort, spontaneous in their interpersonal behavior, and often have common goals. The family, gang, or friendship groups are examples. Generally a primary group is "fun," brings enjoyment of some kind, and functions in a training or supportive capacity. Secondary groups are made up of persons who are apt to be impersonal, rational, contractual, and formal. Members of these groups participate in special capacities and not necessarily as whole personalities. The groups are gathered together as a means to some end and have only intermittent contacts. Examples include a range of associations which include professional, office, community, or bureaucratic interests.[17] It is membership and functioning in secondary or community groups for which the nurse needs to become knowledgeable.

### Problems in Entering a New Group[18]

When the nurse enters a new group, whether it is a professional or a community group, she is faced with four issues which must be resolved before she can be comfortable. The first is that of *identity*. She must decide on a role with which she is comfortable and which is acceptable with the group. What role should I play that is acceptable to me and to the group? The choices include that of an aggressive talker who wants to gain attention, a quiet listener who avoids all risks, a logical thinker who asks pertinent questions, the obstructionist who finds fault with all suggestions, the humorous person who gives a "light touch" to the conversation at appropriate times, and any number of other possible roles. The second issue involves *control, power,* and *influence.* Who are the persons in the group with the most power and control? Which individuals will influence me or vice versa? Therefore, initial group dialogue may be characterized by individuals' testing and experimenting with different forms of influence until they feel acquainted and have come to terms with the basic structure of the group. *Individual needs* and *group goals* are the third issue with which the group

[16]Michael S. Olmsted, *The Small Group*, Random House, Inc., New York, 1959, pp. 21–22.
[17]*Ibid.*, pp. 17–19.
[18]Adapted from Edgar H. Schein, *Process Consultation: Its Role In Organization Development,* Addison-Wesley Publishing Company, Inc., Reading, Mass., 1969, pp. 32–37.

member is concerned. Will the group goals be such that my own personal goals are met? Can I be committed to work toward a group goal if my own need is not attended to? In many groups where group goals are decided but little action evolves, the explanation often lies in the fact that the group's needs as a whole were not requested or discussed; therefore, little member commitment was obtained. Early in a meeting group members often take a "wait and see" attitude until the direction of group activity develops, which reveals that personal interests will be met in some way. Then the members get on the bandwagon. The fourth issue that concerns the new member is *acceptance* and *intimacy*. Will I be liked and accepted by others in the group? Can I be comfortable and respectful of the others? Is the environment conducive to formal or informal behavior?

*[handwritten: ④ Acceptance Intimacy]*

With respect to the four issues involved in entering a new group, there are generally three basic kinds of coping patterns which the membership of the group demonstrate. They are (1) the basically tough, aggressive coping, which is characterized by arguing, cutting down another's points, deliberate ignoring of others, or barbed humor. These behaviors may be manifested in an open, assertive manner or in a subtle, polite manner. Members who are resisting the authority or chairman of the group can demonstrate aggressive coping by setting up the situation with "Let's find out what the chairman wants and then *not* do it." (2) The basically tender, support-seeking coping is demonstrated by those members who try to form an alliance with another group member or who avoid conflict by being supportive of each other. Their support may be based on genuine understanding or a blindly dependent response to the person in authority, to whom they look for guidance or solution of their problems. (3) The withdrawal behavior based on denial of any feelings is characterized by the passive, indifferent kind of response. The attitude of these group members is that feelings are inappropriate in a group discussion, and they withdraw when feelings become apparent. They let others fight an issue while they sit blandly on the sidelines. However, feelings *are* a reality, and until they are brought out into the open, group tasks representative of the entire group cannot be accomplished.

*[handwritten: Coping Patterns; (1) Tough; (2) Tender; (3) Withdrawal]*

When groups have worked through the four issues described and reached the point where all members realize that they are a contributing part of the group, they begin to relax and are willing to pay closer attention to each other. Their cooperation as a group becomes apparent and they are ready to attend to group tasks.

## Content of Group Meetings

When an individual focuses on what the group is talking about, that is *content*. Members of the group may be working toward accomplishing some task or goal which they have established and will demonstrate spe-

*[handwritten: Defn. of Content]*

*Fulfillment of task* (handwritten margin note)

cific behaviors that facilitate this end. The behaviors which aid in the group's fulfillment of its *task* include the following. (1) *Initiating:* a member proposes a task or goal, succeeds in defining a group problem, suggests an idea for solving the problem, or sets target dates for fulfillment of a task. (2) *Seeking information or opinions:* someone requests facts, asks for an expression of feelings, or seeks suggestions or ideas. (3) *Giving information or opinion:* an individual offers facts, provides information which is relevant to the discussion, or gives suggestions and ideas. (4) *Clarifying and elaborating:* a member attempts to interpret ideas and suggestions in order to clear up confusions, defines terminology, or indicates alternatives open to the group. (5) *Summarizing:* someone pulls together related ideas, restates suggestions more succinctly, reviews points that have already been considered, or offers a conclusion for the group to accept or reject. (6) *Consensus testing:* an individual may ask, "Are we ready to decide?" to test if the group is ready to make a decision.[19]

*Maintenance Functions* (handwritten margin note)

Behaviors which enable the group to survive, maintain good working relationships, and also permit maximum use of the resources of the members are called maintenance functions; these include the following. (1) *Harmonizing:* a member attempts to reconcile disagreements, reduces tension, or attempts to help people to explore their differences. (2) *Gatekeeping:* someone tries to keep communication channels open or suggests procedures that will permit sharing remarks. (3) *Encouraging:* an individual will maintain friendly, warm responses to others or will indicate acceptance of others' contributions by nonverbal means (nodding, facial expression). (4) *Compromising:* a member whose original idea was not totally acceptable will offer a compromise, may admit an error, or will modify an idea in the interest of group cohesion. (5) *Standard setting and testing:* someone will test whether the group is satisfied with its procedures or will suggest procedures that are available for testing.[20]

In all groups both kinds of behaviors are observed to some degree and are needed in order to get the job done and to keep the group in good working order. As the nurse becomes increasingly familiar with group work, she will be able to identify each behavior as it occurs.

### Group Process

*Defn. of Group Process* (handwritten margin note)

When an individual focuses on how the group is handling its communication, i.e., who talks how much or who talks to whom, that is *group process.* It refers to the "here and now" of what is happening within the group. Many groups do not wish to look at group process because they are reluctant to analyze their own and others' behavior. If individuals do not wish the group

[19] *Ibid.,* pp. 38–40.
[20] *Ibid.,* pp. 40–41.

process to be studied, it should not be urged. However, if a group is willing to take five or ten minutes at the conclusion of their meeting to discuss *only* the group process as it occurred, it facilitates understanding and openness and promotes cohesion of the group. If group process is to be studied, an observer should be selected whose function is to remain objective and carefully observe the group interaction. When the group is ready to examine and reflect on their process, the observer reports his observations to the group and discussion ensues. The observer does not provide a summary of the discussion, is free to participate in the discussion, and only reports on *process* that facilitated or inhibited the group.

## Leading or Facilitating a Group

In many groups the entire responsibility for leadership is expected to be taken by the chairman. However, if the chairman wishes to involve all members in any group, he can do so. By virtue of their presence in the group, all members can be seen as possessing some degree of responsibility or resourcefulness which must be ferreted out and revealed by the leader. All members ideally need and want to have a commitment toward fulfillment of the task for which the group was organized. Therefore, it is up to the leader to set the stage. Rather than acting as an authoritarian leader, he can consciously act as a *facilitator,* a person who makes sure that the task and process function of the group are carried out effectively. By doing so, he keeps the group process moving smoothly and reminds the members to continue moving toward clearly defined and mutually set goals. He does not dominate or lead but encourages or facilitates all members of the group to assume responsibility for accomplishing the group goals.[21]

*Facilitating Group Discussion*

The task of facilitating a group takes preparation and forethought. Some of the factors and questions that must be considered by the leader are:

**1.** *Preparation.* Why is this group being formed? Will the members become interested and motivated to work toward purposeful goals? What can I say or do that will "catch" their attention? When the leader prepares for the meeting by thoroughly studying appropriate readings, reference materials, and audio-visual aids, ideas for presenting the material in an interesting and provocative way to group members can be her focus. Sometimes a short, appropriate film or tape recording will be effective or, depending on the group, a game or exercise may be the initial way of "warming up" a group and gaining their attention.[22] The ability of the leader to be re-

[21]Elwin C. Nielsen, "Process Groups For Self-Learning and Problem Solving," (unpublished).
[22]William C. Schutz, *Joy,* Grove Press, Inc., New York, 1967, pp. 117–186.

sourceful, original, or creative in the beginning enhances the possibility for gaining the group's attention and ultimate commitment.

**2.**  *Getting Started.* What physical set-up will be most conducive to establishing a comfortable environment? Sometimes the chairs are best arranged around a table or in an intimate circle. The environment should be such that the temperature, light, and ventilation are adequate. If a blackboard, charts, or audio-visual apparatus are needed, they should be set up before the meeting begins. The leader should arrange the room so that it communicates the climate she wishes to establish.

When the group members enter the meeting room, the leader should greet each individual with friendliness and make him feel welcome. When all members are gathered together, the leader should start the meeting by introducing herself and the overall purpose for being together. Time should be taken for all to become acquainted and feel a pleasant friendly atmosphere. An effective method for enabling others to relax and feel free to express their ideas is to state that a way for getting better acquainted is for all members in the group to introduce themselves and tell something about themselves. The leader should always start the introductions with a description of herself and whatever information she wishes the group to know about herself. Dependent upon the length and extent of the leader's self-introduction will be the contribution of each succeeding member's description of self. Groups tend to conform to the norm established by the leader. If the leader divulges quite a bit of appropriate information about herself, group members will feel more at ease in following her lead and revealing pertinent information about themselves, and general group comfort will be facilitated. Sometimes, it is a good idea to have name cards until the members are well acquainted.

**3.**  *Purpose and Objectives.* The general purpose for which the group was formed should then be expressed or reiterated by the leader, and her plan to involve the members should be executed, whether it is a game, a film, or something deliberately provocative. When the time arrives for the group members to discuss, react, or present their thoughts, the leader should ask for an expression of ideas and *facilitate* discussion from that time on. The facilitator's task involves (1) getting an expression of ideas from all members; (2) keeping the conversation centered on the issues of the meeting; (3) promoting the establishing of objectives or goals that are agreeable to all members; (4) encouraging the divulgence of each member's resources or skills; (5) promoting a commitment to the group's goals by all the members. When words or terminology are not clear, the facilitator can ask group members for clarification. If the members of the group expect the facilitator to solve an issue, she can return it to the group by rephrasing or reinterpreting the issue at stake. At periodic intervals summarizing statements of the discussion or important points can be phrased for the purpose of clarifying the progress of the discussion. Tolerance, patience, open-mindedness, and flexibility are important for successful meetings. As all persons in the group are encouraged to speak their ideas, thoughts are formulated and crystallized, are spread to others contagiously, and the group inevitably progresses toward new, sometimes exciting conclusions. By being willing to hear different viewpoints expressed, a flexibility and open-mindedness is facilitated and each member learns.

**4.** *Concluding the Meeting.* The facilitator must be aware of the passage of time and stay within the scheduled limits. It may be advisable to warn the group that only five or ten minutes are remaining. Or the facilitator may summarize the progress of the discussion and ask "What have we decided to do?"; "Have we included everything?" Or she may indicate that the meeting is due to be terminated by asking, "What assignments or tasks do we need to do before the next meeting?" or "When shall we meet again?" If all members have participated verbally in the issues of the meeting or have demonstrated nonverbal interest, there will be a general aura of purposeful activity and involvement that denotes a successful meeting.

## Criteria for Group Growth
To determine if the group is developing into an effective, workable unit which functions smoothly, the following questions can be asked and cogitated upon:

1. Does the group have the capacity to deal realistically with its tasks?

2. Is there basic agreement within the group about ultimate goals and values?

3. Does the group have a capacity for self-knowledge?

4. Is there an optimum use of the resources available within the group?

5. Does the group learn from its experience? Can it assimilate new information and respond flexibly to it?[23]

A successful and satisfying group is one in which all members participate and assume responsibility for functioning in an integrated fashion. Facilitation of such a group is a stimulating learning experience for the leader. The composition of the group does not affect the process of leading or facilitating a group. Professional groups or community groups can be facilitated by a skillful leader who consciously draws out the resourceful-

[23]Schein, *op. cit.,* pp. 61–63.

ness of the members, whether they have lay, nonprofessional, or professional identities. Much of what happens in groups can be attributed to the leadership, particularly if it is creative and flexible.

## COORDINATION OF INTERDISCIPLINARY PERSONNEL

Nursing is a highly diversified occupation and there are some tasks which nurses undertake that are not noted to be their function exclusively. One such task for community health nurses is that of *coordination* of patient care. When working intensively with families, community health nurses learn of a variety of agencies or personnel who are communicating with one or more members of the family constellation and often arrange for a conference of all interested personnel or call the representative of each discipline individually in an effort to coordinate the services given to the family. This particular task is essential and must be *stressed* as an important, vital attribute of community health nurses.

*Coordinating involved people*

When people are drawn together to combine their efforts for a given purpose, this is coordination. *Coordination* is the orderly arrangement of group effort to provide unity of action in the pursuit of a common purpose.[24] In community health nursing the common purpose that is focused upon by the various health representatives is the integration of community health services to the patient or family. Communication among personnel of all community health facilities is essential to share information and discuss what is involved in sustaining or improving the health status of the given patient and family. All too often coordination of health personnel is not initiated spontaneously and duplication or overlapping of services to a family occurs. By assuming the task of coordination with responsibility, the community health nurse contributes to the assurance that continuity of patient care will be achieved.

*Defn. of Coordination*

### Health Teams

In community health nursing the composition of health teams varies according to the purpose for gathering the group and the nature of the personnel attending. Community health teams can consist of professional persons or a combination of lay and professional persons. Some examples of health teams include: (1) a group of community health nurses working in an agency; (2) a group of community health nurses, licensed practical nurses, home health aides, and community aides working in an agency; (3) a community health nurse representing a health department, a social worker representing the department of public assistance, a physician, a school

[24]James Mooney, "The Coordinative Principle," in Joseph A. Litterer (ed.), *Organizations: Structure and Behavior,* John Wiley & Sons, Inc., New York, 1963, p. 39.

principal, a school nurse, an individual representing the housing authority, etc.; (4) a community health nurse and paraprofessional personnel representing a clinic service such as family planning; (5) a community health nurse, a medical nurse representing the hospital, a family member, a family counselor, a school teacher, and other involved personnel; (6) a community health nurse and a group of lay volunteers getting ready to execute a screening test for vision, hearing, or a related health measure.

When the nurse is a member of any health team, she must know her purpose for being included as a participant and must be willing to assume responsibility for leadership when it is needed or implicit. The preceding discussion about "Working with Groups" is applicable to developing effective health teams, particularly if the team meets on a regular basis. The emphasis of health teams should always be focused on their mutual purpose, action directed toward agreed-upon goals, and effort expended toward maintaining working relationships which facilitate satisfactory progress. Sharing of information in a noncompetitive fashion enables all team members to function in a responsible, satisfying manner and expedites the purpose for which the group was brought together.

## Multidisciplinary Conferences

When the community health nurse initiates a plan for a conference of professional persons representing several community agencies to discuss a care plan for a specified family, she must call all the professionals serving the family and invite them to a stated place at a specific time for the purpose of pooling their information about the family. *Arranging a meeting — Role of CHN.* All too often representatives of the various community agencies working with a given family are not called together to unify their purposes and goals in giving assistance. If the conference is to be one in which confidential information is disclosed, the nurse should clear the exchange of such information with the patient by asking him to sign a release-of-information form. In so doing, the patient is made aware that such a conference is in the planning stages and realizes the purpose is to facilitate the integration of health services in his behalf. When talking to the professionals who are being invited to the conference, the nurse should state that the patient has signed a release slip, indicating that it is permissible to bring confidential records and reports. She should also state her expectation of the contribution the professional person will make to the conference, and if he wishes to bring printed materials that will aid in the group's understanding, this would be desirable. If it seems expedient to invite the professional worker's supervisor to the conference, the procedure for doing so correctly should be requested. By being knowledgeable about the organizational structure of allied community agencies and complying to their modus operandi, coordination is facilitated.

*Leading a Group*

A review of the four points in the discussion of "Leading or Facilitating a Group" will give the nurse ideas regarding her plan of procedure for the conference. It is important to remember that all group members should be introduced. Too often in professional groups, the assumption is made that everyone knows each other and this is not necessarily so. Another essential point to realize is that the initiator of the conference must act as the leader or facilitator. When the group is composed of community professional leaders, it is often tempting for the nurse to transfer the leadership of the conference to another person who holds a more imposing position. However, when the nurse is the initiator, she *must* perform responsibly as the leader or facilitator. If she thinks refreshments will serve the function of relaxing the group members, she should plan for and offer coffee and cookies early in the conference. If a blackboard is available and the listing of issues coming out in the discussion seems indicated, the leader should feel comfortable about writing the ideas on the blackboard herself or asking someone else to do so. Regardless of the composition of the group, whether it is made up of eminently more important persons professionally than herself, the nurse leader should perform the tasks of facilitation with confidence and responsibility.

### Coordination with Other Community Professionals

*Communicate*

It is essential that the community health nurse keep open lines of communication with the family physician at all times. This may require several telephone calls or a visit to the physician's office. When the nurse interprets her function with the family to the physician, she can emphasize the nature of her role as a coordinator. She can explain how she was referred to the family, and the contract agreed upon by the family and herself for continued service. She can describe her assessment of the family situation and identify her need for validation of specific information given or activities prescribed by the physician. By bringing out omissions, misperceptions, or incompletions of the family's health knowledge or practices in the home, the nurse can demonstrate the efficacy of her role as a coordinator. By working *with* the physician, making him knowledgeable about the obstacles which are hindering the family's implementation of his recommendations, and the goals toward which she is working, the nurse communicates the essentiality of her function with the family.

It is equally important for the nurse to keep open lines of communication with all allied professionals representing different community facilities who are serving commonly known families. For example, if the family receiving public assistance is on the active roster of the housing authorities and family counseling service, those workers representing allied disciplines should be made aware that the nurse is also serving the family. The main objective for keeping open lines of communication is to work toward com- *Objective* mon, unified goals in serving a family. Otherwise, families are given the opportunity to exploit the services of several community facilities in a number of ways or become confused about the multiplicity of professionals who are communicating varying suggestions. When the nurse starts working with a family, she should inquire about the possibility of other community facilities to whom the family is known. She should make a point of requesting the names of other workers who are serving the family currently and explain that she wishes to talk to them. If it is necessary for the family member to sign a release-of-information slip, the form should be made available and signed at the time of the visit. The nurse can then arrange for a multidisciplinary conference or talk to each professional individually. It is vital that all community workers, professional and nonprofessional, discuss their contact with the family so that common goals are determined and methods of working toward goals are synchronized. Attitudes toward a given family are concomitantly revealed, discussed, and adjusted toward the purpose of accomplishing the mutually accepted goals. To reiterate, the community health nurse is in the best position to initiate and implement coordination of community health services to the patient and family whenever several professionals are involved.

## Coordination with Other Community Nonprofessionals

The utilization of nonprofessionals or paraprofessionals in the medical and nursing ranks is increasing rapidly in our society. With the advent of a wide selection of trained and untrained community workers, it is essential that all community professionals relate in a manner that enhances and enriches the capabilities of these people. The term *nonprofessional* refers to those persons whose tasks are mainly of a technical nature, i.e., licensed practical nurses, nurse's aides. Paraprofessionals refer to those persons within the community who are unskilled, have little formal education but are being trained successfully as assistants in some capacity to professionals, i.e., home health aides, community aides, nutritional aides. Studies have shown that locally selected trainees or paraprofessionals living in impoverished neighborhoods have a strong desire to work and earn a decent living. When they have received on-the-job training, they contribute effectively to a given program because they know a great deal about the persons living in the "hard to reach" neighborhoods who have need for health services. The paraprofessionals can be genuinely open, empathic, supportive, and persuasive of people they serve because they have lived through very similar circumstances. They can overcome barriers of cultural differences, communication difficulties, lack of motivation, and understanding which have often interfered when professionals have dealt with the disadvantaged groups.[25]

Because nonprofessionals and paraprofessionals are demonstrating their effectiveness in the health field, it is essential that professionals recognize and utilize their services to a maximum degree, promote the idea of teamwork, and take advantage of the extra time to perform professional functions which they alone can best fulfill, i.e., managerial tasks or research studies. Relating effectively to nonprofessionals is no different from relating to any other group of people. Nonprofessionals want to be seen and heard, deemed worthy, and considered a part of the team. They generally know their assets and limitations, appreciate recognition of their strengths, and are honest about their limits. They appreciate and want supervision when their competencies are uncertain. Even though they are not so well educated academically as professionals, they have knowledge and attitudes about the local community which are valuable for the professional to know. Often they have an intuition and compelling warmth for the consumer which the professional may not possess. In team meetings the skilled, effective nurse is one who provides a comfortable environment and encourages all members to contribute their ideas whether they have a professional, nonprofessional, or paraprofessional status. It behooves the nurse leader to recognize all of her team members, regardless of their professional standing, as worthy of her respect and interest. By working *with* the nonprofessionals and paraprofessionals and not *over* them, the performance of the team as a whole is enhanced and satisfying.

It is not unusual for professionals to demonstrate lack of enthusiasm toward the skills of nonprofessionals. When a negative reaction of professionals is perceived, it often results from a lack of understanding and acceptance of paraprofessionals in any field of nursing. One way to counteract negative attitudes is to provide the opportunity for professionals to talk openly about their feelings and attitudes in a series of closed sessions. When it is appropriate and timely, their special strengths and capabilities as professionals should be pointed out in conjunction with the paraprofessional's requirement for competent supervision, and a new relationship which is reality-based and very much needed may be started. Emphasis on the responsibility for directing or supervising other personnel to give skilled health services to consumers is highly important and demanding. When done well, the professionals can take pride in the fact that they played an essential role in facilitating expert care to the patient, which restored his dignity, worth, and health.

[25]Wilbur Hoff, M.D., "Older Poor Adults Trained As Home Health Aides," *Public Health Reports,* 83:3:184–185 (March) 1968.

## USE OF CONSULTATION

There are many times when a community health nurse needs consultation. Because she is a generalist, consultation in specialized fields of nursing and closely allied disciplines such as nutrition, social work, psychology, community development, and others is essential and edifying in improving the quality of services given to the consumer. Consultation can be gained from many sources, such as nursing supervisors, clinical specialists, physicians, social workers, nutritionists, specialists for specific disease categories or social conditions, and others.

The consultation process involves three features: (1) the consultee, an individual who has defined a need—something she wishes to know; (2) the consultant, the person with the expertise to fulfill the need; and (3) the problem area with which the consultee wants help. The problem can be a health need of a patient or a community activity in which the consultee is involved. The assumption is made by the consultee that the consultant can fulfill her need, and the consultant assumes that the consultee will be prepared with all the data relevant to the problem.

When the consultee desires help in regard to a problem, she requests an appointment with the appropriate consultant and gathers all data she believes will be pertinent to the consultation. This may involve making a summary of all essential information from the family record and forwarding a copy of the summary to the consultant prior to the appointed time. Or, it may involve reading more-inclusive references pertinent to the problem to enable the consultation to be on a sharing, knowledgeable basis between two professionals.

The success of the consultation is dependent on several factors: whether the consultee (1) has correctly diagnosed her needs; (2) is adequately prepared with all essential data; (3) has adequately communicated her needs to the consultant; (4) has selected the appropriate consultant; and (5) has thought through the consequences of implementing ideas or changes that may be recommended by the consultant.[26] The conversation between consultant and consultee should be two-way, not in one direction only. Ideas suggested by the consultant should be thoroughly explored by both parties as to their feasibility in relation to the specific problem area being studied. Since the consultee is personally acquainted with the problem area, its idiosyncracies and complications, she alone can suspect if an idea will work. When the consultee is helped to see a problem area more comprehensively and is actively involved in reaching realistic conclusions regarding her next steps, she is more likely to feel satisfied with the consultation process and will demonstrate subsequent activities which reveal successful learning. Rather than expecting the consultant to provide answers,

[26]Schein, *op. cit.*, p. 5.

the consultee should anticipate the problem-solving approach to be used, during which the consultant aids in sharpening the diagnosis of the problem area and suggests ideas or alternatives that have not already occurred to the consultee. It is up to the consultee to make the ultimate decision as to what action to take, since she is fully acquainted with the uniqueness of the problem. Inherent in the consultation process is the requirement for openness in discussion, a comfortable, sharing environment, and a bond of mutual respect which facilitates a helping relationship between the two participants.

As the community health nurse learns to make use of a wide selection of available consultants within the community, she develops her own expertise in becoming an exceptional generalist who is recognized by all community specialists. She is the individual who has a grasp of the wholeness of health practices occurring within her particular community.

## SUMMARY
The emphasis on and importance of attainment of relationship skills for community health nurses was stressed as having *high* priority if successful practices with individuals, families, or groups are desired. To be a truly helping person who will be accepted and often appreciated by the consumer, the nurse must possess three characteristics: accurate empathy, nonpossessive warmth, and genuineness. When consumers are asked to describe the kind of nurse they would like to have serving them, they invariably bring out their desire for a nurse with warmth, humor, friendliness, and a special liking for them.

Community health nurses use a variety of different approaches when they work with individuals, families, or groups, Descriptions and examples were given of some specific approaches which can be successfully implemented dependent upon the individualized responses of the individuals, families, or groups.

The coordination role of the community health nurse was stressed as vital to ensure that health services to a family are integrated and purposeful. Someone must bring into a common focus all of the elements of the health-care system which are directly or indirectly involved in giving service to individuals, families, or groups. This means teamwork with professionals, nonprofessionals, and paraprofessionals who are working in the various health facilities in a community. Because the community health nurse is a generalist, she must be prepared to use consultation, which will result in increased expertise for herself and beneficial activities for consumers.

## SUGGESTED READING

Brammer, Lawrence M., and Everett L. Shostrom: *Therapeutic Psychology,* 2d ed., Prentice-Hall, Inc., Englewood Cliffs, N.J., 1968.

Brunetto, Eleanor, and Peter Birk: "The Primary Care Nurse—The Generalist in a Structured Health Care Team," *American Journal of Public Health,* 62:6:785–793 (June) 1972.

Caplan, Gerald: *Principles of Preventive Psychiatry,* Basic Books, Inc., Publishers, New York, 1964.

Carlson, Carolyn E. (ed.): *Behavioral Concepts and Nursing Intervention,* J. B. Lippincott Company, Philadelphia, 1970.

Dunn, Halbert L.: *High-Level Wellness,* R. W. Beatty Co., Arlington, Va., 1961.

Frankl, Viktor E.: *Man's Search For Meaning,* Washington Square Press, a division of Simon & Schuster, Inc., New York, 1963.

Haley, Jay: *Strategies of Psychotherapy,* Grune & Stratton, Inc., New York, 1963.

Jourard, Sidney M.: *The Transparent Self,* D. Van Nostrand Company, Inc., Princeton, N.J., 1964.

Langsley, Donald G., and David M. Kaplan: *The Treatment of Families In Crisis,* Grune & Stratton, Inc., New York, 1968.

Maslow, Abraham H.: *Toward a Psychology of Being,* D. Van Nostrand Company, Inc., Princeton, N.J., 1962.

Otto, Herbert A.: *Guide To Developing Your Potential,* Charles Scribner's Sons, New York, 1967.

Rogers, Carl R.: *On Becoming a Person,* Houghton Mifflin Company, Boston, 1961.

Satir, Virginia: *Conjoint Family Therapy,* Science and Behavior Books, Inc., Palo Alto, Calif., 1967.

Schein, Edgar H.: *Process Consultation: Its Role In Organization Development,* Addison-Wesley Publishing Company, Inc., Reading, Mass., 1969.

Stein, Leonard J.: "The Doctor-Nurse Game," *American Journal of Nursing,* 68:1:101–105 (January) 1968.

Towle, Charlotte: *Common Human Needs,* National Association of Social Workers, Inc., New York, 1965.

Travelbee, Joyce: *Interpersonal Aspects of Nursing,* F. A. Davis Company, Philadelphia, 1966.

Van Sickle, Aileen B.: "Bookshelf For the Community Health Nurse Specialist," *American Journal of Public Health,* 60:4:618–627 (April) 1970.

# 3
# Community Characteristics and Health Practices

Since community health nurses are practicing in a variety of geographical locations, the setting of the local community and factors affecting it must be studied in addition to the health needs of the local residents. Each community, whether urban, suburban, or rural, has its own unique characteristics, strengths, and limitations. As the nurse becomes knowledgeable about the community in which she is working, she enhances her ability to play a significant role in developing awareness of and improving the health practices of its people. As stated by Remillet and Reading, the community health nurse must know the community she serves. She must have accurate knowledge of the age-group percentages, ethnic differences, the dominant culture and subcultures, sociological factors that spawn health problems, the socioeconomic range, the ecologic problems, and the resources for finding solutions once problems have been differentiated from cause. Accumulation of data is only the beginning; application of the findings in order to assess needs further and to participate in realistic decision making to improve the environment for better living follows in logical sequence.[1]

By looking at the field of health as a generalist in nursing, the community health nurse must be prepared to know multiple facets of the community; the health problems, needs, and desires of consumers; health resources, personnel, and facilities; and methods for integrating the health-care system so that all parts complete a whole. When viewed as wholeness of individuals, families, and groups, health opens up many new avenues of approach and responsibility which the community health nurse can meet if she is

[1]June Remillet and Sadie Reading, "Adapting to Changing Community Health Needs," *Nursing Outlook,* 18:10:47 (October) 1970.

creative, ingenious, enterprising, and seeks to act as a coordinating, facilitating agent. In these times of rapid change, the role of the community health nurse must also reflect change to keep up with the requirements of our progressive society.

## THE COMMUNITY

For the purposes of this book a *community* is defined as a group of people with a common characteristic, location, or interest living together within a larger society. Generally, a geographic area is considered to be a community; however, groups of individuals who gather together because of their interest in a particular health problem are also a community. For example, an individual may live in a congested neighborhood of a city and be particularly interested in the drug traffic and drug abuse of the residents and work actively in developing a drug rehabilitation program. This person represents a responsible citizen who is living in a particular neighborhood or geographic setting and participating in one aspect of a health interest, namely drugs. Therefore, the word "community" refers to a geographic location and/or an association of interests. A citizen can live in and work with a variety of communities, dependent upon his dwelling place and scope of interests.

The nurse can focus on all behavior within a community from three points of view: (1) maintenance of the physical and social environment; (2) securing of help and support at times of stress; and (3) strengthening of individuals to gain a sense of self and social worth.[2] The emphasis of her work will be gauged by her perception of the diverse needs of the community citizens with whom she is working. For example, from the first point of view, she may work mainly with the elementary school population in terms of safety and immunizations. The second point of view will be directed toward young married couples with newborn infants who are entering the family system. Low-income families living within a specified housing project may be responsive to the emphasis on the third point of view, particularly when they are ready to participate in community planning and action directly affecting them.

To become acquainted with a given community, the nurse must determine those factors for which she desires more information. She can obtain her data by (1) observations; (2) visiting community facilities; (3) interviewing key community leaders; and (4) reviewing reference materials which describe different factors about the community.

### Observation of a Community

For the nurse who wants to study unofficially a community new to her, a first activity for gaining data is to obtain a map and drive around the local

[2]Donald C. Klein, *Community Dynamics and Mental Health,* John Wiley & Sons, Inc., New York, 1968, p. 10.

community to gain impressions of the housing, spacing of residences, business establishments, industrial establishments, neighborhood services such as grocery stores, transportation facilities, shopping centers, educational facilities, recreational facilities such as parks or playgrounds, health facilities such as hospitals, physicians offices, safety of the environment, number of churches, and the faces of the people. Some of the questions which may come to mind are: How do the people support themselves? Is there evidence of pride in this community? How did this community come into being in the first place? Is there a "mix" of population such as several nationalities and races, extremes of wealth and poverty, extremes of young and old? Do the people seem preoccupied, busy, impersonal, friendly, prosperous, poor, old, young?

After gaining early impressions, a suggested second activity is to purchase a local newspaper and scan the contents. Does it reflect national, state, and local news or does it concentrate on folksy items? What is the nature of the advertisements in the paper? Are there editorial comments that give a sense of the attitudes of the residents? Are there any health items reported? Are there announcements of local meetings or reports of local agency activities? Are there meetings or facilities that the nurse may want to visit?

By getting a "feel" of the appearance and interests of the community, the nurse can map out subsequent activities she wishes to engage in. She can formulate questions in her mind for which she wants answers so that the ultimate goal of getting well acquainted with the community includes purposeful and informative activities. A well-informed community health nurse must know the characteristics, idiosyncrasies, and attitudes of her community. It takes time for a new nurse to become well informed but a carefully planned, informal study facilitates the process.

When visiting the homes of consumers of health services, the nurse must take note of space, safety factors, water, heating, sewage disposal, light, cleanliness, sanitation, ventilation, furnishings, food-storage facilities, bathing and toilet facilities, sleeping arrangements, play areas, yards, and gardens. The assumption must never be made that the possession of an automobile or a television set signifies evidence of an adequate income. At one time a television set was considered a luxury item; however, the appearance of one in the home is no longer a criterion for determining the solvency of the consumer.

## Community Facilities within a Community
The nurse must be cognizant of the numbers and locations of educational, religious, business, industrial, and recreational facilities within a community, but the *health facilities* are of particular interest to her. Many com-

munities have booklets or directories compiled by a coordinating or planning agency which list the names, telephone numbers, and addresses of a wide variety of community resources, the purpose for which they were formed, the services they offer, the source of financial support, the eligibility requirements for consumers, and the fees. Such a booklet or carefully compiled handbook organized with health-services information is essential data for the community health nurse to have at her disposal at all times. Frequently the directories have a classified index, which assists in locating needed services according to a given category, such as welfare assistance, services for unmarried mothers, handicapped children and adults, vocational training, special education for special conditions, services for the aging, and many more categories. The classification is done to facilitate the location of needed information with a minimum of time.

By visiting those community facilities in which the nurse is particularly interested, she becomes personally acquainted with professional workers, the implementation of health services, and the referral system, and she has the opportunity to initiate a reciprocal relationship that will give impetus to future teamwork with allied disciplines. Until the nurse has a comprehensive knowledge of available community resources and facilities, she often does not feel adequately prepared to practice her role of coordination and referral.

## Key Community Leaders

Every community has formal and informal leaders who hold positions of power, influence, or status in terms of facilitating or hindering community actions. It behooves the work of the community health nurse to become acquainted with the key community leaders, because they have influence in the field of health. The leaders can be found in local government as elected or appointed officials, businesses, educational systems, religious structures, or health and welfare organizations. When investigating a local community structure it is clarifying to secure an organization chart which outlines the lines of authority and position. From the chart formal leaders of the specific organizations under scrutiny may be identified, such as the local mayor, sheriff, judge, school principal, health officer, or welfare director. Informal but significantly influential leaders may also be found in occupations or professions such as industries, banks, clergy, medicine, and law. Associations representing service clubs, labor unions, political party organizations, communication media, community councils or boards, voluntary health organizations, housing authorities, fraternal groups, cultural groups, and minority groups are additional sources for finding key community leaders.

With timing and a sensitivity for gaining appropriate knowledge from all available sources, the power structure of the local community can be determined and future plans for activities involving the services of key citizens can be filed mentally as the nurse becomes oriented to the community. As the need arises, she is then able to contact appropriate samples of individuals to organize, plan, implement, and evaluate needed health programs, provide effective and successful services to consumers, and broaden the interpretation of nursing services to the general public. An example of a direct method which was used by one student nurse to become acquainted with the leadership of a small rural community involved a visit to the local bank and inquiring of the banker, "Who represents the power structure in this town?" The banker thought momentarily, then replied, "I guess you would say that I do!"

### Reference Sources about a Community
Depending upon the type of data desired, sources of information about a local community can be found in the library, in books and periodicals, in historical societies or archives, newspaper offices, directories, diaries, public records, town records, community development or planning agencies, church records, vital statistics offices, and other reference locations. An additional means for securing data is to interview older residents, key community leaders, and political figures or to question a cross section of local citizens or consumers of health services. "Mini" studies are one method of gaining data. They can be conducted in a variety of ways, such as constructing two or three pertinent questions and asking a selected portion of the local population about a selected interest area. For example, the data collector could ask a small sample of high school sophomores, "Do you think law and order exists in this community?" "What does law and order mean to you?" "To whom would you go if you wanted better enforcement of law and order?" By securing answers to these questions from a representative sample, the data gatherer would know the concern of male and female high school sophomores about the issue of law and order, the meaning of the term, and who they consider reference sources. The findings would give an indication for further investigation of the problem or redirection toward a focus more pertinent to the high school population.

### The Health System within the Community
In many communities, according to Sanders, there are five types of health structures found within the health-care system.[3] However, a sixth type has emerged in recent years which is designed to meet the needs of consumers who have not been serviced adequately by the five existing systems. The

[3]Irwin T. Sanders, "The Community: Structure and Function," *Nursing Outlook,* 11:9:642–643 (September) 1963.

sixth structure includes the proliferation of free clinics, community service centers, and neighborhood health stations which have come into being, often with the assistance of the Office of Economic Opportunity, and focus primarily on the needs of minority or low-income groups. The six health structures are closely intertwined, yet distinct enough to be studied separately by those nurses who wish to serve as coordinators and collaborators with all of the structures. The five health structures described by Sanders are: (1) private office practice of professionals, namely the physician or group of physicians working in the office or clinic setting; (2) group health care, in which consumers buy medical and health services by becoming members of facilities set up for that specific purpose; (3) large hospitals and clinics with their own boards and clientele; (4) public health agencies that protect, administer, and perform more preventive than curative health services for the consumer; and (5) those facilities and personnel who sell treatment products and appliances required, such as pharmacists, orthopedic supply houses, and similar establishments. Each of the health subsystems requires a different network of organized activity and therefore operates within an individualized organizational structure, which may be loose-knit or tightly coordinated.

Each health structure fulfills community expectations of a specified sort and conducts its affairs within certain codes of operation.[4] Nurses work in most of the health subsystems and give special services concurrent with the health structure and abide by the code of operation expected within that particular structure. Each health subsystem has basically similar expectations for the functioning of the nurse, but the manner in which she performs her tasks varies according to the structure and setting. In the sixth health structure, which was described as a burgeoning number of community health centers, neighborhood multiservice centers, free clinics, or similarly named stations which have come into existence because of needs of consumers, nurses either volunteer their time or are employed by organizations or consumers who receive funding from governmental sources. In the centers in which consumers are participating actively in the determination of health services, nurses play a different role than in any of the other five health structures. Primarily they are working *with* the consumer of health services, rather than *for* him, and this entails a redirection in focus in many ways. As described by Milio, the nurse sometimes must play a subtle role, or nonvisible one, in order to accomplish a desired objective.[5] Or the nurse must be able to account for her activities in a way that makes sense and is relevant to the consumer.[6]

[4]*Ibid.*, p. 643.
[5]Nancy Milio, *9226 Kercheval: The Storefront That Did Not Burn,* The University of Michigan Press, Ann Arbor, 1970, p. 31.
[6]Kate R. Lorig, "Consumer-Controlled Nursing," *Nursing Outlook,* 17:9:52 (September) 1969.

It is an important task of the community health nurse to be cognizant of all facets operating within the health-care system in her given community, to be knowledgeable about coordination practices and procedures with other nurses and professional personnel working in the health structures, and to be able to interpret and link all six health structures in an understandable and intriguing way to the consumer. Because the consumer is demanding to be heard about his right for health-care services, the nurse must utilize increasingly the opportunity to enlarge the consumer's knowledge of the health-care delivery system and work with him to develop effective methods for gaining appropriate, official attention to community health problems in need of correction.

## SOCIAL CLASSES IN THE COMMUNITY

Every community is made up of a variety of components which constitute its structure. In general, the citizens have a vague awareness of the composition of their community, but upon questioning reveal a lack of specific knowledge about any one component. Because of the nature of her work, the community health nurse will enhance her skill in dealing with individuals and families if she is curious and investigative about selected components existing in the community. The composition of each community has its own structure and personality, which is not duplicated by any other community; when the nurse becomes knowledgeable about the discrete social classes in existence she provides herself with vital essential information.

When talking with citizens of a given geographic location, there is often a denial of social classes existing within their community, yet an existence of a parenthetic upper-, middle-, and lower-class stereotype description is generally acknowledged and understood. Social classes are differentiated by their degrees of prestige, education, income, residence, and access to products and services in the community. They are unorganized groups. People are born into them, marry into them, or otherwise enter them from adjacent social classes. Within them, people tend to associate with each other more than with others outside their social class. On the average, people of different social classes vary in aesthetic tastes, in the type of books and magazines they read, the way they vote, the size of their families, the way they spend their leisure time, and even in their sex morality.[7]

In our changing society the characteristics identifying social class are constantly fluctuating, so that clearly defined criteria for determining social class are becoming less distinct and the merging of social-class characteristics can be likened to tentacles reaching out to cover the outlines of formerly clearly identifiable rocks. For the purposes of community health nurses, it

[7]Roland L. Warren, *Studying Your Community*, The Free Press, New York, 1965, p. 351.

is valuable to maintain a curiosity about the changing nature of the social-class system, to keep up-to-date with current events, happenings, and research studies in order to meet health needs of new groupings of citizens as they occur, and to relate with understanding, acceptance, and readiness to the wants of the consumer.

Of import to the nurse is awareness of (1) her own method for classifying families in terms of social class and avoiding the stereotyping based on unvalidated data; (2) her own feelings of withdrawal or superiority based on past personal experiences; and (3) the family's receptivity cues to her general services. When she is cognizant of general behaviors and attitudes representative of each social class and her own personal reactions to a social-class image, she is better able to identify strengths and weaknesses of a given family with objectivity and work in an effective, understanding, and facilitative manner. By recognizing the family as possessing characteristics representative of an identified social class, but also exhibiting unique characteristics which cannot be classified, the nurse is helped to view the family as a distinct entity rather than squeezing it into a poorly fitting, preestablished mold.

Community health nurses are commonly thought to come from a middle-class orientation and do much of their health practice with the lower classes. Of interest are the great variety of studies that have focused on the nurse image as seen in the context of social-class perspective. Simmons reported that in general the evaluation of nurses becomes consistently more favorable as the opinions move from higher to lower socioeconomic groups.[8]

Watts compared selective characteristics of lower- and middle-class people and described the lower-class person as being oriented to the present rather than the future and taking pleasures as they are available rather than planning for a future he cannot visualize. The middle-class person looks to the future and is willing to defer gratifications by planning ahead and saving for desired goals. He values cleanliness, work, and self-discipline.[9]

In regard to health activities, studies have been reported in professional health journals and books indicating that members of the lower classes have a high percentage of illnesses and are dissatisfied with the medical care available to them.[10] They have less information and knowledge about disease and are more likely to hold irrational ideas about illness, rely on folk medicine and fringe practitioners, and delay seeking medical

[8]Leo W. Simmons and Virginia Henderson, *Nursing Research, A Survey and Assessment,* Appleton-Century-Crofts, Inc., New York, 1964, p. 179.

[9]Wilma Watts, "Social Class, Ethnic Background, and Patient Care," *Nursing Forum,* 6:2:155–162 (Spring) 1967.

[10]Evelyn Millis Duvall, *Family Development,* 2d ed., J. B. Lippincott Company, Philadelphia, 1962, pp. 85–86.

treatment.[11]  It is generally accepted that medical care is not as readily available to the lower classes as to the middle and upper classes in the present health-care system. Members of the middle and upper classes know more about the dynamics of illness and health and are more aware of medical care resources for prevention and treatment of sickness. They make use of available resources in a climate of social acceptance.[12]

There are general differences of behavior required of the nurse when associating with the different social classes of people. Some of the perceptions of the nurse are described as follows. When working with the lower classes, nurses often prefer the families who are responsive to suggestions, seem to value her teaching and friendship, and demonstrate changes in health practices concurrent with her influence. The apathetic families described in Chap. 4, such as low-income families, tend to be frustrating to the nurse because she is unable to determine if her work with these families has any influence whatsoever. A greater, more intensive effort must be made by community health nurses to study lower-class, multiproblem families because the health needs are so great and new innovative methods for giving nursing services to these families must be created. The use of role-playing techniques has been strongly recommended by many professional workers because it is appropriate to the style of this population. Role-playing is action oriented, concrete, visual, and sometimes game like.[13] It is certainly a method with which nurses are acquainted, yet it is used little with families. In Chap. 4 an elaboration of ways for working more effectively with low-income families is given. When working with middle-class families, nurses again prefer the responsive families who are interested in health information and teaching on a curing and prevention basis. The fact that middle-class families are often better educated than lower-class families requires the nurse to be prepared always to give an intellectual explanation of any symptom within her domain of knowledge about which there is an inquiry. When a middle-class family member is better educated than the nurse, this sometimes causes anxiety feelings within the nurse which may deter her effectiveness in creating a professional image. With upper-class families, the nurse is sometimes relegated to the status of servant or domestic and responds according to her perception of this station in life. With all social classes it helps to be thoughtfully prepared before making a contact, so that the best approach is used, all avenues for alternative plans are explored and ready in case a change of plan is required, and the nurse feels comfortable and secure.

[11]David Mechanic, "Illness and Cure," in John Kosa, Aaron Antonovsky, and Irving Kenneth Zola (eds.), *Poverty and Health,* Harvard University Press, Cambridge, Mass., 1969, p. 207.

[12]Duvall, *op. cit.,* p. 85.

[13]Salvador Minuchin, Braulio Montalvo, Bernard G. Guerney, Jr., Bernice L. Rosman, and Florence Schumer, *Families Of the Slums,* Basic Books, Inc., Publishers, New York, 1967, p. 37.

## COMMUNITY ORGANIZATION FOR HEALTH PRACTICES

By becoming actively involved in health programs, problems, needs, and desires as evidenced by a particular community, the nurse broadens her scope of health practices, which include additional skills such as teaching, leading, managing, collaborating, speaking, writing, and analyzing. By participating in community action, she becomes knowledgeable about methods of public relations, politics, and social legislation. She knows which community meetings to attend by becoming aware of their agendas and is prepared to articulate with health facts as needed during the meeting. The enlarged scope of nursing within the community encompasses many components of health interests and requires many additional skills the nurse of the past did not possess. Since time and energy of individual community health nurses have practical limits, it is essential that each community health nurse select her own particular health interest and devote time, energy, and commitment to the *one* health component within the widely diverse health programs in operation in the community. An ideal goal in each community would be to have a nurse—not the same nurse—representing nursing interests on every planning or advisory committee of the existing health-care system in that community.

Learning about community organization is best done by working actively in community health work. Until a person gets acquainted with the individualistic climate and interests of his community and is identified and accepted as serving the community, he cannot become an effective leader or facilitator in advancing the health goals of the community. Ross defined *community organization* as a process by which a community identifies its needs or objectives, orders these needs or objectives, takes action in respect to them, and in so doing extends and develops cooperative and collaborative attitudes and practices in the community.[14]

### Community Organization Process

The first step of the community organization process is to *identify needs or objectives.* Methods for determining the health needs of a given community can consist of surveys, house-to-house or street interviews, identification of observable health problems, study of weekly or monthly health statistics, or questionnaires via the communication media. When exploring ideas with citizens it is advisable to discern their health *wants,* as opposed to their health *needs,* in order to be assured of the support of a substantial number of citizens regarding any potential health issue that may be selected. Ideally, the movement toward a health objective should be instigated by the citizens or at least receive their enthusiastic endorsement so that motivation toward

[14]Murray G. Ross, *Community Organization,* Harper & Row Publishers, Inc., New York, 1955, p. 39.

action is already inherent. The *ordering of needs or objectives* is primarily setting priorities and focusing on the most urgent health need or desire first. When a health issue is selected that represents the citizens' wants, commitment and action will be secured early with minimum prompting from any health expert. People have always known of health *needs* which would be beneficial for them, but few individuals respond to "You should have this" or "You need this" unless they *want* it. For example, a community may tend to be apathetic and unconcerned about the general drug traffic problem on which the communication media is concentrating until several local high school students from respectable homes in their own community are picked up and jailed for possession of illegal drugs. Then the citizenry is truly alerted, aroused, and ready to take action in any advised direction that will resolve the problem. Progress cannot be made in the community any faster than the understanding and consent of the concerned group of citizens.[15] *To develop the will and confidence* to work at the selected needs or objectives, persons representing the community must become *involved* with the health issue. The more intimately associated they are with the gathering of data and planning for action, the more widespread will be the network of influence and concern that disperses to other interested citizens. When a core of persons are selected, volunteered, or influenced to join a task force about a particular health issue in which they are deeply concerned, they represent the *human resources* in the community who will deal with the needs or objectives. It is advisable that the concerned group represent a valid cross section of citizens and agencies in the community, that some key influential persons be included, and that a professional individual with expertise in knowledge about the selected health issue be asked to serve as a consultant when needed. By expecting committee members of the task force to be involved, the gathering of a wide variety of resources within and without the community evolves in surprising directions when the group is allowed to be innovative and creative. The capacity of local citizens to solve problems and help themselves has unlimited potential, and the task of the facilitator need only be aimed at exerting indirect leadership and giving support whenever required by the group. Workers should assume the responsibility and get the credit for their community action. When they have decided on the appropriate *action* to take in terms of the health issue, they should feel a commitment or confidence about it and be ready to adapt the action as necessary so that unforeseen events which may occur will be managed smoothly and with flexibility. It is very important that *collaborative and cooperative attitudes and practices* in the community be in operation during the entire community organization process. It is essential that lines of communication remain active, open, and effective—a requirement which

[15]Clarence King, *Working With People In Community Action,* Association Press, New York, 1965, p. 82.

is more easily stated than accomplished. When citizens learn to work together and develop teamwork, they are equipped to cope cooperatively and skillfully with future problems as they arise. As pointed out by Ross, the existence of differences of opinions, tensions, and conflicts often give life and vitality to a movement. The conflict can be handled destructively or constructively. When dealt with constructively, increased understanding, tolerance, and strength are developed in the community. When the attitudes of persons allow for cooperative and collaborative work, they learn to endure, welcome, and move comfortably with diversity and tension.[16]

The role of the health professional who is facilitating the community organization process in regard to a specific health issue is one of working *with* the citizens, encouraging the development of all the essential elements in the process, making use of consultation as necessary, serving as a worker in the background rather than the forefront, and strengthening the capacity of the local citizenry to function as a team toward accomplishment of the goals and objectives to which they have committed themselves.

It must be pointed out that the steps of the community organization process are not necessarily followed in order. Sometimes early action will hasten the development of the other elements in the process. What is essential is that all activities have a purpose, that the positive and negative alternatives are considered before acting upon them, and that the community group is continuously evaluating or judging the evolving events that occur as movement progresses toward the established goals.

## A Community Project

An example involving a group of senior baccalaureate nursing students in community health nursing who wanted to witness the establishment of a drop-in center for teen-agers in the community in which they were working is cited to show how the community organization process is learned by means of actual experiencing. The students felt a deep concern about the alienation of youth and the potentiality of a drug abuse problem in the local community. They felt that if a drop-in center for teen-agers were available where they could "come and rap," perhaps some teen-agers might be prevented from resorting to drugs.

Their first steps in proceeding to identify the needs of the community in regard to youth were to investigate the existence of resources currently in operation. They found that the youth in the community had no "constructive" recreational facilities and there were no resources dealing with the drug problem. There were facilities for youth in nearby communities; however, because of the rivalry of community competition, the youth did not feel

[16]Ross, *op. cit.*, p. 49.

welcome in nearby community facilities. The next activities of the nursing students were to interview a cross section of local community citizens. They interviewed school teachers and administrators, psychologists, police, clergy, representatives of the local coordinating and planning agencies, and a member of the YWCA. The nursing students returned from these interviews either depressed or enthusiastic, depending upon to whom they talked. As they discussed their goal and experiences among themselves, regardless of the up-and-down swings of emotion, they became increasingly convinced that a drop-in center was desperately needed in that community. An empathy for the plight of the local teen-agers was particularly poignant at that stage of the community organization process. An opportunity arose to attend an evening community meeting sponsored by the local YWCA in relation to the need for a drop-in center in the community. The director and two high school students from a nearby community facility were on the agenda to explain their organization, purpose, and functions. During the meeting the local citizens were informed that all that was necessary to start a drop-in center was a group of interested young people and a house, and other details could be worked out thereafter. The discussion during the meeting accepted the assumption that a drop-in center was needed; however, the securing of a house and the financial and legal implications involved a risk with which no one wanted to deal. As the meeting terminated on an indecisive note, a young woman counselor of the local community recreational center volunteered her services to work toward the goal of a drop-in center. At a subsequent meeting with the counselor, the nursing students were advised to contact a clergyman who had expressed an interest in the project. It was at this point that the nursing students were searching for potentially productive local resources to deal with their objectives. They were also vacillating in emotions about the behavior of local citizens at meetings. With uncertainty, but with hope, they met with the local clergyman who had with him a public school counselor and physical educational coordinator. In their report of this meeting they described the discussion as follows:

> We discussed the drop-in center in abstract terms. Father ____ and Mr. ____ mentioned influential people in the community who might be of some aid to our project. Father ____ stated that if he was going to help us financially, he wanted to know more about how we were going to be organized. He mentioned lawyers, incorporating the center, and made what we thought to be a relatively simple organization a very complex endeavor. However, his assistance was vital in making us aware of the problems that would arise.

A series of meetings were held with the clergyman and school counselor at regular intervals thereafter, and an increasing number of local citizens were drawn into the project, including a lawyer, a judge, a policeman, a Catholic clergyman, a local businessman, a physician, representatives from the local school district, local service clubs, and the local coordinating agency, as well as local high school students. All aspects of planning and implementing the project were discussed thoroughly. The nursing students learned many things, including the following: (1) the importance of planning which envisions all obstacles, possibilities, and events that may aid or infringe upon the project. (2) How citizens behave and talk when dealing with a controversial project during community meetings—the desire of some citizens to become involved changes when they are asked to assume some responsibility. (3) Action seems slow when a large number of citizens are involved. (4) When asking for support, words must be carefully chosen; for instance, if comparison is made with facilities of nearby communities, citizen response is inclined to be negative. (5) Influential persons are essential because of their emotional support, financial backing, and knowledge about existing local politics. (6) Risk taking is involved in any project and some citizens assume more responsibility and risk than others. (7) Organization is a must; all procedures are best anticipated in advance and planned for before implementation of action takes place. (8) There is an orderly procedure involved in establishing a center, which takes into consideration the need for rules and regulations, criteria for eligibility of staff workers, an advisory board, a board of directors, and other considerations. (9) With a firm foundation, a newly established center is less vulnerable to negative legal procedures or negative public opinion.

A center was opened in the local community eight months after the first nursing students became actively involved in initiating the establishment of such a facility. The nursing students participated actively in the community organization process. In their evaluation of their activities they stated:

> The students' efforts in organizing this project have had a tremendous influence on our ideas about how to organize a community, how to contact key people in the establishment, and how to become involved. As nurses, we find that our training and our individual personalities can lead us far from the emergency room or the operating room of a large hospital, and very much into the community to work with the people with whom we live. We can work at any level of community organization, in that we have the ability to recognize problems, to make people aware of them, and then to do something about them.

## SUMMARY

In becoming acquainted with any given community, the community health nurse must study its characteristics purposefully. The composition of each community has its own structure and personality, which is not duplicated by any other community. Information is gained about a community by making direct observations, visiting community facilities, interviewing key community leaders, and reviewing reference materials which describe the community under study. The nurse is able to identify a health-care system in every community and existence of several social classes of citizens. To be an effective health worker, the nurse must participate actively and knowledgeably in the community organization process in order to represent health interests and advance health practices beneficial to the citizens of the community.

## SUGGESTED READING

Barry, Mildred C., and Cecil G. Sheps: "A New Model For Community Health Planning," *American Journal of Public Health,* 59:2:226–231 (February) 1969.

King, Clarence: *Working With People In Community Action,* Association Press, New York, 1965.

Klein, Donald C.: *Community Dynamics and Mental Health,* John Wiley & Sons, Inc., New York, 1968.

National Commission on Community Health Services, *Health Is a Community Affair,* Harvard University Press, Cambridge, Mass., 1966:

Ross, Murray G.: *Community Organization,* Harper & Row, Publishers, Incorporated, New York, 1955.

Wade, Serena E.: "Trends In Public Knowledge About Health and Illness," *American Journal of Public Health,* 60:3:485–491 (March) 1970.

Warren, Roland L.: *Studying Your Community,* The Free Press, New York, 1965.

Traditionally the family has been the unit of service for the community health nurse. However, the orientation and practice of individual nurses for years has varied on a continuum from patient-centered to family-centered, dependent upon the nature of the family system and the illness of the identified patient. Unfortunately, it is too easy to *speak* words like "family-centered," "caring," and "continuity of care" yet behave in *actions* differently from what the descriptive words suggest. Sometimes the nurse may consider that she is using the family-centered approach when she draws all of the family members together for the goal of understanding and assisting the identified patient of the family to make a more satisfactory recovery. A *truly family-centered approach* is one in which the nurse meets and assesses *all* of the family members, either individually or as a group, is cognizant of the developmental role, power, and influence position of each family member, identifies the interactional patterns used by the family, and works with the family, including all members, to achieve a higher level of coping ability or health. The methods used for the family-centered approach are discussed in Chap. 5.

## THE FAMILY

The common meaning of the word "family" is generalized to be the nuclear family, a structural unit composed of a man and woman who are married and have children. However, in view of the living patterns and kinship systems of people of different cultures and the emerging pattern of communal living among the youth of America, the family can also be considered a primary group possessing certain generic characteristics in common with all small groups.[1] These characteristics are

[1] F. Ivan Nye and Felix M. Berardo, *Emerging Conceptual Frameworks In Family Analysis,* The Macmillan Company, New York, 1966, p. 63.

mainly relationships with a high degree of intimacy, extensive communication, and common goals. When viewed in this manner, the family can be seen as a miniature society, with a culture all its own.[2] The concept of family tends to be a fluid one because of the accelerating changes occurring within the societies of the Western Hemisphere. One-parent families, communal families, extended families living in a single residence, and other groups residing together in single dwellings must all be viewed in a common context, the nature of which supplies the nurse with her frame of reference, the family-centered nursing approach. For the purpose of this book, the family is the nuclear family or the primary group living and interacting together intimately in a common residence.

### The Systems Approach

When the family is viewed from a systems approach, its role as a basic component of society is seen as a complex, many-faceted one. A system is an organized or complex whole—an assemblage or combination of things or parts forming a complex or unitary whole.[3] The world is made up of many systems, including social, biological, physical, and environmental systems. Parsons identified a social system as a plurality of persons or social roles bound together in a pattern of mutual interaction and interdependence. It has boundaries that enable us to distinguish the internal from the external environment, and it is typically imbedded in a network of social units both larger and smaller than itself.[4] The family is an open system which sustains relationships with other systems in the total transactional field and is interdependent and independent at the same time. When using the systems approach, the family's position in society can be identified in simple or complex terms. It is helpful to visualize a system by drawing a large circle and placing elements, parts, and variables inside the circle as components.[5] Circles representing components can be separate, touching, or overlapping depending on the strength of the attracting forces in operation among the components. For purposes of simplicity, the position of the family in relation to the health-care system in the community can be illustrated as shown in Fig. 4-1. Each circle represents a subsystem which has boundaries but will admit individuals from other subsystems as necessary. It is possible for the community health nurse to act as a representative for any of the health subsystems, serve as a liaison agent with the family, and coordinate

[2] *Ibid.,* p. 140.
[3] Fremont E. Kast and James E. Rosenzweig, *Organization and Management,* McGraw-Hill Book Company, New York, 1970, p. 110.
[4] Talcott Parsons and Robert F. Bales, *Family, Socialization and Interaction Process,* The Free Press, New York, 1955, pp. 401–408.
[5] Warren G. Bennis, Kenneth D. Benne, and Robert Chin, *The Planning of Change,* Holt, Rinehart and Winston, Inc., New York, 1961, p. 203.

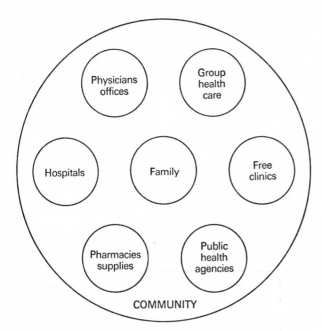

**Fig. 4-1**  Health-care systems in the community.

the health-care delivery system in the community so that it has meaning and purpose to the family.

From another perspective, which includes a multidisciplinary approach, the family may be drawn as one of many social systems within the community with the possibility of having transactions with other systems on a frequent or infrequent basis. The community health nurse can act as the liaison agent for a dysfunctioning family and coordinate or integrate transactions with other participating social systems so that the family's equilibrium and coping abilities are eased. The illustration of social systems from a multidisciplinary approach may be drawn as shown in Fig. 4-2. The particular role of the community health nurse as a coordinator of services in the figure below can be elaborated from the following hypothetical example. The community health nurse was referred to the family initially through the department of public assistance because the mother was pregnant and was not seeking prenatal care. Following an appraisal of the family on a home visit, the nurse assessed the family as a dysfunctional one because of the evidences of marital strife, the lack of health care of older children, the lack of prenatal care for the mother, and the complaints regarding insufficient clothing and poor transportation facilities. After the nurse determined short- and long-term goals to be attained, immediate plans to talk with or make referral to personnel in each of the pictured social systems were instituted.

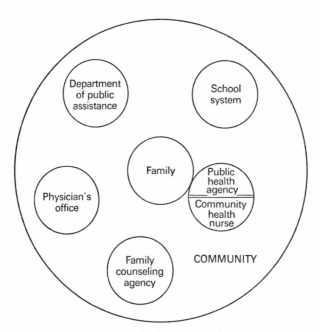

Fig. 4-2  Social systems in the community.

For example, the nurse wanted to speak to the caseworker of the department of public assistance to share her observations and assessment of the
family with the worker. She wanted to know if the data gathered were
complete and if a cooperative effort by the caseworker and nurse would
reap better results than working separately or discretely in predetermined
subject areas. By conferring with the school nurse and teachers in the
school system, the nurse wanted to learn if the school had been alerted to
the health condition of the children of the family. Again, by a unified effort
of all professionals concerned with family members, a change would be
effected more easily if the family received concerted special attention. A
first priority of the nurse was to refer the mother of the family to a private
physician for prenatal care. She planned to call the physician chosen by the
mother to advise him of the current health status of the mother and the fact
that continued supervisory visits would be planned during the antepartum
and postpartum periods. When the mother and father of the family indicated
a readiness to seek marital counseling, it was the plan of the nurse to call
the family counseling agency to alert them to the nature of family problems
and the fact that she had been guiding the family to seek additional assistance. Eventually, as the designated social systems within the community
became acquainted with the family, a multidisciplinary conference of all
representatives of the social systems would be arranged by the nurse to
integrate and implement the health care needed by the family. By picturing

the social systems involved with the family, the nurse clarified the coordination aspect of her role.

## Structure of the Family

The family structure is made up of individual members and the roles they play in interacting with each other. A *role* is defined as a goal-directed pattern or sequence of acts tailored by the cultural process for the transactions a person may carry out in a social group or situation.[6] No role exists in isolation but is always patterned to adjust in a complementary or reciprocal manner with the role partner. In general, the assumption is made that a nuclear family consists of a male who enacts an instrumental role and a female who fulfills the expressive role function. The instrumental role is one which emphasizes the performance of tasks and decision making and communicates power by the thinking, logical, perceptive approach. The expressive role emphasizes support of the instrumental leader and conveys power through the ability to mediate and influence feelings and emotions of others. In every small group there are persons who demonstrate either instrumental or expressive roles. The structural relationships in a family vary according to the particular mode of family organization, social class, or culture. Thus, various manifestations of family structure are seen in terms of role behavior. The structure and role behavior of members of a given family must be determined by the nurse before she can decide intelligently on the best method for initiating a health activity. It is sometimes clarifying for the nurse to draw her perceptions of the family structure in terms of circles and orbits of closeness or influence. When the center of the circle is considered as demonstrating the most power, placement of family members can be tentatively arranged from that perspective. A stable family unit may be drawn as shown in Fig. 4-3. Because the baby is more dependent and seems to receive more attention than the school-age child, he is placed close to the mother and father, who work well together in a complementary fashion as shown by the overlapping circles.

A family in which the daughter is favored by the father and the son favored by the mother may be drawn as shown in Fig. 4-4. The daughter is close to the father and more distant from the mother, as is the son from the father. The mother and father work closely together, but not always in a complementary fashion as seen by the circles that do not overlap. Any number of ingenious pictures of family structures can be devised by the nurse as she gathers evidence regarding the role behaviors of family members. The pictures may change as the nurse's assessment of the family structure deepens. Sometimes families themselves will respond to the idea of picturing their placement in the family system when given the assignment.

[6]John P. Spiegel, "The Resolution of Role Conflict Within the Family," in Norman W. Bell and Ezra F. Vogel (eds.), *The Family,* The Free Press, New York, 1960, p. 363.

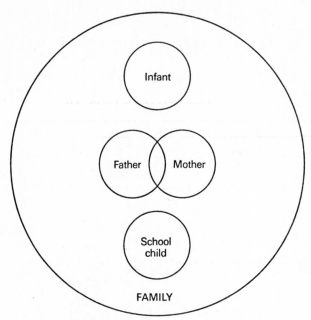

Fig. 4-3   A family unit.

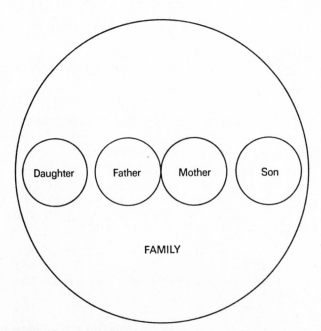

Fig. 4-4   A family unit.

## Function of the Family

In view of controversial opinions about the continuing existence of families as familiarly known in society, the function of the family assumes major importance.[7] It may be that the traditional concept of families should not be the focus of attention as much as the change or diversity of family functioning and structuring. Parsons stated that the functions of the family in a highly differentiated society are performed for the benefit of the personality rather than on behalf of the society. Families are necessary because the human personality is not "born" but must be "made" through the socialization process.[8] When babies are born and raised in their own distinct family environment, they learn to cope with the world by identifying with or in opposition to models with whom they have been intimate all their early years. Each child picks up individual characteristics from the adult models, mother and father. It is fascinating to observe small children at play and witness the behavior that is unconsciously mimicked from either the mother or father. Children learn to perceive the world through the adult models in their environment, and they remember best the *actions* which gained their attention rather than adult words. Therefore, when adults rely on words to create an impression, they are often producing an inconsistency that is not understandable to a child. For example, when a mother cautions her child never to run across the street without first looking to the right and left for the presence of vehicles, and later runs across the street herself without following her own directives, the child takes note of this. The performed act has a much greater impact on his memory than the words. When he is disciplined for running across the street without looking to the right or left, he tends to regard the punishment as unjust.

Hill outlined basic requirements for family survival, continuity, and growth. These included seven tasks:

*[handwritten: Family Survival Continuity Growth]*

1.  Reproduction: planning and controlling family size
2.  Physical maintenance of family members: providing food, clothing, shelter and medical care
3.  Socialization of offspring into functioning adults, capable of assuming adult family roles of husband-father, wife-mother
    *a.* Organization of explicit expectations for children and adults
    *b.* Organization of family objectives to which members are subordinate
4.  Allocation of resources and division of duties and responsibilities
    *a.* Allocation of authority, including prestige, and designation of accountability
    *b.* Allocation of economic income and output

[7]See Alvin Toffler, *Future Shock,* Random House, Inc., New York, 1970.
[8]Parsons and Bales, *op. cit.,* p. 16.

*c.* Division of labor: specialization of roles to secure performance of essential family jobs

*d.* Division of time: scheduling of tasks and services

**5.** Maintenance of order within the family and between the family and outsiders

   *a.* Within the family: meeting the emotional needs of members and determining types and intensity of emotional-affectional ties among members; channeling of sex drives; providing means of communication among members

   *b.* Between family and outsiders: developing methods of articulating with other groups and the larger social structure

**6.** Maintenance of family morale and motivation to carry out family tasks: providing a system of rewards and punishment to keep members at family tasks; development of equilibrating and inspiring mechanisms for upset or discouraged members

**7.** Development of methods for orderly recruiting and releasing of group members: incorporating of adopted children, stepparents, kin, guests, and servants into family group; releasing members at adulthood to jobs and marriage[9]

The mastery of these seven tasks by families varies widely. The nurse can be of greatest assistance to families when she can identify the tasks which need strengthening, enlist the interest of family members in clarifying their own resources and methods of coping, and teach methods of problem solving and interaction skills adapted to the family and facilitative of family recuperative strengths.

**Developmental Tasks**
Families and individuals change and develop in different ways, according to the nature of their individual living processes, family interaction, and stimulation by the social milieu. Each family member and each family is unique in its complex of age-role expectations in reciprocity.[10] The family as a small-group system is interrelated in such a manner that change does not occur in one part without a series of resultant changes in other parts.[11] As stated by Lederer and Jackson, the family is a unit in which all individuals have an important influence—whether they like it or not and whether they know it or not. The family is an interacting communications

[9]Reuben Hill, "Challenges and Resources For Family Development," Iowa State University Center for Agricultural and Economic Development, in *Family Mobility In Our Dynamic Society,* The Iowa State University Press, Ames, 1965, p. 255. (Reprinted by permission.)
[10]Nye and Berardo, *op. cit.,* p. 210.
[11]*Ibid.,* p. 203.

network in which every member influences the nature of the entire system and in turn is influenced by it.[12]

The family role pattern constantly changes as each member grows, develops, and matures according to his age and cultural role expectation. The developmental task concept takes into consideration the human needs of the individual and the cultural demands made upon him. It is defined as a task that arises at or about a certain period in the life of an individual, successful achievement of which leads to his happiness and success with later tasks, while failure leads to unhappiness in the individual, disapproval by society, and difficulty with later tasks.[13] For example, one developmental task of the preschool child is to learn to develop physical skills appropriate to his stage of motor development.[14] When he learns to button his coat or tie his shoes before going to school, he gains the approval of his mother, feels pleased with himself, and is challenged to try new skills. A developmental task of the teen-ager is to achieve a satisfying and socially accepted masculine or feminine role.[15] When a teen-age girl does not perceive herself as sexually attractive or lovable, has few girlfriends and no boyfriends, she is unhappy and all of her behavior reflects her dissatisfaction with herself. Her adaptation to all subsequent events in her life is affected and often dysfunctional if the developmental task is not satisfactorily resolved. Duvall lists in detail the developmental tasks of individuals for each age level in the life cycle in her book, *Family Development*. She states there are ten ever-changing developmental tasks which are faced by every individual. They are:

1. Achieving an appropriate dependence-independence pattern
2. Achieving an appropriate giving-receiving pattern of affection
3. Relating to changing social groups
4. Developing a conscience
5. Learning one's psycho-socio-biological sex role
6. Accepting and adjusting to a changing body
7. Managing a changing body and learning new motor patterns
8. Learning to understand and control the physical world
9. Developing an appropriate symbol system and conceptual abilities
10. Relating one's self to the cosmos[16]

[12]William J. Lederer and Don D. Jackson, M.D., *The Mirages of Marriage,* W. W. Norton & Company, Inc., New York, 1968, p. 14.
[13]Evelyn Millis Duvall, *Family Development,* 2d ed., J. B. Lippincott Company, Philadelphia, 1962, pp. 31–32.
[14]*Ibid.,* p. 230.
[15]*Ibid.,* p. 294.
[16]*Ibid.,* pp. 40–41.

In addition to individual developmental tasks, there are family developmental tasks, which are the responsibility of the family as a whole if they are going to grow and develop in a healthy, satisfying manner. The family developmental tasks keep changing as the family grows, adjusts, and matures from a beginning family, which starts with the marriage, becomes a small group when children are born, allows outsiders to enter the family system when children marry, and becomes an aging family nearing the end of the family life cycle. Duvall lists nine ever-changing family developmental tasks that span the family life cycle. They are to establish and maintain:

1. An independent home
2. Satisfactory ways of getting and spending money
3. Mutually acceptable patterns in the division of labor
4. Continuity of mutually satisfying sex relationships
5. Open system of intellectual and emotional communication
6. Workable relationships with relatives
7. Ways of interacting with associates and community organizations
8. Competency in bearing and rearing children
9. A workable philosophy of life[17]

The defined developmental task concepts for individuals and families according to their stage of human growth are extremely helpful for the community health nurse to use as guidelines when working with individuals and families. If the nurse can assist or encourage an individual or family to gain a satisfactory achievement of a developmental task that has been causing difficulties, she has facilitated growth, happiness, and movement toward maturity or self-actualization. It must be remembered that the individual himself must master the developmental tasks that he faces, but he cannot do it in isolation.[18] If an alert community health nurse identifies the juncture at which an individual or family may be stalemated in his or their developmental task progression, she can serve as an essential, facilitating change agent when it is most needed.

A successful, viable family is one that has a balanced division of labor, a father-led system of authority, a mother who is upwardly mobile, a respect for autonomy, strength in problem solving, and a husband and wife who thoroughly accept both their conjugal and parental roles.[19] An emotionally

*Defn. of Successful Family*

[17] *Ibid.*, pp. 478–505.
[18] *Ibid.*, p. 42.
[19] William A. Westley and Nathan B. Epstein, *The Silent Majority,* Jossey-Bass, Inc., Publishers, San Francisco, 1969, p. 35.

healthy individual is one who has dealt and is dealing in a satisfactory manner with the conflicts inherent in each stage of development.[20] Community health nurses visit all families, functional or dysfunctional, with the intent of facilitating or assisting them to achieve satisfactory adjustments to life events which are temporarily causing tension or disturbance. During the normal life cycle of a functional family, the nurse is always ready to lend assistance when a new baby arrives in the family, a preschool child is ready to enter school for the first time, or a preadolescent is entering the age of puberty. Her frame of reference reflects the developmental task concepts and appraisal of physiologic and psychological growth and development of individuals from infancy to old age. She is prepared to give anticipatory guidance or assist families undergoing the state of crisis.

## FAMILIES REPRESENTING SOCIOECONOMIC GROUPS
It has been said that the community health nurse works with *all* families in need at whatever stage of development or period of adjustment they are undergoing in their family life cycle. She is a helpful assistant when the family has special problems for which they are not adequately prepared, such as illnesses, accidents, birth of handicapped children, emergence of undesirable health or social conditions, and personality disorders. Since the nurse is a generalist, she views the family objectively from the perspective of wholeness. She identifies the coping patterns of the given family, the degree of discomfort they are experiencing, and is able to direct their energies, when they are ready, toward community resources and facilities which most closely meet their requirements. She also directs her own energies to those professional consultants within the community from whom she needs special instruction and guidance in assisting the family to cope better with explicit problems. Families representing socioeconomic groups are described in subsequent paragraphs to alert the nurse to her style of interaction and implementation.

### Low-income Families
The community health nurse visits all socioeconomic groups, but the low-income groups receive a proportionately large concentration of her time and services because of their high incidence of chronic diseases, multiple environmental hazards, high birth rates, high infant mortality rates, poor health standards, multiple social problems, and often inadequate delivery of health-care services. These groups are generally identified as poverty families, multiproblem families, hard-core families, disorganized families, or

[20] *Ibid.,* p. 48.

disadvantaged families. They are often families plagued by many serious problems, which they are unable to handle by themselves or through the services made available in the community, and they come repeatedly to the attention of community agencies in a negative connotation.[21] These families realize that health is an important reality for them but they often do not avail themselves of preventive health programs. Because community health nurses are very familiar health workers to these families, it is essential for the nurses to understand their life styles and implement methods of approach that will be successful in changing their health practices. Much research has been done in recent years from which nurses can profit as they experiment with new ways of developing self-esteem in these families and changing destructive health patterns to more acceptable, amenable practices.

Families of poverty are found in every community. Many of them reflect a design for living which Lewis has characterized as the culture of poverty. Regardless of their race, creed, color, culture, or setting, they have a life style which shows remarkable similarity in the structure of their families, in interpersonal relations, in spending habits, in their value systems, and in their orientation in time. To demonstrate the culture of poverty, the social order of a population in general must be one in which members prize the value of thrift and work toward the accumulation of wealth and property and the advancement of upward mobility. In such a society, the individuals of a low economic status tend to be seen as personally inadequate and inferior.[22]

Once the culture of poverty has come into existence in a society, it tends to perpetuate itself. The family does not cherish childhood as a specially prolonged and protected stage in the life cycle. Initiation into sexual activity comes early. With the instability of consensual marriage the family tends to be mother-centered and tied more closely to the mother's extended family. The female head of the house is given to authoritarian rule. In spite of much verbal emphasis on family solidarity, sibling rivalry for the limited supply of goods and maternal affection is intense. There is little privacy.[23]

Irelan described four distinctive life themes which are manifested in lower-class behavior. These include (1) fatalism; (2) orientation to the present; (3) authoritarianism; and (4) concreteness. When individuals have persistent fatalistic beliefs regarding unavoidable or uncontrollable external forces in their lives, a sense of powerlessness and resignation emanates, which acts as a definite deterrent to any efforts to break a chain of unfortunate circumstances. They receive their "hard luck" as their fate. Because of

[21]L. L. Geismar and Michael A. La Sorte, *Understanding the Multi-Problem Family,* Association Press, New York, 1964, p. 33.
[22]Oscar Lewis, *La Vida,* Random House, Inc., New York, 1966.
[23]*Ibid.*

their basic need for survival (physiological and safety needs), they are oriented to the present rather than the future. They spontaneously take their pleasures and discomforts immediately or in the "here and now" rather than defer any gratifications to a future time. They believe in the rightness of existing systems and in strength as the source of authority. By simplifying life experiences, they classify people as either weak or strong and will use authority, rather than reason, as the basis for decision making. The theme of concreteness deals with an emphasis on material rather than intellectual things. Because these individuals are preoccupied with tangible, day-to-day problems, they understand best any activity or emotion which is concrete and visible. They value action that has results or gives tangible rewards.[24]

In looking at their goals in life, they want the same things that any *"American Dream" —* other citizen in America wants[They want to improve their life by acquiring security, material comforts and luxuries, and social values which appeal to *work towards* all individuals.]Their drive toward better occupations and more income is *the top.* often based on escaping the discomforts of life in poverty. They want better housing, living conditions, and education. They value the opportunity to escape routines and pressures of day-to-day existence. Their desires are similar to the desires of any other social class; however, their life experiences have been such that their expectations for reaching toward their goals have been limited drastically. It is at this juncture that the community health nurse can play an active role in eliciting the feelings and desires of family members, encouraging the development of a plan of action which is conceivable to the family, and supporting and enabling the implementation of a plan so that success is achieved. To do this, the nurse must start with minute goals that are achievable and have the strong possibility for culminating in a positive direction. Success breeds success and families in poverty must begin at a level that they can see, understand, and trust. Oftentimes this means that the nurse must spend considerable time in developing the self-esteem and self-confidence of the individuals with whom she is working before they are ready to move toward a projected desired goal, even though it may be a minute one.

It must be emphasized that not all poor families exhibit characteristics of the culture of poverty. There are stable lower-class families who are cohesive and function as integral parts of the society. The fathers are employed in steady positions as semiskilled or unskilled workers, and have an elementary-school level of education. In these homes the intellectual stimulation for the children is rather low. These families profit from the attention of the nurse but must not be managed or categorized in the same classification as the families who demonstrate the poverty culture.

[24]Lola M. Irelan, *Low-Income Life Styles,* U.S. Department of Health, Education and Welfare, Government Printing Office, Washington, D.C., 1966, pp. 7–9.

It cannot be overemphasized that each family with whom the nurse comes in contact must be assessed *individually.* Textbook profiles and research studies point out important, significant data with which the nurse should be familiar to aid in her understanding and implementation of purposeful nursing actions. For example, the levels of social functioning are spelled out in detail for families classified as inadequate, marginal, and adequate by Geismar and La Sorte,[25] and descriptive characteristics which will help the nurse to work with disorganized and disadvantaged families are elaborated upon by Minuchin et al.[26] The ultimate success of the nurse's work depends on the synthesis of her knowledge of facts and data about families, her ability to relate, and the individuation of her nursing efforts with each family situation.

*Success*

### Health Perceptions of the Poor

*Health Status*

Poverty is a health hazard because of crowded or deteriorated housing, inadequate nutrition, and insufficient medical care. Consequently, low-income families are more vulnerable to ill health and less able to cope with it. They are often ignorant about causes, treatment, and outcomes of various diseases. They are not informed or particularly concerned about preventive measures. They accept poor health conditions as inevitable, such as dental decay with ultimate loss of teeth. Physical discomfort is a way of life and only when one becomes incapacitated and unable to fulfill daily responsibilities does he regard himself as "sick." Therefore, treatment is sought at a late stage of development, in contrast to early detection of disease symptoms. Many low-income families do not participate in health activities or programs available in the community, including preventive type of programs. They do not conceive of themselves as having a voice in community concerns since they lack contact with community organizations and among themselves. They tend to practice self-medication and when they need medical advice, they ask friends, neighbors, or the druggist's advice. They feel a distrust of physicians and clinics, particularly if they sense that they are evaluated as being inadequate or uncooperative or are treated as impersonal objects. They tend to set higher value on concrete physical improvements such as better housing, better transportation, or improved household equipment than they do on health.[27]

### Working with the Poor

The nurse is better able to relate with the poor if she understands some of their behavior patterns and attitudes. She must be willing to experiment

[25]Geismar and La Sorte, *op. cit.,* pp. 205–222.
[26]Minuchin et al., *op. cit.,* pp. 192–242.
[27]Irelan, *op. cit.,* pp. 51–62.

with new ways of implementing nursing activities and health teaching, since nursing actions in the past few years have not always ended in success when applied to low-income families. When knowledgeable about characteristic patterns of behavior as described by studies dealing with the poor, the nurse is better armed to adapt her approach to the specific needs of the particular family with whom she is working. When she realizes that low-income families value material things, she will readily accept the fact that they are more action-oriented than verbally oriented. When talking with *(Action Oriented)* an individual who uses speech as a means of direct, specific communication rather than an elaboration of thoughts or intellect, she will realize that she must create a mutual understanding which does not rely on words alone. This forces her to use her ingenuity and creativity in selecting an approach which will have meaning for the family. The use of tangible rewards, demonstrations, active participation with tasks, role-playing, or acting out behaviors or games are some approaches that may be more effective than words for the patient.

By being observant of the communication patterns of low-income families who are disadvantaged, the nurse can learn essential data which will have bearing on her subsequent activities. She will become aware that family members do not expect to be heard. No one really listens. If someone responds to a statement, it is not necessarily along the lines of the preceding communication. A high tolerance of interruptions and changing of subject material is demonstrated; therefore, a subject is rarely carried to any conclusion. Noise and motor activities often take precedence over the continuation of a subject being discussed. The mother is the central pathway for most transactions among family members when they are all together. Spouses rarely talk to each other but engage in "parallel" type of conversation that is directed to a third party or to the children. The mother's messages to the children are mostly in terms of "don'ts." She rarely gives a message which emphasizes any positives to the children. Children learn to pay attention to the person rather than to the content of the message received.[28] Consequently, the children do not talk in long sentences or express their desires by words alone.

Because the intellectual stimulation at home is limited, the concepts of time, size, and shape have to be dealt with in terms of familiar objects and words. For example, children may have to be taught that a ball is a "circle," or a clock is a "square." It is not unusual that parental control is at times confusing, because of inconsistency in being at one moment completely authoritarian or at the next moment powerless. The ambivalence with which discipline and punishment of children are exercised in the home can be witnessed frequently. Often there is little evidence of commercial toys in the

[28]Minuchin et al., *op. cit.,* pp. 201–206.

home, and the means by which children improvise playthings or give their attention in play can be instructive to the nurse. If no regular mealtime routine is practiced in the home, conversation at the dinner table or a parental focus on table manners is unknown.[29]

As the nurse assesses the behavior and communication patterns of a given family and synthesizes data gained from an appropriate textbook or research study, she will be prepared to try new methods of implementation which will be stimulating to the family. For example, she can set a goal to encourage spouses to talk directly to each other or alert the mother regarding her predominantly negative messages to the children. Her method for drawing the attention of family members regarding her goal may be through role-playing, psychodrama, or role-reversal games. By bringing observed patterns of behavior to the attention of family members, the nurse has a starting point from which to determine if they want to do anything about it, and if so, to plan with the family regarding the best way of implementation.

It sometimes happens that family members express a desired goal which is too global, so the task of the nurse requires restricting the goal specification to a dimension possible for the family to attain. For example, a mother might express a desire for her eight-year-old son to stop wetting the bed, since this behavior causes her to be continuously annoyed and irritable with him. In order for the nurse to implement successful activities with this goal, she must elicit detailed information from both the mother and the eight-year-old son. She must be assured of the desire of both to attain the stated goal. By requesting all data related to the problem, gaining the individual perceptions of both mother and son regarding the causes of the problem, and discussing the activities each will feel able to carry out, a plan for eliminating the enuresis for one night only out of the week can be the stated beginning goal. Gathering baseline data before implementing a plan of action is always desirable. See Chap. 5 for an elaboration of the behavior-modification method.

Nurses must remember that the poor are distrustful of outsiders and have been exploited often, so considerable time and attention has to be given early to developing trust and a relationship in which communication has meaning for both the family and the nurse.

### Middle- and High-income Families
Many professional workers, including nurses, come from a middle-class orientation and are familiar with attitudes, values, and behavior patterns of middle-income families. Some of the characteristics descriptive of middle-class values are the desirability of the accumulation of material wealth, a

[29]Sol Adler, *The Health and Education of the Economically Deprived Child,* Warren H. Green, Inc., St. Louis, Missouri, 1968, pp. 17–20.

belief in work and thrift as necessary attributes, an acceptance of upward mobility as indicative of success and progress, a future orientation for gratification of desires, and the importance of education. Children raised in a middle- or high-income family learn to express themselves with language which communicates observations, thoughts, and feelings. Curiosity is cultivated and questions are answered by parents. Children are raised in an environment which includes the stimuli of books, magazines, newspapers, toys of all sizes and shapes. Mealtimes are regular and attention is given to table conversation and proper use of eating utensils.[30]

In essence, the delivery of health care in any community is structured for and utilized mainly by middle- and high-income groups because they are the people who are alert and responsive to early disease symptoms, are able to pay for services, and expend much energy in participating as planners and organizers of beneficial community services.

## Working with Middle- and High-income Families

For nurses working with middle- and high-income families, the task of encouraging preventive health services is often made easy because of the acceptance and responsiveness of the consumer. The basis for a relationship may differ from that in low-income groups because the consumer is frequently well-educated and has a cognitive understanding and natural desire to learn about any phenomenon under study which captivates his interest. For the consumer who prizes intellectualism, the nurse must prepare differently than for the customer who wants the concrete, pertinent facts and no more. Many middle-income family members have as great a need for strengthening their self-esteem as low-income families. However, some seem to have a high propensity for utilizing defense mechanisms, which makes the development of a therapeutic relationship difficult and time-consuming, yet essential. Defensive people respond to openness and honesty and can be convinced about an idea if it is presented in a logical manner which gives recognition to all the arguments or barriers opposing the idea. The necessity for the nurse to assess the consumer in terms of her interests, personality, background, and education is vital as the nurse *plans* her teaching content and methods of approach on subsequent visits. Often it is not difficult for the nurse to recognize the need for a relationship with the middle-income family member if the consumer is friendly, receptive, and responsive—and most middle-class families are amicable. However, occasionally a family member is encountered who is hostile, openly questioning, highly educated, or unmistakably defensive, and the nurse tends to want to withdraw rather than pursue the difficult course of developing a relation-

[30]*Ibid.,* pp. 17–20.

ship. The nurse must be encouraged to plan carefully her strategy with the challenging patient in a way that is convincing to the consumer. This requires extensive educational and psychological preparation on the part of the nurse, but she is rewarded by broadening her own educational and experiential background and by strengthening her belief in herself. If she maintains an open, honest style and refuses to react emotionally to any intentionally provocative statement by the consumer, nine times out of ten, she can "win" the patient.

## FAMILIES REPRESENTING CULTURAL GROUPS

To gain an understanding of families representing cultural groups, the meaning of culture is described, followed by a discussion of selected families representing cultures upon whom the focus of attention has been centered in recent years. The overview of families of other cultures as contained in this chapter represents only a "taste" of the vast amount of information that is currently available in a cross section of popular and professional books and periodicals.

### Meaning of Culture

The concept of culture refers to those specific ways of thinking, feeling, and acting which differentiate one group from another. Culture varies in its patterns and meanings as represented by different groups who have been studied. Each group has developed its own way of life based on modifications and adaptations occurring through the course of history in the particular setting in which the group lived. The design for living of any particular group is transmitted to the children of the group directly and indirectly as they grow, develop, and learn to adapt to their physical environment and the people who act as their models and teachers. Culture serves as a subtle and systematic device for perceiving the world.[31] It stands for the way of life of a people, for the sum of their learned behavior patterns, attitudes, and material things.[32]

Every culture is of paramount importance to its possessor. It is a universal tendency for human beings to accept that their way of thinking, acting, and believing is the right way and to rate one's own culture as generally superior to others. Each individual has no choice but to function in the culture of which he is a part. It exercises a strong influence in the way individuals perceive themselves and others. As stated by Hall, culture is a mold in which we all are cast, and it controls our daily lives and behavior

---

[31]Benjamin D. Paul, *Health, Culture and Community,* Russell Sage Foundation, New York, 1955, p. 467.

[32]Edward T. Hall, *The Silent Language,* Copyright, 1959, by Edward T. Hall. Reprinted by permission of Doubleday & Company, Inc., Garden City, New York, p. 31.

in many unsuspected ways. Culture hides much more than it reveals, and it hides most effectively from its own participants.[33] It is not because of any difference in the basic nature of man that the cultures of different ethnic groups differ so much from one another, but because of the differences in the history of experiences which each group has undergone.[34] Because man relies on learned behavior or culture for survival, it is this acquired guidance that enables him to adapt to change.[35]

Since the community health nurse talks and works with such a wide variety of cultural groups, she must be constantly alert, consciously obser-vant, sensitive, accepting of all differences, and curious about the behavior patterns and life styles that are revealed in her presence. There is much to be learned about other cultural groups, and according to Hall, much about our own culture.

### Cultural Shock

When an individual visits a new country for an extended period of time or returns to his own country after a long absence, he is apt to feel a "culture shock," a removal or distortion of many of the familiar cues one encounters at home and the substitution for them of other cues that are strange.[36] The person experiences great differences that exist between himself and the people with whom he is working. He regards all things as strange and incomprehensible and may feel that he is not communicating to another in an understandable fashion because of the inconsistent response of his listener. In adapting to the new dimension in life to which the individual has been exposed, he must be ready to develop esteem in others who are different from him, and at the same time maintain his own sense of integrity and worth. The process of developing esteem for others who are different begins with getting to know the other person, by being willing to talk his language, using his particular jargon or phrases appropriately when their meaning is understood, and finding out his interests. It sometimes takes effort and involves periods of frustrations, but the ultimate outcome is satis-fying and broadening to one's experience when dealt with successfully.

Frequently, selected groups of student nurses undergo culture shock when they are exposed to completely new patterns of family living, an experience which often occurs in community health nursing. They see and talk with families whose culture is greatly different from their own. For many nursing students, the actual experience of entering a dirty, insect-ridden, poverty-stricken home is a highly charged one. She may have intellectual-

[33] *Ibid.,* pp. 38–39.
[34] Ashley Montagu, *The Biosocial Nature of Man,* Grove Press, Inc., New York, 1956, p. 81.
[35] Benjamin A. Kogan, *Health, Man In a Changing Environment,* Harcourt Brace Jovanovich, Inc., New York, 1970, p. 34.
[36] Hall, *op. cit.,* p. 156.

ized these conditions for some time, but coming upon the actual situations at a time when she may think that she has seen all and is wise to the world and its ways can be shattering.[37] The nurses must be allowed to talk freely in discussion groups about their initial impressions, followed by encouragement to look for factors in the strange home environment that will reveal the family's strengths. As the nurses adjust to the reality of accepting differences in family living patterns, they facilitate their productiveness in implementing effective nursing services.

### The Cultural Gap
The success of any health teaching is dependent upon the way in which it is understood, accepted, and implemented by the learner. The fact that there may be a gap or difference between the culture of the family and that of the nurse must always be remembered. Until the health worker or teacher understands the sociocultural patterns of the families she is serving, what purposes they serve, why they persist, and how they change, she will be unable to transmit health information which she believes to be desperately needed by the family. If the health teaching or activity is incompatible with the family's idea of illness and curing, the obstacle and challenge of changing their beliefs and practices must be attended to first. This necessitates many contacts with the family during which an understanding of their beliefs as the basis for their reluctance to change is gained, trust is developed as the family members accept the health worker, and the subsequent relationship of family members and health worker eases the willingness to change. Cultural values give meaning and direction to life, and it is doubtful if anyone ever really changes culture. What happens is that small, informal adaptations are continually being made in the day-to-day process of living.[38] Until the nurse has a hint of the cultural value which seems to be impeding her progress toward a desired goal with a family, she is working as though blindfolded. It is essential for the nurse to elicit the family's perception of their health problems and needs, to *avoid* making assumptions based on her *own* values, and to implement further actions based on an accurate understanding of the family's physical, mental, and emotional resources and the value they place on health. This takes effort, patience, and ingenuity. Health practices and adaptations may sometimes be initiated by appealing to pride or suggesting a gain in prestige. Long-term goals have a better chance of being implemented if they are combined with tangible measures to meet immediate health needs. For example, if the nurse has a goal for convincing the mother of a family of the necessity of immunizations

*Avoid making assumptions*

[37] Elaine C. Gowell, "Helping Student Nurses to Become Involved," *International Journal Nursing Studies*, 7:225–234, Pergamon Press, London, New York, November, 1970.
[38] Hall, *op. cit.*, p. 90.

for her children, she will hasten the deadline for her long-term goal if she attends to immediate illnesses, dental, clothing, or nutritional needs of the children. Early, tangible proof of her concern for the children will aid in convincing the mother of the family that the nurse is in earnest and genuinely cares about improving the overall health status of the family. Consequently, in due time the mother may be motivated to seek immunizations or practice health measures as advised by the nurse.

Sometimes the values of both the health professional and family can be met by making use of means of adaptation and compromise. For example, for the adamant elderly Scandinavian male who stubbornly insists on the use of kerosene dressings for his leg ulcers, the nurse can agree that kerosene is useful for superficial skin burns because of the property of being oil-based, but for present purposes she can indicate firmly that she will use it only around the healthy skin edges. For the leg ulcers, she will use only the prescribed medication as ordered by the doctor.

It is good to remember that an individual, regardless of his culture, wants to be recognized as an entity, a being who serves a purpose of some kind. When he is seen, heard, and made to feel that he has an impact of some kind on the person with whom he is communicating, then he knows he is in contact with a real person. If the nurse communicates a genuine desire to get to know the other person by learning the meaning of his words, which are different, his customs, his foods, his dress when different, and his interests, an enduring rapport is often initiated. Universal inquiries that are responded to with warmth after two participants have established a mutual feeling of trust are "What was your early childhool like?"; "How did you meet your husband or wife?"; "Tell me about the country where you were born"; "What are your favorite foods?"; "Tell me about the holidays or celebrations that you particularly love." By eliciting descriptions of events that the patient has experienced, the nurse becomes involved in a mutual exchange which is informative of the patient's culture, habits, attitudes, and values and serves as a basis for future conversations about health practices. The nurse broadens her scope of knowledge about learned behavior and perhaps gains a curiosity which will someday prompt a desire to visit the country or locale about which the patient is speaking.

*[handwritten margin note: Self-Worth]*

*[handwritten margin note: Mutual Involvement]*

## Black Families

Many books have been written recently that are informative and descriptive of the black people in America. A major factor which causes the black culture to be different from other cultural groups who have migrated to America involves the severance of traditional ties with the native land. The black man was brought to America forcibly and was completely cut off from his past. He was robbed of language and culture. He was forbidden to be an African and never allowed to be an American. While other cultural non-black groups passed on proud traditions to their children, black people were unaware of a sense of worth about the values and rituals which they shared. The culture that was born during the days of slavery passed from generation to generation, and the black people consequently developed constricting adaptations which continue to persist as contemporary character traits.[39]

The black family is first of all an extended family. Relatives share the responsibilities of child rearing and members of the family often come to the aid of a troubled member.[40] The black man uses music and language, with a particular emphasis on double meanings, to give him a feeling of identity and group unity. Blacks today continue to follow the patterns of slavery times. By appearing to accept the ethnic stereotypes that are intended to depreciate them, they turn these stereotypes to their own group purpose. The idea that Negroes have natural rhythm was originally used by whites to depreciate any musical creativity observed among blacks. Today this stereotype is embraced by black people and elaborated in the creation of a singular music which the white cannot create and which he can neither play nor understand. In the concept of "soul," black people agree that they can sing and dance and experience music in a way that whites cannot. They also agree that Negroes have a kind of animal-like capacity to excel in athletic events, as well as having sexual superiority.[41]

The life of many Negroes has been one of social chaos. Oppression and discrimination have played a major role in causing the destruction of the family structure, insecurity caused by crime, insufficient education, the lack of proper health standards, and the signs of various antisocial activities such as illegitimacy, drug usage, and alcoholism. Defense mechanisms such as apathy, self-abasement, work slow downs, and escape into boisterous hedonism are not uncommon behaviors among blacks. Grier and Cobbs describe the Negro family as weak and relatively ineffective because it has not been allowed the rights and privileges of protecting its members.[42] The black male is expected to maintain a family, educate his children, and provide the normal conveniences of modern living, even though he is more likely than his white counterpart to be unemployed, earn less money, and pay more for housing. Constant failures in his attempts to be a successful provider are great blows to his manhood. Often his wife is forced to work to add to the family income.[43] As parents, the man and wife teach their children what the world is like, how it functions, and how *they* must function

[39]William H. Grier and Price M. Cobbs, *Black Rage,* Basic Books, Inc., Publishers, New York, 1968, pp. 22–24.
[40]*Ibid.,* p. 87.
[41]*Ibid.,* pp. 105–106.
[42]*Ibid.,* p. 71.
[43]A. Ludlow Kramer, *Race and Violence In Washington State,* Report of the Commission on the Causes and Prevention of Civil Disorder, 1969, p. 24.

if they are to survive. All too often the children have the hope and desire to succeed in the world but because of futile and dangerous competition, they are unable to fulfill their ambitions.

Billingsley described in detail the three social-class groupings of Negro families. About ten percent of Negro families may be considered upper-class because the men are highly educated, are in high-income brackets, have secure careers and adequate comfortable housing. About forty percent of all Negro families are middle-class as distinguished by educational, income, and occupational achievement and styles of family life. Half of all Negro families are in the lower classes. Of these, there are the "working nonpoor," the "working poor," and the "nonworking poor." The "working nonpoor" are the families with the males working as semiskilled, unionized laborers in industries. The "working poor" represent families whose males work in unskilled and service occupations with marginal incomes. The "nonworking poor" are those families who receive the most publicity and who comprise fifteen to twenty percent of Negro families. These are people who are unemployed or intermittently employed, supported by relatives and friends or by public welfare.[44] The *majority* of *poor Negroes* live in nuclear families headed by men and not by women and are self-supporting rather than supported by public welfare.[45]

When studying the "nonworking poor," the lower-class Negro family, the existence of a matriarchal pattern is frequently found. Many black families are headed by the woman because opportunities for welfare payments are better for the female-headed household. The woman is often overburdened by many children and substandard living conditions. Her attitude toward her child may be one of ambivalence or indifference. Discipline tends to be inconsistent, but the child is expected to meet high standards of behavior and is severely punished when he fails to meet them. Activities are impulse-determined and consistency is totally absent. The children are often given more freedom outside the home and form important peer-group contacts early in life. The influence of the peer-group association often has more significance to the child than that of his parents because of the sense of importance and the identity of being a "gang" member.[46]

A black norm of behavior has developed which involves a profound distrust of white citizens and of the nation. The black person has learned to protect himself from physical hurt, cheating, slander, humiliation, and outright mistreatment by the official representatives of society. For his own survival, the black man views every white man as a potential enemy until

[44]Andrew Billingsley, *Black Families In White America*, Prentice-Hall, Inc., Englewood Cliffs, N.J., 1968, pp. 8–9.
[45]*Ibid.*, p. 139.
[46]Martin Deutsch, Irwin Katz, and Arthur R. Jensen, *Social Class, Race, and Psychological Development*, Holt, Rinehart and Winston, Inc., New York, 1968, p. 204.

proved otherwise and sees every social system as set against him unless he personally finds out differently.[47]  This in part explains the many pent-up resentments and latent frustrations felt by the blacks and being expressed in many overt and covert ways, according to Martin Luther King.[48]

For the white nurse visiting the black family, verbal and nonverbal evidences of the resentments and frustrations are easily detected if the nurse is sensitive and alert to cues. Many of the traditional nursing behaviors in home visits, which had a logical basis for existence initially, are being interpreted in a different way by Negroes. Standeven cited the example of the community health nurse's routine in placing a newspaper under the nursing bag. The blacks saw this action as indicating their home was particularly repelling and dirty, and the nurse was avoiding contamination of herself and the bag.[49] Members of the black family are particularly sensitive to cues of behavior. They do not like a friendly, charming manner if it seems phony, but respond with warmth and consideration of the nurse after they are convinced that she accepts them as having value and truly desires to be of assistance. There is much for the white nurse to learn about blacks, and the best teachers are blacks themselves, whether they are black nurses or black families. If the nurse concentrates first on initiating an empathic relationship, the resultant dialogue between the two involved persons will enhance their knowledges of each other, their adaptations of behavior, and result in positive exchanges which may be beneficial to both nurse and patient.

*Develop Empathic Relationship*

The health status of black groups is complicated by environmental conditions, unemployment, and lack of money to obtain medical treatment. Residents of racial ghettos have a high incidence of major diseases. The infant mortality and prematurity rate is higher for Negroes than for Caucasians. The rate of illegitimacy is high among the poor. One of the many tasks of the nurse is to increase the knowledge and sensitivity of black families about available health-care facilities such as medical and dental services, hospitals, and clinics dealing with family planning, abortion counseling, immunizations, child health, drug abuse, nutrition, prevention, and many other health-related problems. She also must be prepared to cope with the problems of little cash, transportation, baby-sitting problems, and erratic hours since these obstacles often stand in the way of attendance to health-care needs for blacks and their families. The black consumer has become active in exercising his right for health care and is increasingly convinced that he must do his own thing in health. In other words, he must play a major role in the design and management of health-care programs for blacks.

*Health Status Complications*

[47]Grier and Cobbs, *op. cit.,* p. 149.
[48]Judson R. Landis, *Current Perspectives on Social Problems,* Wadsworth Publishing Company, Inc., Belmont, California, 1969, p. 108.
[49]Muriel Standeven, "What the Poor Dislike About Community Health Nurses," *Nursing Outlook,* 17:9:72–73 (September) 1969.

According to Milio, Negroes want to learn to be self-sufficient in meeting their health needs and appreciate efforts from white persons only when the goal is directed toward independent self-care for blacks. In striving for the "black is beautiful" concept, they are building their self-respect and gaining confidence in their own abilities to successfully determine and cope with the intricacies of modern living.[50]

## Indian Families

Increasing attention is being given to American Indian culture and the role of the Indian in our current society. Since different tribes live in various locations of the United States, information about local Indian families must be obtained from literature specifically describing the local tribe and from the Indian people themselves. There are a great variety of Indian tribes who have their own histories, languages, customs, religions, and traditions. In addition, strong Indian leaders and war chiefs of the past hold a revered place in the memories of their people and symbolize the great tradition of the Indian people. As described by Deloria, individual tribes show incredible differences. The single aspect of major importance is tribal solidarity. Tribes that can handle their reservation conflicts in traditional Indian fashion generally make more progress and have better programs than do tribes that continually make adaptations to the white value system.[51]

There are many differences between the white culture and the Indian culture, and also among widely scattered Indian groups. A ritual or value of one tribe may not necessarily be accepted as essential by another tribe. The different geographical settings and cultural characteristics of various tribes complicate the work of health workers because transference of knowledge about one Indian tribe will not necessarily be valuable when working with a different tribe. This fact is frustrating because the health worker must start anew with each tribe with whom she works. Consequently, the health worker when working with Indian families in a local community must become acquainted with the values and beliefs of that specific Indian community. This takes time and patience. One example of a difference between two distinct tribes in terms of their responses to the implementation of health care by professionals is cited to demonstrate that the values of each tribe must be understood and dealt with as individual to that particular tribe. In a Pueblo reservation it was found that when parents were expected to transport their own children with health problems to clinics and hospitals outside the reservation, they gained a clearer understanding of the health services provided to the children and followed through with the recom-

*[handwritten margin note: Values differ from tribe to tribe.]*

---

[50]Milio, *op. cit.,* pp. 191–195.

[51]Vine Deloria, Jr., *Custer Died For Your Sins,* The Macmillan Company, New York, 1969, p. 28.

mended health care much more dependably.[52]  On a Tulalip reservation, however, the community health nurse was seen as more helpful if she brought concrete health services to the Indian child on the reservation or personally transported the child outside the reservation to the clinics and hospitals providing the health services.[53]

*Leadership*        Indian people place absolute dependence on their leaders and expect them to produce. Because leadership is taxing, physically and emotionally, the usefulness of the leader is sustained only as long as he is able to withstand the pressures of leadership over a dependent people.[54] Indians welcome the future but don't worry about it. They like to meet other tribes, have a good time, and learn to trust one another. However, they reserve the right to change their minds about an issue whenever it serves their own purposes. Indians know the human mind intimately. They savor innuendo and inference and can dwell for hours on slight nuances that others completely miss. Because of this, Indians know the Indian mind best of all.[55]

*Health Status*        The health status of Indians in some aspects is more appalling than that of the blacks. The infant mortality rate is the highest in the nation, with infants dying of influenza, pneumonia, respiratory conditions, gastroenteric and parasitic diseases. The life expectancy of the Indian is less than that of all other races, and the suicide rate is triple the national rate. Suicide alone among Indian youth has caused great concern in recent years and for one tribe in western Washington led to the development of a progressive youth program in an attempt to forestall an epidemic of suicides among teen-

*Leading Diseases*        agers. Leading diseases among the Indians are otitis media, tuberculosis, trachoma, anemia, and dental caries. A high incidence of lethal accidents, cirrhosis of the liver, and alcoholism also occurs with Indian populations.[56]

*Need for teaching*        Because of crowded housing, unsafe water, unsatisfactory waste disposal facilities, lack of nutritious food, and adherence to practices hazardous to health, the nurse has much health teaching to do *after* she has overcome the initial barrier of coming into the midst of the Indian people as a helping person and gone through the long procedure of becoming acceptable.

For the community health nurse working with Indian families on a Western reservation, Aichlmayr brought out the importance of starting a health program based purely upon the Indians' statement of need and desire and of being accepted as equals in a mutual endeavor. The concepts of social prestige, age, anonymity, time, patience, and generosity as per-

[52]Lucille J. Marsh, "Health Services For Indian Mothers and Children," Children's Bureau, Division of Indian Health, Public Health Service *Children* (November-December) 1957.
[53]Rita Hoeschen Aichlmayr, "Cultural Understanding: A Key to Acceptance," *Nursing Outlook*, 17:7:23 (July) 1969.
[54]Deloria, *op. cit.,* p. 214.
[55]*Ibid.,* pp. 215–220.
[56]Hilda Bryant, "Bad Health Adds to Indians' Woes," *The Red Man In America.* Reproduced by the information and editorial offices of the State Superintendent of Public Instruction, Olympia, Washington, by permission of the Seattle *Post-Intelligencer* (January) 1970, pp. 15–17.

ceived by Indians were gradually learned by the nurses over a time period of fifteen months. Indian people value sincerity, honesty, and absolute trustworthiness.[57] Similarly, as all people on the face of the earth, Indians are human beings who respond positively to treatment by helping persons when they are dealt with as having dignity, honor, and value. Regardless of race, color, culture, or creed, human beings have the universal need to be recognized and interacted with as worthy individuals.

*Self Worth*

## Families of Other Cultural Groups

In each local community there are often families representing a given culture who can be found in residential pockets, neighborhoods, or cul-de-sacs. They may be groups of Chicanos, Orientals, Scandinavians, Puerto Ricans, Filipinos, Italians, Jews, and other groups representing a country, a particular section of the United States, or religious creed. Each group has its own distinct culture in addition to some assimilation of United States culture. The task of the nurse is to become acquainted with each cultural group and attempt to understand the manifestations of behavior about which she is curious. Each family has characteristics and behaviors which need to be assessed before any effective action or teaching can take place. To learn more about a cultural group, the nurse can begin by inquiring about their foods, since people prefer to eat their own kind of food and often enjoy sharing their particular likes and individualized patterns of eating with others. She can ask about the manner of dress and admire distinctive clothing such as the sari of the women of India or the pina cloth of the Filipino. Historical tales can be requested about the early beginnings of the culture such as the Puerto Rican history or the ancient civilization of the Aztecs. Descriptions of recreational festivities that have special meaning can be elicited, such as the bullfights of the Mexican and Spaniard, the Bon Odori of the Japanese, or folk dance festivals of the Scandinavian. She can request clarification of the roles of family members, such as the male dominance or machismo exercised in Mexican and Hindu homes. The meaning of religious procedures of Italians or Jews can be elicited in terms of the marriage ceremony or upbringing practices of the children. Clarification of beliefs about health practices that seem impractical, ritualistic, or incongruent to the nurse can be requested. Always, the nurse must remember that when asking additional information about a cultural group, she must transmit genuine and sincere interest in the activities and practices of the family. If she can promote a liaison with the family based on mutual understanding of existing behavior patterns, a solid basis for teaching and counseling about practical and acceptable health practices is eased. Underlying the

*Foods*
*Dress*
*Historical Tales*
*Recreation*
*Religion*

[57]Aichlmayr, *op. cit.*, pp. 20–23.

*Planned Change Wanted*

*Change occurs p̄ therapeutic relationship established.*

implementation of any desired health action is the implicit suggestion to both nurse and family that planned change is wanted. Consent to change is most easily acquiesced when a mutual understanding and agreement occurs between nurse and family. Preparing a family for change often takes time and patience and is most easily accomplished when a therapeutic relationship has been developed simultaneously with the strengthening of the family's readiness.

## SUMMARY

The family has traditionally been the unit of service for the community health nurse as a means for focusing on all members of the family toward achieving higher levels of health or wholeness. The family was defined as a nuclear family or primary group living and interacting together intimately in a common residence. From the perspective of a systems approach, one of the roles of the community health nurse was described as that of coordinating the health-care systems and social systems within the community with the health needs of the family. The nurse also assesses the structure of families, the functions, and developmental task levels of families and individuals within the family. Interacting with families representing different socioeconomic positions requires careful preparation by the nurse, as she plans to implement successful activities with each family according to their values, beliefs, and culture. Low-income families frequently cope with multiple health problems and health hazards of a different nature than middle- and high-income families. The existing health behavior and health needs of families representing cultures unfamiliar to the nurse are studied in order to facilitate changes of health practices which will be desirable, acceptable, and beneficial to the family. For examples of people deserving improved health services, families of the black culture and Indian culture were described.

## SUGGESTED READING

Aranda, Robert G.: "The Mexican American Syndrome," *American Journal of Public Health*, 61:1:104–109 (January) 1971.

Bell, Norman W., and Ezra F. Vogel: *The Family*, The Free Press, New York, 1960.

Billingsley, Andrew: *Black Families In White America*, Prentice-Hall, Inc., Englewood Cliffs, N.J., 1968.

Deloria, Vine, Jr.: *Custer Died For Your Sins*, The Macmillan Company, New York, 1969.

Duvall, Evelyn Millis: *Family Development*, J. B. Lippincott Company, Philadelphia, 1962.

Geismar, L. L., and Michael A. La Sorte: *Understanding the Multi-Problem Family*, Association Press, New York, 1964.

Ginott, Dr. Haim G.: *Between Parent & Child,* The Macmillan Company, New York, 1965.

Grier, William H., and Price M. Cobbs: *Black Rage,* Basic Books, Inc., Publishers, New York, 1968.

Hall, Edward T.: *The Silent Language,* Doubleday & Company, Inc., Garden City, N.Y., 1959.

Herzog, Elizabeth: *About The Poor: Some Facts and Some Fictions,* U.S. Department of Health, Education and Welfare, Children's Bureau, 1967.

Huessy, Hans H., Carlton D. Marshall, Elizabeth K. Lincoln, and John L. Finan: "The Indigenous Nurse as Crisis Counselor and Intervener," *American Journal of Public Health,* 59(11):2022–2028 (November) 1969.

Irelan, Lola M.: *Low-Income Life Styles,* U.S. Department of Health, Education and Welfare, Government Printing Office, Washington, D.C., 1966.

Langsley, Donald G., and David M. Kaplan: *The Treatment of Families In Crisis,* Grune & Stratton, Inc., New York, 1968.

Lederer, William J., and Don D. Jackson: *The Mirages of Marriage,* W. W. Norton & Company, Inc., New York, 1968.

Leininger, Madeleine M.: *Nursing and Anthropology: Two Worlds to Blend,* John Wiley & Sons, Inc., New York, 1970.

Levine, Sol, Norman A. Scotch, and George J. Vlasak: "Unravelling Technology and Culture In Public Health," *American Journal of Public Health,* 59:2:237–244 (February) 1969.

Lewis, Oscar: *Five Families,* Basic Books, Inc., Publishers, New York, 1959.

Liebman, Samuel: *Emotional Forces In the Family,* J. B. Lippincott Company, Philadelphia, 1959.

Messner, Gerald: *Another View: To Be Black In America,* Harcourt Brace Jovanovich, Inc., New York, 1970.

Minuchin, Salvado, Braulio Montalvo, Bernard G. Guerney, Bernice L. Rosman, and Florence Schumer: *Families Of the Slums,* Basic Books, Inc., Publishers, New York, 1967.

Nye, F. Ivan, and Felix M. Berardo: *Emerging Conceptual Frameworks in Family Analysis,* The Macmillan Company, New York, 1966.

Sussman, Marvin B.: *Sourcebook In Marriage and the Family,* Houghton Mifflin Company, Boston, 1968.

Tapia, Jayne Anttila: "The Nursing Process in Family Health," *Nursing Outlook,* 20:4:267–270 (April) 1972.

"The Sick Poor," *American Journal of Nursing,* 69:11:2423–2454 (November) 1969.

Toffler, Alvin: *Future Shock,* Random House, Inc., New York, 1970.

Walker, A. Elizabeth: "Primex—The Family Nurse Practitioner Program," *Nursing Outlook,* 20:1:28–31 (January) 1972.

# 5
# The
# Home
# Visit

The home visit has been the principal means by which community health nurses have interacted with families. The home continues to hold emphasis as a desirable setting because family interactions, patterns of coping, and life styles are best revealed in a familiar environment. However, community health nurses are increasingly making use of telephone and office visits, particularly if the busy schedules of the family or nurse cannot be synchronized at mutually agreeable times. Also, community health nurses are realizing the efficacy of group meetings in which health teaching can be given to a group of persons, discussed by the group from the standpoint of their individual and different viewpoints, and accepted by the group as each individual clarifies and adapts his thinking based on perception of the messages given and received. In group work, the nurse is able to work with numbers of people. In home visits, the interaction is often on a one-to-one or three-way basis, depending on how many family members are home. The nurse must be prepared to do both individual and group work and sometimes may wish to diversify her methods of working with the family by talking with individual members occasionally on a one-to-one basis and meeting with the entire family at other appointed times.

## FUNCTIONS OF THE COMMUNITY HEALTH NURSE

The functions of the community health nurse were accepted in 1964 by the Public Health Nursing Section of the American Nurses Association as consisting of five processes which could be used to achieve results. These processes were:

1. Assessing: identifying the need for the act

**2.** Planning: arranging for the methods and techniques necessary to meet the assessed need

**3.** Implementing: taking the action required to carry out the plan to meet the need

**4.** Evaluating: testing the outcome of the actions against previously determined criteria

**5.** Studying and researching: searching for knowledge in a systematic way[1]

An elaboration of the meaning of the functions is outlined as follows:

Assessing

*Function I.* Identifies present and potential needs and resources related to the health of individuals, families, and the community
A. Uncovers health needs and problems through observation, interviews, analysis of records, and use of vital data
B. Observes, explores, and evaluates the patient's physical and emotional condition, reaction to drugs or treatments
C. Considers age, sex, culture, economic status, or geographic location that may influence the incidence or prevalence of health problems
D. Recognizes attitudes that influence individual and community health
E. Estimates the ability and readiness of individuals and families to recognize and meet their own health needs
F. Identifies the availability and utilization of community resources
G. Evaluates the urgency and complexity of the need in determining priority of action

*Function II.* Shares in identifying present and potential needs and resources related to the agency's program and the nurse's job responsibilities
A. Appraises community health and social needs and resources for interpretation to administrative and planning groups
B. Appraises the adequacy of community health nursing services in her district in relation to community needs and agency program
C. Determines through her contacts with patients, families, members of related disciplines, and others, the extent of their knowledge of the agency's program
D. Estimates the effectiveness of intra- and extra-agency communications

---

[1]The American Nurses Association, Public Health Nursing Section, *Functions and Qualifications in the Practice of Public Health Nursing,* New York, 1964, p. 27.

E. Participates in the exploration and identification of her own needs in relation to the job

Planning

Function I. Plans for the comprehensive nursing service to individuals and families in their homes

A. Interprets nursing and other services of the agency to patients and families as a part of planning

B. Plans with the individual, family, physician, and other concerned members of the health team for care which is appropriate

C. Plans with other individuals and agencies for continuity of patient care

Function II. Participates in planning for community health nursing service in special settings such as schools, places of employment, nursing homes, and similar institutions, hospitals, clinics, and health conferences

A. Helps develop and arrange for community health nursing services in special settings

B. Develops plans for group teaching to meet the special needs of various groups

Function III. Contributes to planning for the development and operation of the community health agency

A. Contributes to the development of philosophy, purposes, policies, and procedures of the community health nursing services in the agency

B. Participates in planning nursing aspects of new and ongoing programs

C. Contributes to the preparation and revision of the nursing budget

D. Participates in planning the administrative procedures of the nursing office

E. Participates in planning continuing education programs for agency personnel

Function IV. Participates in planning with other agencies for community health programs

A. Advises or participates in community group planning related to nursing and health

B. Plans with professional organizations and civic groups for the improvement and advancement of the practice of nursing and community health

Implementing

Function I. Helps provide comprehensive nursing service to individuals and families in their homes

A. Gives skilled care to patients requiring part-time professional nursing service and teaches and supervises the family and other members of the nursing team

B. Interprets extent and limitations of available nursing service
C. Gives preventive and therapeutic treatment under medical or dental direction and teaches positive health measures
D. Utilizes her understanding of behavior patterns in giving nursing service
E. Initiates nursing measures to prevent complications and to minimize disabilities
F. Helps the individual and family to develop attitudes that permit them to make optimum use of available resources and health facilities
G. Helps the family accept and assume its responsibility for providing and arranging care and guides it toward self-help
H. Helps the patient and family understand implications of the diagnosis and recommended treatment consistent with their readiness and with the knowledge of the physician
I. Helps individuals and families to utilize their capabilities and make the best possible adjustment to their limitations
J. Helps individuals and families understand patterns of growth and development and encourages attitudes and actions that will promote optimum health for each individual
K. Aids in effecting changes in the environment or in the organization of activities for the elimination or modification of health hazards
L. Communicates with other professional workers regarding the individual and family and refers pertinent information to the appropriate agency
M. Participates in conferences with other disciplines to coordinate services and plan joint action
N. Assists the physician and dentist with examiniations and treatments when nursing skills are required
O. Obtains laboratory specimens, performs diagnostic tests when indicated, and interprets the significance of the results to individuals and families when authorized
P. Participates in recruiting, training, and supervising volunteer workers
Q. Maintains necessary records and reports

*Function II.* Provides community health nursing service in special settings
A. Gives direct or consultative nursing services in such settings as schools, clinics, hospitals, or places of employment
B. Provides nursing service, on a demonstration or temporary basis, to convalescent and nursing homes and similar institutions
C. Carries out inspections of institutions when delegated by the licensing authority for the purpose of making nursing recommendations
D. Participates in the teaching of selected individuals and groups

*Function III.* Participates in the development and operation of the community health agency

A. Keeps the agency informed about changes in the community and in nursing practice which may have an effect on the program
B. Assists with the orientation and guidance of new staff members, volunteers, citizen committees, and boards
C. Participates in the public information and promotion activities of the agency

*Function IV.* Participates in community health programs

A. Teaches basic principles of healthful living in relation to changing needs of individuals in all age groups
B. Provides for or encourages others in the community to provide for group instruction related to health
C. Represents the agency in her professional organizations and community groups when so designated
D. Interprets to the community the need for the meaning of health laws and regulations and reports violations to the appropriate authority
E. Participates in community health surveys, epidemiologic studies, and other organized health programs
F. Interprets health and welfare needs to appropriate community groups

Evaluating

*Function I.* Appraises performance

A. Evaluates the effectiveness of her nursing service to individuals and families
B. Evaluates the effectiveness of her service in health programs in special settings
C. Contributes to the evaluation of workers for whom she shares supervisory responsibility
D. Uses available help to study and evaluate her own job performance and plan for continuing professional growth

Studying and Researching

*Function I.* Engages in surveys, studies, and research

A. Identifies problem areas related to her functions in assessing, planning, implementing, and evaluating
B. Participates in defining problems for study
C. Participates in the conduct of surveys, studies, and research related to her clinical and functional responsibilities

*Function II.* Applies pertinent research findings[2]

[2]*Ibid.,* pp. 9–12.

It is obvious that not all community health staff nurses will carry out every detail of these functions, for the scope of the nurse's work and her responsibilities will be governed by the agency's program. Each community health nursing agency determines its program and obligations to the community in relation to the community's needs, interests, and resources.

Community health nurses will need to continue defining and redefining their functions. The results of research in medicine, nursing, and the natural and social sciences, and the implementation of new health and social programs will have implications for broadening the responsibilities of the community health nurse and the scope of community health agencies.

## COMPONENTS OF A HOME VISIT

In this chapter all the processes involved in making a home visit are described. The definition of the family, its structure, functions, developmental task status, and position as a unit in the society of social systems was outlined in Chap. 4. When making a home visit, the community health nurse is faced with many functions, immediate or latent, which include preparation for the visit, her introduction to the family, contract with the family, assessment, plan, implementation, evaluation, and written summary. These functions occur on every home visit, but the depth of purpose and emphasis changes as movement toward an agreed upon goal by family and nurse becomes more resolute. The ultimate objective of the nurse is to assist the family's advancement toward wellness or an acceptance of their present reality as exemplified by their improved coping skills, increased self-confidence, and attainment of better levels of health. *Wellness,* as defined by Dunn, is an integrated method of functioning that is oriented toward maximizing the potential of which the individual and family are capable, within the environment where he or they are functioning.[3] When the family and nurse agree that essential and desired goals have been reached satisfactorily, then the nurse has accomplished her purpose as a helping change agent.

## PREPARATION FOR A VISIT

There are two acceptable methods used by nurses when preparing for a visit. The first method consists of thorough preparation and assimilation of all data before making the first home visit, and the second method postpones the gathering of related data until the first home visit has been made and initial impressions have been received by the nurse. The first method requires a careful reading of the family folder in order to become familiar with the family constellation and the unique considerations of cultural, eth-

[3]Halbert L. Dunn, *High Level Wellness,* R. W. Beatty Co., Arlington, Virginia, 1961, pp. 4–5.

nic, religious, and social conditions. By reading all the nursing notes thoroughly, an impression is gained about past events and successful and unsuccessful maneuvers which have occurred between the family and former nurses. Talking with other nurses or personnel from related fields who know the family also helps the nurse to form a mental image of the situation for which she is becoming prepared. The second method consists of a brief perusal of the family folder to make note of the family constellation and reason for the referral or continued visits. A conscious effort is made to avoid reading nursing notes or talking with personnel who are acquainted with the family before making the first home visit. When the second method is used, the nurse is dependent upon her individual skills of on-the-spot observation, assessment, and the family's feedback of events that have occurred in the past as seen from their perception. After gaining a picture of the situation from the family's point of view and her own appraisal of cues which occurred on her first home visit, the nurse consequently reads the family folder and nursing notes thoroughly and talks to all individuals who are acquainted with the family to ascertain if all viewpoints coincide. It is a matter of individual preference and knowledge of one's own style of proceeding which determines the method selected by the nurse. The nurse who prefers to make her own assessment believes that the first method gives an unconscious predetermined bias, which may be deceiving and difficult to overcome. The nurse who relies on the first method believes she is more thoroughly prepared for any occurrence which may arise and will respond more successfully with tactics that may be attempted by the family.

When the family has a telephone, the nurse has the opportunity to call and arrange for a home visit at an appointed time. She introduces herself and gives the reason why she wants to visit the family. By making an appointment in advance, the nurse and family member become psychologically prepared for the visit. Also, the nurse is assured that someone will be home when she makes the visit, and the family has been allowed the courtesy of arranging a time interval most suitable for them.

## INTRODUCTION TO THE FAMILY

When the time comes to knock on the door or ring the doorbell, it always is a moment of uncertainty for the nurse. She knows *why* she is making the visit but never is certain what tableau will be revealed when the door is opened. Feelings vary as the nurse waits for the door to open. One student nurse described her thoughts as follows:

> (knock, knock) As I stood outside the door, I could hear the radio playing within, and various images of stubborn, suspicious, frightened, or confused countenances flashed across my mind; I hoped to meet any or none of them as best I could.

Unless the nurse is well known to the family, the first step in her visit is to introduce herself, stating clearly her name and that of her agency. She explains the reason for her visit and the source of the referral for the visit if that is necessary, e.g., "Good morning, Mrs. Brown, I am Miss Jones. I am the community health nurse from the Ocean County Health Department. Your physician, Dr. Smith, asked that we call on you about your pregnancy." Or, Good morning, Mrs. Brown, I am Miss Jones, the community health nurse from the Ocean County Health Department and Ocean City Visiting Nurse Service. I came in response to your telephone request this morning to visit your little boy who has a cold." The introduction or social phase will vary with the situation, but warmth, friendliness, and expressed interest on the part of the nurse will help her to establish rapport with the family and to develop a relationship on which to base effective teaching later.

The social phase of the visit cannot be overemphasized, because it is during this time that the family member becomes acquainted with the nurse as having the potential for being a warm human being and not another official professional entity who must be treated with awe, respect, and compliance. When anxiety is moderately high for the nurse and the family member, recall of all the words that were spoken during the home visit is limited. When comfort and relaxation occur, facilitated during the social phase of the visit, then the professional content of the visit has more possibility of being remembered and the family member and nurse are better able to absorb the implications of subsequent interactions.

## CONTRACT WITH THE FAMILY

When working with a family, it is essential that the family members and the nurse know the purpose of the nurse's visits, that there is a mutual agreement to work toward a desired end or goal, and that both family members and nurse will direct their activities or abilities toward the achievement of the mutually determined goal. In essence, a *contract* is made in which the family and the nurse are involved. As a consequence of the contract, both know the goal or goals toward which they are striving, both realize what is expected of them as participants, and both will know when the contract has been completed.

For families who have had nursing visits in which contracts have not been made, there is often an uncertainty about the reason for nursing visits. They find the nurse a pleasant person, attempt to meet her needs by telling her about their past illnesses or reasons for failure to attend clinics, and after her visit resume their life patterns as always.

It is difficult to establish a contract that is mutually acceptable to family members and the nurse when the family has little knowledge of the nurse's scope of abilities. If the nurse is seen as one who only gives shots, baths, and direct nursing care, then an interpretation of the current change in nursing focus must be explained in a way that makes sense to the receiver of the information. The ability of the nurse to secure needed professional information from appropriate professional sources, coordinate the activities of all community professional specialists who show interest in the family, or teach the family about practical methods of improving health or wellness are some of the early "selling" reasons for nursing visits. Later, when the family and nurse have established a relationship in which each trusts the other and knowledge of each other's potential has been experienced, the contract can be adjusted to reflect a more accurate direction toward the agreed upon goal.

Examples of contracts which can be agreed upon by family members and nurse are (1) to gain a better understanding of the various methods of birth control; (2) assistance in toilet training the preschool child successfully and with minimum trauma; (3) support in a weight-reduction program; (4) interpretation of the team activities of professional personnel in special clinics who meet with family members regarding special problems; (5) assistance in preventing frequent respiratory diseases in infants and children; and (6) strengthening the feeling of competence of the mother of the family about her task of mothering one or several children. Nursing students have had success with contracts primarily aimed at assisting the student to learn the complex factors involved in adjusting to an existing health problem. The families who are responsive to a contract of this nature engage in and enjoy a reciprocal relationship with the nurse in which both are learning and benefiting.

## THE NURSING PROCESS: ASSESSING

Nurses are accustomed to assessing the patient's needs based on a medical and nursing model and can often identify many more needs than can a patient. However, unless a patient also sees a need as one that exists and for which he desires help, there is little point in making the assessment.

Assessment is a continuous process which becomes more accurate as knowledge of the consumer deepens. As defined by Harpine, *nursing assessment* is the continuous, systematic, critical, orderly, and precise method of collecting, validating, analyzing, and interpreting information about the physical, psychological and social needs of a patient, the nature of his self-care deficits, and other factors influencing his condition and care.[4] While determining patient needs, the nurse will concentrate only on those

---

[4]Frances H. Harpine, "Assessing the Needs of the Patient," in Helen Yura and Mary B. Walsh (eds.), *The Nursing Process: Assessing, Planning, Implementing, and Evaluating,* The Catholic University of America Press, Washington, D.C., 1967, p. 22.

needs which she can influence or change by her nursing intervention. She will seek to know the patient as a distinctive person so that she may utilize her self and her abilities as a therapeutic agent as effectively as is possible.

All persons have needs, but which needs will the patient confirm as indeed existing and with which he will accept assistance from the nurse? For low-income families, the needs which have to be focused upon early are often the physiologic and safety needs, whereas with middle- and high-income families the needs for love, belonging, esteem, or self-actualization may be the ones that are most urgent and in need of attention. All persons, regardless of social class, periodically regress in their individual fashions toward seeking satisfaction for the more basic physical needs when they indulge in overeating or lose their appetite, seek additional sleep or have insomnia, or reveal similar manifestations of stress.[5] The ability to assess and observe the patient with his present reality makes use of the nurse's senses, her knowledge of hierarchy of needs, and her ability to relate to the patient's verbal and nonverbal cues in a facilitative manner. As she observes and makes note of cues, she must share and explore her perceptions with the patient to ascertain if he is in agreement with her perceptions.[6] Sometimes, the patient has difficulty expressing his desires and must be helped by the nurse to articulate his needs. A facilitative way to do this is to state, "You look worried. Are you concerned about something that I am unaware of?" Or the nurse may say, "Sometimes it is difficult to ask for help because we all like to think we can handle our own affairs. However, there are times when each one of us needs the help of another, and I sense that you may feel that way now. Is this true?" By admitting that we all are human beings and have moments of need, a relationship is facilitated in which each participant feels a greater freedom to exchange his own inner meanings with the other person involved.[7] When the nurse is authentic, she excludes the possibility of seeing the patient as a problem and herself as a person who can solve the problems. She tries to be responsively aware so that the patient, in turn, can be authentic and reveal his true concerns.[8]

Obstacles which tend to blunt the perceptions of nurses and deter the attainment of accurate assessments of patients and families have been experienced by all nurses and must be watched for as undesirable behaviors. The first one is taking a partial view of the person, labeling or stereotyping that person with descriptive labels such as uncooperative, slow, immature, incompetent, and so on. Once the judgment has been made or the label attached to the patient, the nurse tends to miss other positive or negative attributes which may change her mind about the person. All people

[5]Sister Kathleen M. Black, "Assessing Patients' Needs," in Yura and Walsh, *op. cit.*, p. 8.
[6]Harpine, *op. cit.*, p. 22.
[7]Black, *op. cit.*, p. 17.
[8]*Ibid.*, p. 18.

have likable and dislikable characteristics and an attempt should be made to view all persons as accurately as possible.

A second obstacle is that of viewing the patient as a thing instead of a person. All too often in nursing and medicine, patients have been referred to as a room number, a bed number, or a diagnosis. In fact, sometimes the common practice of calling a person a patient is discriminatory and not always beneficial for the person. When the person is viewed as an object, it is all too easy to deal with him purely as the receiver of nursing ministrations and to deny him the choice of accepting or refusing procedures that are designed to help him whether he sees it that way or not.

A third deterrent is viewing the person who is the patient in terms of his potential to meet the nurse's needs, rather than the nurse's potential to meet his. This obstacle has to do with the esteem needs of the nurse and her natural desire to be influential and successful with the person receiving her assistance.[9] It is difficult for the nurse to know that the patient can be helped yet have the patient refuse nursing service or observe the patient as demonstrating no improvement in spite of nursing ministrations. It is also sometimes difficult to accept the fact that the patient no longer requires nursing services and is competent to make his own decisions. For example, a student nurse during a routine visit to a young mother with a new baby was shown the diaper rash of the baby, which was causing the mother considerable concern. The nurse instructed the mother carefully and thoroughly about the care of the buttocks, and in the event that no improvement was demonstrated, referral to a well-baby clinic was given. The nurse promised to return in a week. Three days later, the student nurse felt a compelling urge to visit the young mother and baby to see for herself if the diaper rash was better or not. After a vigorous conflict within herself, the nurse decided that her *own* need to see the mother and baby must take second priority to the knowledge that the mother had been carefully instructed, had understood, and was probably competent to manage the situation. On the home visit the following week, the nurse received the report from the mother that the diaper rash had cleared after the mother implemented the instructions she had received from the nurse.

### Factors in Assessing the Family
On the initial home visit to a family many early impressions are secured, which form the initial basis for the ongoing assessment. As data are gathered and assembled continuously during subsequent visits the nurse becomes better acquainted with the family and responds to the assessment process similarly to that of assembling a jigsaw puzzle. The early pieces of

---

[9] *Ibid.,* pp. 14–15.

the jigsaw puzzle give one an early image of the completed picture, but while sorting and trying the various pieces for size, there are frequent periods of puzzlement and frustration. Until all the pieces are in place, a complete understanding of the picture is not reached. Families are like jigsaw puzzles in that sometimes it takes several months before an understanding of the mechanisms operating within families is gained by the nurse. Early impressions are important but not always accurate. Therefore, the nurse must be flexible, patient, and willing to adjust her assessment as new data are revealed over the course of time.

To make a comprehensive assessment of the family is time-consuming and must involve all of the following factors on a superficial or detailed basis. When specialized information is needed in addition, many nursing texts and professional periodicals are available that describe more specifically the data required for special diagnoses and conditions. These factors include: (1) the family's physical and environmental status, including the medical history and present health of each family member, with special consideration of housing, number of rooms in relation to size of family, ventilation, cleanliness, sanitation, source of water supply, sewage disposal, and general safety, e.g., fire protection. (2) The family's cultural background, which is important to the nurse in her understanding and appreciation of the needs of the patient and family. What are the family's attitudes and practices with regard to religion, medical care, nutrition, and eating habits? To what degree does the family participate in the life and activities of its neighborhood and wider community? (3) The economic factors, including the occupation of the family breadwinners and the family's approximate income. The latter is helpful to the nurse when she assists with budget problems and purchasing. It will help her to determine, also, the family's eligibility for medical and dental care in clinics if it is needed and there is no medical insurance. (4) The developmental levels of family members, including ages and levels of achievement, both physical and mental. (5) The psychological factors, including family relationships both within and without the home, the emotional tone of the family life, and patterns of family behavior and intrafamily relationships, e.g., parent-child relationships and sibling relationships. (6) The educational, vocational, and recreational interests of its members. Knowledge of these interests is important in the nurse's appraisal of the family because she plans her teaching according to the apparent knowledge, educational background, interests, and levels of understanding of the family members. An appreciation of the recreational needs and interests of the family and the facilities available in the neighborhood and community for meeting them is helpful to the nurse. Does the family plan its recreation together? Does their church meet some of these needs through church clubs and classes? What other community resources are available? a library? a playfield? a zoo? (7) The family's use of resources within the community. Is the family knowledgeable about resources available within the community? Are they willing to visit the resources? Are they ready to avail themselves of needed services or would they like the nurse to serve as a liaison agent initially?

In order to provide a family health service, the nurse must be alert to the health and welfare needs of all the members. For this reason she explores the many facets of family life in order to try to answer the questions, "What information do I need so that I can plan constructively with this family?" and "Which family need or needs should be given top priority immediately?"

## Assessment Tools

It is always sound nursing practice to make use of screening devices, tests, or measurements whenever possible to determine more accurately what the nurse suspects based on her early observations or intuitive hunches. An essential tool for assessing the basic reflex patterns of newborns, infants, and preschool children up to three years is the reference *A Developmental Approach to Casefinding,* by Una Haynes.

This booklet describes the reflexes, how to elicit them, and how to appraise the baby during the bathing procedure. A wheel device for quick recall of developmental skills in conjunction with age in months is included with the booklet.[10]

A second excellent tool is the *Denver Developmental Screening Test,* which evaluates the gross motor, fine motor, adaptive, language, and personal-social areas of a child's functioning from birth to six years of age. It is easy to administer and utilizes participation of the parent during the testing procedure. Most parents respond with great interest to this screening device and are motivated subsequently to assist the child in practicing the skills that are in need of further development.[11]

It is essential for community health nurses to maintain ongoing curiosity about research studies reported in professional journals. In this way the nurses remain up-to-date and knowledgeable about new screening devices and procedures which more accurately assess the health needs of patients and families.

## NURSING DIAGNOSIS

After gaining essential data about the family and determining a contract with the patient and/or family about the need which has immediate priority,

[10]Una Haynes, *A Developmental Approach to Casefinding,* U.S. Department of Health, Education and Welfare, Social and Rehabilitation Service, Children's Bureau, 1967. (For sale by the Superintendent of Documents, U.S. Government Printing Office, Washington, D.C. 20402.)

[11]Manual, form, and kit are available from *LADOCA,* Project and Publishing Foundation, Inc., E. 51st Ave. and Lincoln, Denver, Colorado 80216.

the nurse is then faced with making a nursing diagnosis that will form the basis for her plan and implementation of nursing intervention. Durand and Prince defined *nursing diagnosis* as statement of a conclusion resulting from recognition of a pattern derived from a nursing investigation of the patient or family.[12] By making a diagnosis the nurse sets the stage for her subsequent activities with the patient and/or family.

The following example very briefly illustrates an assessment of a family made by a student nurse and her subsequent nursing diagnosis.

> It wasn't until after I made my initial visit that I realized that health encompassed more than just the physical and mental, but included the social, cultural, environmental, and socioeconomic factors. . . . Identifying the medical needs of the family was not difficult since this was one of the mother's major concerns for herself and the children. The mother was very open and willing to talk about her own ailments, which were many, and the medical care needs of the children. . . . The family's economic situation was precarious, which had an effect on the follow-through of medical needs. . . . Focusing on the mental health of the family made me acutely aware of how the manner of communication can deeply affect the mental attitudes of family members toward each other. I was able to make a home visit when the mother and father were home. Even in my presence, it was quite apparent that these two people annoyed each other. The father was very intolerant of the mother's naive concepts about the subject we were discussing at the time. The mother likewise voiced her anger toward the father on a separate occasion. The mother views the father as a very egocentric individual and feels rejected by him. The problem with both of these people is that they do not have the appropriate outlets upon which to release their anger. They are unable to discuss their feelings on a rational, adult level; consequently, they use their children to release their anger on. It comes through in their communication to the children. I am sure they are unaware of how their communication is perceived by the children or anyone else. They sound intolerant, impatient, and very angry. . . . The nursing diagnosis for this family is the mother and father's destructive communication patterns which affect and expand family health problems, influencing all members of the family.

## NURSING SERVICES AND FEES

The nurse describes the purpose and philosophy of the agency and explains that its services are available to all in the community according to their health needs. If, however, the agency is private or nonofficial, a combination agency, or an official agency that charges for some services, she explains the fee schedule for services.

Although these services of the agency are available to all in the community according to their health needs, today's concept (first expressed by

[12]Mary Durand and Rosemary Prince, "Nursing Diagnosis; Process and Decision," *Nursing Forum,* 5:4:50–64, 1966.

the old woman in the London slums) that patients and families pay for services as they are able has become fairly well established and accepted. Most people wish to pay what they can, and agencies have found that patients and families tend to value nursing services and teaching more when they pay at least something for them.

In discussing the fee schedule with the family or patient, the nurse keeps the following points in mind:

I.   The actual cost to the agency of the visit, including costs for travel, professional nursing services provided, equipment used, overhead expenses (e.g., rent, light, and telephone), and the necessary personnel in addition to the nurse, i.e., administrative, supervisory, and secretarial personnel.

2.   The family's ability to pay for nursing service. This is based on a consideration of the family's overall income and fixed expenditures, e.g., food, rent, utilities, and financial commitments such as insurance. When the patient is the wage earner, it is to be expected that the family income will be markedly reduced. In such situations, some families may be unable to pay the full fee but might find it possible to pay on a partial basis.

3.   The type of illness and the nursing care needed. If the illness promises to be short, requiring two to three visits, a full fee might be indicated, but if it appears that the illness may be long, such as cancer or disability following a stroke, the nurse must consider the probable number of visits necessary and then evaluate with the family their ability to pay under the circumstances.

4.   The fee schedule is flexible and may be adjusted easily to the family situation.

5.   Many families today have certain types of medical insurance that provide for nursing services. Often they are not aware of the provisions in their policies.

When a family requests a nursing visit on an appointment basis in order to meet their convenience, the full "cost-of-visit" fee or more is charged by some agencies. On the other hand, if the family can adjust to the nurse's plans for the day, the full fee or less may be charged.

Most official agencies make no charge for visits for nursing service, demonstrations of nursing care, or teaching when the request was made because of a communicable disease; when the visit is for the purpose of supervising maternal and child health or handicapped children; when families are faced with problems of mental or emotional difficulties or mental retardation; or when the visit is a first one that has not been requested by the patient or family.

If a fee is to be charged for a first visit to a new family, and for later visits, the patient, family, and nurse discuss the fee, but before making a final decision, the nurse may wish to discuss aspects of the situation with her supervisor. Sometimes a patient or family, prompted by an appreciation of the nurse's help, will want to pay more for the services than their budget actually allows.

Generally speaking, nurses find it very difficult to discuss fees with patients and families. They recognize that their visits merit payment but are reluctant to evaluate their services in terms of monetary value. Establishing fees tends to be considered a cold, mercenary task and talking about money conflicts with the nurses' view of themselves as warm, helping persons. For this reason, nurses have responded favorably when some official agencies have hired a person whose title is that of fee clerk. The fee clerk's primary task is to visit all new families who have been accepted for nursing services, interpret the agency's policies in regard to fees, and establish a fee for services that is satisfactory to the family. Whenever the nurse reports a change in the family's financial status after the initial encounter, the fee clerk visits again to adjust the fee according to the ability of families to pay. In many agencies a graduated fee schedule based on family income is used as a guide for determining a fair fee.

Every three to five years, community health nursing agencies conduct "cost-of-visit" studies. The findings will reflect the current cost of each visit made by the nursing agency. On the basis of this information, the fee is adjusted. Established fee schedules are helpful to the nurse as she interprets the agency services to the family.

## MEDICARE AND MEDICAID

In 1965, the United States Congress passed legislation setting up the health insurance plan, now known as Medicare and Medicaid, under Titles XVIII and XIX, to be administered under Social Security. It was intended to provide much of the expense for hospitalization, laboratory tests, home health services, extended-care facilities, and medical bills for patients sixty-five years of age or older who voluntarily subscribed to the plan. Agencies providing these services, e.g., hospitals, laboratories, nursing homes, and community health nursing agencies, were required to meet the Federal government's specific conditions before being certified to accept patients.

Although the Medicare legislation was passed in 1965, patient benefits commenced in July, 1966, with services from hospitals, home-care agencies, and laboratories. In January, 1967, extended-care facility service was added. All but two states agreed to participate in this program, the benefits of which may be extended to the medically indigent if desired.

The Federal government's specific requirements for participating home health agencies, such as visiting nurse associations, subdivisions of local or state health departments, or combination visiting nurse associations and health department agencies, in their service to patients included:

**1.** Being primarily engaged in providing skilled nursing service and other therapeutic services to patients in the home.

**2.** Having policies established by a group of professional personnel with the agency and including one or more physicians and one or more registered professional nurses and providing professional supervision by physicians and nurses.

**3.** Maintaining clinical records on all patients. Services of allied professional groups such as physical therapists, speech therapists, and occupational therapists were also to be made available to patients, subject to the requirements of the Medicare plan.

Medicare and Medicaid should not be considered as static programs. Their requirements have continued to develop and change, depending somewhat on the economic, social, and political climate in each state. New programs and practices have been devised to meet specific needs and new conditions and some old ones have been discarded, having proved to be ineffective. It is anticipated that legislation will be passed by Congress at some date for a national health insurance plan that will meet the medical, nursing, and health needs of the nation's entire population at a reasonable cost. This will demand a tremendous amount of comprehensive planning and thought on the part of all concerned. Nurses must utilize the opportunity to contribute their ideas because of their present experience in working with Medicare, Medicaid, and other Federal medical programs.

## THE NURSING PROCESS: PLANNING
When sufficient data about the health needs of a patient or family have been gained and a contract with the family established, the nurse is faced with the necessity for planning. A plan is the method of action or the blueprint for activity based on the resources available and the goals desired.[13] Of primary concern is the patient with his knowledge, capabilities, customary patterns of coping, resources, needs, desires as he sees them and as the nurse sees them. The nurse must also consider her own knowledge, capabilities, ways of coping, resources, needs, desires, as well as her limitations, which may have a bearing on the attainment of the patient's desired goals.[14] The setting of the patient must be viewed from a realistic and

---

[13]Joan Nettleton, "Planning To Meet Patient Needs," in Yura and Walsh, *op. cit.,* p. 44.
[14]*Ibid.,* p. 47.

objective standpoint to ensure that desired goals have the potential for successful fulfillment.

While talking about realistic goals the patient desires, the nurse can give valuable assistance by suggesting practical, short-term and long-term goals. The long-term goals exemplify the ultimate objectives desired by the patient, whereas the short-term goals represent the graduated steps marking progression toward the desired long-term goals. When short-term goals are attained, they build confidence that the next goal can likewise be achieved. For example, for the mother who wishes her son to be toilet trained, the long-term goal is independent self-care in toileting for the son. The short-term goals may be (1) determining the boy's physiologic and psychological readiness for toilet training; (2) ascertaining the boy's present toileting patterns; (3) setting up a toileting procedure which is feasible for the mother and son and includes rewards or positive attitudes for activities done successfully; and (4) determining a measuring method or chart for observing frequency of success. Early expectations should be minimal, then show progress as the boy develops skill in his toileting activities. Charts with gold stars can often be motivating stimuli for preschool children. When toileting accidents occur infrequently, then the mother realizes that the long-term goal has been achieved.

It is important that the family and nurse plan toward desired goals together because goals decided upon are a prelude to action for both family and nurse. Dependent upon the health-care needs of the family, the goals may be directed toward care of sickness and handicaps or health teaching and counseling.

## Care of Sickness and Handicaps

For those patients needing physical care, the nurse plans her administration of nursing procedures and treatments prescribed by the physician and also includes an inventory of all medications used by the patient to ensure that the drugs are being taken properly as ordered and are having the desired effect. The nurse remains up-to-date on rehabilitation and exercise measures and plans for execution of activities for daily living for those patients who desire to acquire new self-help skills. For those patients on special diets, she obtains a history of their nutritional practices and plans for implementation of ideas which seem practical and geared to the patient's needs, desires, and limitations.

Frequently the nurse will need to adapt nursing equipment and procedures to the home situation; she can encourage family members to work with her in improvising many articles to contribute to the patient's safety and comfort, such as a back rest from a cardboard carton or a wheelchair made by attaching castors to the bottom of each leg of a sturdy chair. The use of disposable, self-help, and low-cost equipment is always an important consideration. Utilizing transfer procedures which ease the difficulty of moving a patient from one object to another or from one room to another is sometimes a major feat to accomplish in the setting of some homes.

Many ideas for assisting the patient with personal grooming and eating may be found in current nursing periodicals and pamphlets. On occasion, families work out helpful ideas for the comfort and safety of the patient that will contribute to his independence. They should be encouraged to do this, and appreciation should be shown for their efforts.

During bedside nursing activities, the nurse has the opportunity to observe the patient and assess his condition. She may note also the degree of understanding the family has for the situation. Whenever possible, she should delegate certain responsibilities to family members so that they may participate in the care of the patient, such as assembling equipment for a bath or a treatment. She shows one or more of the family members how they may care for the patient in her absence and observes them in a return demonstration. Family members will watch closely the nurse's techniques, even when she is not consciously teaching. The care she takes with the contents of her nursing bag, with her handwashing, and with the use of equipment is of great interest to them.

Patients and families like to know what is causing the patient's distress, so interpretations of the medical phenomena underlying the disease process are appreciated when explained in an understandable manner. Also, explanations of the treatment, its purpose, its length, and what can be expected as an end result are important in enlisting the intelligent cooperation of the patient and family members.[15] If the patient is faced with a choice of two acceptable treatment plans, he should be allowed to make the decision regarding the treatment plan he desires after he has been made cognizant of the benefits and limitations of both plans. At all times in community health nursing, the resourceful nurse is prepared for situations requiring adaptability and flexibility. As reported in a study by Johnson, a limiting factor in the delivery of nursing care that was documented repeatedly was the variability of patients' reactions to services rendered by nurses.[16] To meet unexpected challenges successfully takes skill, planning, ingenuity, acceptance of risk, and the belief that all persons have potential talents just waiting to be tapped.

### Health Teaching and Counseling
Much of the work of community health nurses consists of teaching and counseling patients and families about better ways of coping with health problems so that they are able to increase their competency in dealing with

[15]Letha Hickox, "Planning To Meet Patient Needs," in Yura and Walsh, *op. cit.*, p. 65.
[16]Walter L. Johnson, *Content and Dynamics of Home Visits of Public Health Nurses*, Part II, American Nurses' Foundation, Inc., New York, 1969, p. 124.

their health needs and desires. The utilization of patient and family strengths and resources requires involvement of the patient and family in the plan of care. Also, an effective relationship of the nurse with the family must be developed before success can be assured.

In health counseling the approach varies with the family. In one family, the nurse may feel the direct approach will serve the best purpose. In another family, one of the members may be able to assume leadership and make plans and decisions with little assistance from the nurse other than encouragement and support.

Anticipatory guidance is an important part of health counseling. A guided discussion of probable happenings or events provides an opportunity for clarifying ideas, for lessening anxiety, and for constructive teaching. By anticipating the occurrence of an expected event, various ways of handling the event can be explored so that when it actually happens, few surprises transpire. For instance, the nurse can explain objectively to the expectant mother the mechanics of labor and delivery, using a birth atlas or similar teaching material. This also may provide the mother with emotional support, so that she may be better prepared to accept the experience of her delivery.

New methods for teaching and counseling families appear constantly in books and professional periodicals. Some of them are easily adapted for use in community health nursing. Methods which should be considered when planning for selected families, dependent upon the nurse's assessment of the situation and her knowledge of the implementation of the method, are described briefly as follows:

**1. The operant conditioning or behavior-modification approach**    The behavior-modification approach is used widely in schools, institutions, and homes for children and adults who have special learning needs, such as those persons with distinct handicaps or who are retarded. For the community health nurse assisting the mother in the home in helping the identified patient to acquire necessary new skills or acting as a liaison agent between special schools and the home environment, an understanding and application of operant conditioning methods is essential.

According to an operant point of view, an individual tends to behave in certain ways as a result of events which immediately follow his behavior. One tends to repeat behaviors that have been rewarded. An operant response is simply a behavior which is governed by its consequences. For the nurse who is observing specific behaviors in a patient, emphasis is placed on noting those events or occurrences which immediately precede and immediately follow a behavior of interest. To become completely knowledgeable about the occurring events requires *direct observation* of patient interactions and behaviors by the nurse. As the nurse watches, she observes antecedent events, behaviors or responses of the patient, and consequent events which give her cues as to which conditions produce a positive or negative behavior in the patient.[17] By recording her observations and the frequency with which the observed behaviors occur, she has a base of knowledge from which to plan for effective intervention. The basic premise of the operant method is that behaviors can be shaped in patients by the consistent use of reinforcers. Reinforcers are rewards, behaviors, or events which increase the probability of the desired response. Reinforcers are used to strengthen, weaken, or shape behavior.

When the nurse visits a family with a child who is in need of assistance with his growth and development pattern and may respond to the behavior modification method, she must interpret the method and its purpose to the parents, enlist their interest and cooperation, assess the child's functional level of development, and plot on a chart the variability in the child's achievement of self-help skills in daily living—feeding, toileting, dressing, play, discipline, sleep, and motor development.[18] When she has assembled the data about the child and family, it is advisable to consult with behavior modification experts, decide whether to attempt to work with the family on a concentrated basis herself, or refer the child and family to an appropriate community facility which will give a comprehensive and complete indoctrination of the method.

If the nurse has been encouraged to proceed with the family herself, she must confer with the parents regarding the one behavior which they would like strengthened or weakened first. By selecting one behavior, the nurse is then ready to make direct observations and write down precise baseline data about the behavior. By giving herself specific time intervals on several different days for data gathering, a base rate of the frequency of the selected behavior is gained, in addition to the antecedent events which stimulated the behavior. Also, ideas are accumulated about which reinforcers of the behavior have positive or negative results. When sufficient data have been charted, the nurse is ready to work out a plan of action with the parents regarding the shaping of the desired behavior. See Table 5-1 as an example for recording data. By showing the parents the frequency with which the behavior occurred in conjunction with the antecedent events, a plan of action can be devised where agreement will be reached whether to strengthen or to weaken the specific behavior. A reinforcer will be selected which the parents and nurse will use consistently to shape the desired behavior. At selected time intervals, the nurse will observe and chart the behavior to measure if the plan of action is demonstrating progress. The successful use of the behavior modification method requires frequent con-

[17]Linda Whitney Peterson, "Operant Approach to Observation and Recording," *Nursing Outlook,* 15:3:28–32 (March) 1967.
[18]*Ibid.*

**TABLE 5-1**  How to write down the observed baseline data of the feeding abilities of a five-year-old retarded child during one mealtime.

SETTING:  Five-year-old retarded child was sitting at luncheon table. Soup, crackers, and applesauce were in small dishes on the table. The time was 12 noon.

| ANTECEDENT EVENT | BEHAVIOR | CONSEQUENT EVENT |
| --- | --- | --- |
| 1.  Mother gave graham cracker to child. | 2.  Child grasped cracker with left hand and ate entire cracker. | 3.  Mother smiled and said, "You liked that, didn't you?" |
| 4.  Mother offered a spoonful of soup of a thickened consistency to child. | 5.  Child opened mouth expectantly, took food, and swallowed all of it. | 6.  Child looked expectantly for next spoonful. |
| (After several spoonfuls) | | |
| 7.  Mother offered spoonful of soup to child. | 8.  Child opened mouth, took food, and held it in mouth. | 9.  Mother said, "You've had enough of that, hmm?" |
| 10.  Mother was talking to nurse and not feeding child for several minutes. | 11.  Child spontaneously picked up spoon awkwardly, dipped it into applesauce dish, and successfully maneuvered the spoon to mouth and swallowed the applesauce. | 12.  Mother did not notice child's behavior until nurse said, "Good girl! You fed yourself some applesauce." |
| 13.  Mother offered spoon to child and said, "Here, take another spoonful of applesauce." | 14.  Child refused spoon, would not touch it, and cried. | 15.  Mother said, "OK, I'll feed you." |

sultation with personnel who are skilled in using the method, a team approach with the parents, and patience of the nurse, since predictability of child response is variable.

The method can be modified for use with many families who desire to change specific behaviors in "normal" children. Since the use of positive reinforcers (rewards, praise) is less common than the use of negative reinforcers (criticisms, punishment) in the average American home, the operant conditioning method can be successfully implemented to shape desired behaviors in children by instructing parents to use effective positive reinforcers in a consistent pattern with the children. For example, to shape a desired behavior, the parents can be instructed to consistently notice and praise their son every time he hangs up his coat after school. On the days when he does not hang up his coat, the parents can be instructed to consistently give him a chore that he does not find attractive. In this way, the shaping of the desired behavior is secured as the boy realizes the consequences of the original act. An excellent self-help type of book for parents to use who want to teach their children desired behaviors is *Living With Children*, by Patterson and Gullion.[19] The ingenious community health nurse is able to adapt the use of the method to the capacities of a family after she has observed significant family behavior patterns and interpreted an attractive means for implementing the method in a way that catches the interest of parents.

**2. The family therapy approach**   Family therapy is a procedure that makes use of a true group, a primary group. The sphere of intervention is not the isolated individual patient but rather the family viewed as an organismic whole.

> Family psychotherapy ... is a procedure that makes use of a true group, a primary group; the sphere of intervention is not the isolated individual patient, but rather the family viewed as an organismic whole.... It is developing a body of knowledge, ... illuminating those processes by which the family supports or damages individual development and also those by which the individual supports or damages family development. ... It is evolving a specific system of therapeutic intervention, disclosing how the family method may be related to and combined with other means of supporting the goals of family life. ... It merges the efforts of treatment with the goals of prevention of illness, maintenance of health, and education in the problems of family living.[20]

Community health nurses can make use of a modified form of family therapy when they accept the premise that an individual can change and adjust his behavior in a healthy manner only when the family system allows it. In other words, for one person's behavior to change, the responses of family members must likewise change. The basic procedure in family therapy is to gather the family members together to talk about their relationships with each other.[21] By so doing, the nurse is able to view family interaction patterns and reactions of individual family members to each other. Until the nurse has met the entire family and made an assessment of the family's interaction system, she cannot hope to change coping behaviors of any individual family member with any pronounced degree of success.

19Gerald R. Patterson and M. Elizabeth Gullion, *Living With Children*, Research Press, Post Office Box 2459, Station A, Champaign, Illinois 61820, 1968.
20Nathan W. Ackerman, Frances L. Beatman, and Sanford N. Sherman, *Expanding Theory and Practice In Family Therapy*, Family Service Association of America, New York, 1967, pp. 4–5.
21Penny Kossoris, "Family Therapy," *American Journal of Nursing*, 70:8:1730–1733 (August) 1970.

Virginia Satir makes use of a growth model for families based on the idea that people's behavior changes through process and that the process is represented by transactions with other people. Growth occurs when the system permits it. The therapist is intimately involved in the transactions, and anything he may offer the patient or family to expedite learning and exchange is utilized to help them grow within the context of the relationship. This model requires willingness of the therapist to be experimental, spontaneous, and flexible. The goal of the growth model is to teach people to be congruent, to speak directly and clearly, and to communicate their feelings, thoughts, and desires accurately. The therapist serves as an example of an active, learning, fallible human being who is willing to cope honestly and responsibly with whatever confronts him, including his own vulnerabilities.[22] The implementation of a family-therapy approach on a modified basis by the community health nurse can be an exciting learning experience for both the family and the nurse. One thing to be remembered by the nurse in the implementation of the family-therapy method is that she should not talk solely on a one-to-one basis with any member of the family; she should serve mainly as the facilitator and instigate interaction of family members with each other, and not with the nurse. If family members will direct open, honest statements to each other, communication patterns are more congruent and the nurse can interpret the intent behind the statements in such a way that they are nonthreatening and understandable to the other family members. Also, in this climate the presence of a third party, the nurse, often helps some family members to say things that they are unable to utter usually.

Whether or not the nurse actively participates in the family-therapy method or acts as a coworker with a qualified family therapist, she should be able to identify family interactional patterns which are dysfunctional as described by Satir. These families should be directed or guided toward treatment with family therapists or family-counseling facilities. Much of the work of community health nurses is of a preparatory nature and consists of helping dysfunctional families to become aware of ineffective or destructive interactional patterns and motivating them to seek expert help, since they are often unhappy families and have multiple health problems.

Satir described the use of "family-system games" based on her classification of interaction patterns as either open systems or closed systems. *Closed systems* are those in which every participating member must be very cautious about what he or she says. The principal rule seems to be that everyone is supposed to have the same opinions, feelings, and desires, whether or not this is true. In closed systems, honest self-expression is impossible and if it does occur, the expression is viewed as deviant or "sick"

[22]Virginia Satir, *Conjoint Family Therapy,* rev. ed., Science and Behavior Books, Inc., Palo Alto, California, 1967, pp. 182–183.

by other members of the group or family. The *open system* permits honest self-expression for the participating members. In such a group or family, differences are viewed as natural and open negotiation occurs to resolve such differences by "compromise," "agreement to disagree," or "taking turns." In open systems, the individual can say what he feels and thinks and can negotiate for reality and personal growth without destroying himself or the others in the system.[23] By the use of simulated games, Satir helps families to see and understand the nature of their own family system and experience the movement from a pathologic system of interaction to a growth-producing one. She elicits the family's feelings, responses, and body reactions to the games, each other, and the interactions. She urges family therapists to be open, flexible, enthusiastic, and innovative.[24] By being knowledgeable about Satir's approach to families and willing to try some of the suggested exercises, the community health nurse can adapt and improve her own style of interacting successfully with families. When the nurse initiates role-playing games in the family setting, unexpected insights are gained by all participating members. Often the games are fun and stimulating and create a lighthearted atmosphere, which is therapeutic in itself. New approaches and ideas are often received with enthusiasm by families, particularly if they are implemented skillfully and appropriately and if the results bring forth new insights.

**3. The transactional analysis approach**    Transactional analysis offers a systematic, consistent theory of personality and social dynamics and an actionistic, rational form of therapy which is suitable for, easily understood by, and naturally adapted to the great majority of patients.[25] Its goal is to help people to be their true selves. Transactional analysis identifies three ego states inherent in each person. The ego states are systems of feelings which motivate a related set of behavior patterns.[26] They are called the parent, adult, and child ego states within each individual. The child ego state is represented by spontaneous, rational, and irrational feelings. The child expresses genuine feelings of joy or anger and speaks in words and thoughts saying "*I am.*" The child can be a good or bad child. The parent ego state is represented by fixed feelings of right or wrong behavior, acceptance of traditional values. The parent moralizes and judges others and speaks in words and thoughts, saying "*you* are." The parent can be a good or bad parent. The adult ego state is represented by responsible, rational, and predictable feelings. The adult is nonjudgmental and always in the process of learning. The composition of each person's ego states varies

[23]*Ibid.,* p. 185.
[24]*Ibid.,* pp. 188–189.
[25]Eric Berne, *Transactional Analysis in Psychotherapy,* Grove Press, Inc., New York, 1961, p. 21.
[26]*Ibid.,* p. 17.

according to his past and early childhood experiences, but perceptible predominant characteristics can be identified by other persons when they take note of verbal transactions and nonverbal behavior. When a person does not interact openly and makes use of "games," these cues suggest that the individual is masking his true self and is possibly unaware that he has a distinctive identity. For the person who consistently and spontaneously acts according to his feelings, the child ego state is dominant. When the person tends to be inflexible and judgmental, the parent ego state is dominant. When a person consciously takes an objective viewpoint and acts according to a logical perception of the situation, the adult ego state is dominant.

Transactional analysis classifies four possible life positions that can be held with respect to oneself and others. They are interpreted in detail by Harris in a book which is easy reading for nurses and consumers.[27] The life positions are:

1. I'm ok—You're ok.

2. I'm not ok—You're ok.

3. I'm not ok—You're not ok.

4. I'm ok—You're not ok.

The life position "I'm ok—You're ok" is the healthy situation and is the goal toward which all persons in transactional analysis therapy strive. However, the predominant majority of people hold the life position "I'm not ok—You're ok." As explained by Harris, this is the universal position of early childhood, being the infant's logical conclusion from the situation of birth and infancy. Since all infants are naturally dependent and *must be* cared for by adults, the not-ok-ness is a natural conclusion about themselves. In this position the person feels at the mercy of others and seeks recognition and approval from others.[28] It is the people who hold the life position "I'm not ok—You're ok" of whom the community health nurse must be cognizant. By explaining the simple interpretation of the three ego states and the life positions that the majority of people hold, new insights often are gained which help the person to understand a great deal more about himself. He is naturally drawn to remember his early childhood, the role of his parents in his life, and the conclusions he reached about certain emphasized beliefs which he had accepted at face value once upon a time, yet later questioned when he weighed the facts rationally and thoughtfully. For example, a child may have been told by a parent that if he handled frogs, he would get warts

[27]Thomas A. Harris, *I'm OK—You're OK,* Harper & Row, Publishers, Incorporated, New York, 1969.
[28]*Ibid.,* pp. 43–45.

on his hands. However, as he observed other children handling frogs and eventually ventured to pick one up himself, he found out that he and other children did not get warts. Consequently, he no longer believed a statement which he had accepted at face value formerly.

The belief is held by transactional analysts that each individual is responsible for his own feelings. Feelings are internal and cannot be manipulated by external forces unless the person allows and responds to the outside forces. The individual *chooses* his feelings. When the going gets rough, each person runs back to familiar territory or familiar feelings which he used in early childhood. A necessity for all persons is "stroking," recognition, or attention. As infants and children, any stroking, positive or negative, was sought as long as attention of some kind was gained. Most persons are well aware of negative strokes, since the present society tends to be negatively oriented and criticisms are much more easily given by others than praise or recognition. As adults, symbolic positive strokes are solicited and acquired by receiving compliments, recognition of achievements. Positive strokes are better than negative ones or conditional ones. Conditional strokes are those that imply, "I'll approve of you *if.*" When interacting with individuals and families, positive strokes, not conditional ones, designed to strengthen the recipients should be used at every appropriate opportunity by the nurse.

Transactional analysts make use of another idea which is practical and catches the interest of the consumer. The idea is that of trading stamps, which are collected daily in order to obtain an object or reward that one desires. The trading stamps in transactional analysis represent feelings; good feelings are identified as gold stamps and bad, hurt, or resentful feelings as brown stamps. Gold stamps are collected by giving and receiving tangible positive recognition and earning desirable achievements. Brown stamps are collected by giving and receiving insults, feeling injured or put upon. Brown stamps can be collected dishonestly and are often accompanied by a feeling of triumph. When a book of brown stamps or an accumulation of angry feelings is collected, a person is entitled to have a temper outburst free of guilt, or with several books of brown stamps, a divorce or extramarital affair can be claimed free of guilt. For those persons familiar with the trading stamp idea in transactional analysis, the labeling of a behavior as gold or brown stamping has lasting meaning and can often be conveyed in a nonthreatening manner. For the community health nurse who chooses to use a modification of the transactional analysis method with families, the interpretation of the basic beliefs and language are easily conveyed and understood and provide a nonthreatening climate for growth-promoting interaction. The goal toward which the nurse would work in using this method is assisting the patient or family to become their true, genuine selves and rely less on behaviors which mask their identity.

**4. The epidemiologic approach** Epidemiology has often been considered the study of factors determining the occurrence of communicable diseases in populations. However, the study has broadened to include *all* diseases, whether communicable or not, and health behavior of groups of people. Epidemiology consists of a methodological investigation of disease or health behavior occurring in human groups for the purpose of discovering factors essential to or contributing to disease occurrence or unhealthy behavior and developing methods for prevention of disease or unhealthy behavior. The epidemiologic method is closely related to the problem-solving method, which is generally used with individuals rather than with groups. Epidemiology is more method than a body of knowledge and in essence is similar to the detective approach of gathering clues or data, making hypotheses or deductions, and finding solutions. The epidemiologist mainly uses two methods for study of data, observational and experimental. By observation the investigator simply makes note of circumstances and events in the normal pattern of life. By analysis the investigator searches for association between disease occurrence or unhealthy behavior and the possible causative influences.[29]

Customarily, the community health nurse serves as an associate with epidemiologists in the study of diseases and investigation of all related data. However, by using the epidemiologic approach on a small scale with families or groups, it is proposed that the community health nurse play the role of principal investigator in seeking out solutions for diseases or health behaviors occurring in a given family or group and stimulate family or group members to serve as associates in bringing out related data. For example, a small but effective epidemiologic study could be done of a family or group who are faced with the problem of obesity or a high incidence of home accidents. In dealing with the obesity problem, a detailed history of amounts and types of food ingested by the family or group members for a period of three days to one week would provide data that could be analyzed thoroughly in terms of nutrients and calories. In addition, characteristic habit patterns associated with mealtimes and snacktimes could be studied, and antecedent events which seem to cause undesirable consequent behaviors could be observed. If the group or family members are participating as associates in the epidemiologic study, they may be encouraged to bring out facts related to eating, such as the ingestion of more food following hostile interactions with others or early childhood training which taught them to clean up their plates rather than have food wastage. When all participants are alert for possible causative factors of eating, a great amount of significant data can be secured, which will lead to ideas of possible hypotheses

[29]John P. Fox, Carrie E. Hall, and Lila R. Elveback, *Epidemiology, Man and Disease,* The Macmillan Company, New York, 1970, pp. 7–16.

to be tested. The nurse serves as the detective or agent in search of significant clues from all possible perspectives, including physical, emotional, and
social. By playing the role of detective, she must have a comprehensive
knowledge about the variety of factors which may lead to obesity. When a
definition of the nature and significance of the problem is obtained about
all the participants and all important data are collected, classified, and
appraised, a hypothesis can be tentatively formulated for testing. Future
practical activities based on the hypothesis can be planned and implemented for a determined time period and ultimately, an evaluation of the
results of the study can be decided. For the group studying the causation
of obesity, the testing of a hypothesis focusing on mealtime practices and
habits may lead to more successful results than one related to ingestion of
superfluous calories. By involving all family or group members in the detective game, curiosity is stimulated and motivation to change behavior is often
self-induced.

In the case of a family or group having a high incidence of accidents,
the nurse can introduce the idea that accidents don't happen, they are
caused by what people do or by what they fail to do.[30] This idea alone may
arouse the group to do some reflective thinking and serve as a stimulus for
further study. If the family or group responds with the desire to lessen the
occurrence of accidents, each person can be asked to determine the frequency of his accidents and describe completely the events occurring
before and during the last accident in which he was involved. Environmental, psychological, and stress factors representing hazards in each described situation can be elicited and studied by the group in search of
commonalities. They may formulate a hypothesis based on the relationship
of stress to personal psychological characteristics which culminate in accident proneness in individuals. By becoming more knowledgeable by means
of references about the characteristics of persons who seem to be accident-
prone, by attempting to reduce the number of stress- or risk-producing life
events, and attempting to control unsafe reactions, acts, and behavior, the
group may test their hypothesis by tabulating the frequency of accidents
occurring to them after four weeks of discussion and study compared to
their first frequency estimates. By accepting the fact that accidents occur
when alertness, efficiency, skill, or judgment of persons is temporarily im-
paired, subsequent behavior can be made more conscious and perhaps
"safe." The epidemiologic method provides a more interesting approach to
accident prevention than lectures about safety. The nurse when acting as
a stimulator of ideas and promulgator of learning has more satisfactions and
is more apt to see learning internalized by her family or group.

[30]Albert Chapman, "The Anatomy of an Accident," *Public Health Reports*, 75:630–632 (July) 1960.

**5. The paradoxical communication approach** The community health nurse may make use of paradoxical communication as a last resort when all other approaches have failed or as a mode of communication to which a specific type of patient will respond best. A *paradox* is a term describing a directive which qualifies another directive in a conflicting way, either simultaneously or at a different moment in time.[31] For example, in order to persuade a patient to change undesirable symptomatic behavior, he must be told to do something and that activity should be related to his problem in some way. For a person complaining of persistent insomnia, a directive can be given to spend each night reading books that the patient has put off reading and, to ensure against falling asleep, to stand up at the mantle and read all night. After several nights of reading while standing up, the insomnia problem may be cured and this was accomplished by the patient himself. The emphasis of treatment was placed on the patient's activity rather than on his symptomatic behavior.[32] By directing the patient's attention to activities which must be accomplished and avoiding the suggestion of ceasing the symptomatic behavior, the therapist poses a paradox in the patient's mind of retaining the symptomatic behavior or following directives that are not always attractive to the patient. This method of giving action-type directives related to symptomatic behavior commits the patient to either giving up the symptom or following the directives as given by the therapist. The paradoxical communication method has interesting implications, particularly for childlike persons who want to change symptomatic behavior but cannot resist the desire to rebel when told or ordered to do something. If the nurse utilizes the paradoxical communication approach, she must know her patient well enough to predict how the patient may respond to a direct suggestion. If the nurse is almost certain that the patient cannot resist rejecting an order, she can consciously give a directive which is opposed to the goal she wishes for the patient. This method often works with small children.

A student nurse accidentally stumbled upon this method of communication with the mother of a child who was diagnosed as needing a tonsillectomy to alleviate a hearing loss. The nurse had made repeated weekly visits to persuade the mother to make an appointment for the surgical procedure. Upon each home visit the mother had some legitimate excuse which had caused a postponement in scheduling the surgery. At last the frustrated nurse gave up and told the mother to forget the whole thing. In all probability the child would manage all right without a tonsillectomy. The following week the nurse visited the home and learned that the child had had the surgery and was recuperating nicely.

[31]By permission of Jay Haley, *Strategies of Psychotherapy*, Grune & Stratton, Inc., New York, 1963, p. 17.
[32]*Ibid.*, p. 49.

### Planning Care and Coordination with Others

As a member of the health team serving the patient and family, the community health nurse must be constantly alert to the necessity for conferring with the other interested members of the team. These members include the physician, social workers, nurses in other settings, teachers, and any number of allied community workers and health aides. By initiating communication by means of the telephone, prearranged personal discussions, or scheduling a multidisciplinary conference, all team members can be made cognizant of agreed upon, common objectives by which all will abide in their work with the patient and family. Planning a successful intervention with and for the patient and family involves teamwork, maintenance of an open exchange of information, sharing of resources among team members, and agreement regarding the primary responsibilities of team members and ultimate goals toward which all are working. Planning with other professional and nonprofessional workers is essential and requires time and effort expended to maintain open channels of communication. By following a carefully designed plan of action which has been individualized for the patient and family, successful interventions and satisfying relationships are more likely to be attained by all persons involved.

### THE NURSING PROCESS: IMPLEMENTING

Implementing a nursing care plan implies that a careful assessment and planning process has been accomplished and activities for or in behalf of the patient and family are now available which will contribute to their comfort and well-being or facilitate their coping behaviors as related to their specific health problems. Implementation is an ongoing activity or series of activities which necessitates evaluation in order to determine the effectiveness of nursing care. Action is taken with the expectation that if the planned action is followed, an expected result will occur. The evaluation process may indicate a need for reassessment and replanning or a modification of the plan of care. Implementation of nursing care includes all the activities of the nurse in carrying out the nursing care plan designed to enhance the well-being of the patient and family.[33]

While carrying out a plan of action, the nurse must be constantly aware of (1) a therapeutic use of self with the patient and family; (2) knowledge of physical, psychological, and social manifestations of pathology, deviancy, or wellness; (3) opportunities for teaching, supervising, or guiding persons toward better coping patterns of health; and (4) evaluation of the total effect of the implementation activity.

---

[33]Mildred Wesolowski, "Implementation of the Nursing Care Plan," in Yura and Walsh, *op. cit.*, pp. 78–79.

## The Process of Effecting Change

A persistent goal to which all nurses are committed is to influence change in patients or families in the direction of improved health or wellness. However, what motivates a person to change? Will a person change when he sees no reason to do so? Will he change when others want him to do so? Will he change when he himself believes he wants to do so but cannot resist the pull of forces compelling him to pursue his old habit patterns? Effecting change is much more easily talked about than accomplished. According to Wheelis, *we are what we do.* The actions that we *do* describe our character to others. The fact that the action is repeated over and over reinforces the description that others have ascribed to us. When we *say* that we are one thing but *behave* or *act* in opposition to what we say, others take note of the behavior and believe the behavior rather than the words. Because we tend to maintain behavior or actions that are familiar and customary, we resist change.

All persons have potential for change and can change when they *choose* to do so. Therefore, if a person is suffering or uncomfortable with a health problem, he must recognize that it is a problem that is causing him to suffer or be uncomfortable, and he must be ready and willing to do something about the problem before a change can be effected. Since we are what we do, if we want to change what we are, we must begin by changing what we do. A new mode of action is often difficult, unnatural, unpleasant, or anxiety-provoking and in order to sustain the change, a considerable effort of will is required. Change will occur only if such action is maintained over a long period of time.[34] Consequently, the role of community health nurses in assisting patients or families to effect change can be enumerated as: (1) reach an agreement with the patient or family about the health problems that are causing difficulties and they desire to change; (2) assist the patient or family in determining the new behavior or action which will help them to attain their goal; (3) provide constant reinforcement for the patient's or family's behavior or actions which have been adjusted in the direction of meeting their goal; and (4) maintain contact with the patient or family for an extended period of time and continue to encourage and strengthen them in their new behavior until their goal has been attained and maintained to the satisfaction of all concerned. At the same time that the nurse is working with the patient or family to effect change, she must also be utilizing her relationship skills, cognitive knowledge about the particular health problems which are the focus of attention, interactional skills, and predictive skills in anticipating the probability of success in the venture undertaken by the patient, family, and nurse.

[34]Allen Wheelis, *The Desert*, Basic Books, Inc., Publishers, New York, 1970.

## Barriers to Change

Some barriers which may be encountered by the nurse as she attempts to effect change with patients or families may be: (1) faulty perception regarding the patients' or families' readiness to change. The nurse may believe that the patient desires to change when in reality the patient is only being momentarily compliant to the nurse's persuasiveness or wishes to appear worthy of the nurse's attention. (2) The language used by the nurse may be unfamiliar to the patient or family and rather than ask for an explicit interpretation, the consumer may elect to pretend an understanding of the issues involved. (3) The emotional content of the messages between the patient or family and the nurse may be missed, avoided, or inaccurately interpreted as being irrelevant to the issue under discussion. When the nurse detects an emotion in the consumer that is not completely understandable in terms of the words being spoken, she must state verbally her uncertainty about what she is sensing or perceiving. For example, she may say to a patient who is using bullet-like speech and staring pointedly out the window, "You seem disturbed about something and I am not sure if I understand the message you are giving me. Are you angry with me?" By so doing, the patient is given the opportunity to express or interpret his emotion, whether it is directed at the nurse or another target. (4) Too many suggestions for change may be offered by the nurse, resulting in an overload of information for the consumer to manage. (5) The timing may be poor, inconvenient, or incomprehensible to the consumer. (6) The patient or family may misinterpret the messages of the nurse, or vice versa. To avoid misinterpretations of messages it is good practice to request the consumer to give feedback on what he has heard from the nurse. This is called perception checking. When a verification of the message received is indeed the message intended by the sender, then the communication is clear to both parties. (7) The patient or family may arbitrarily desire the right to refuse, regardless of the idea, because of the element of power. If the nurse is able to accept this type of consumer as he is and assess his behavior characteristics, she can engage in an encounter in such a way that the consumer retains control but is provoked to *think*. Nothing is gained if the nurse enters the game of one-upmanship with the consumer.

## Stress and Crisis

In an earlier chapter an emotionally healthy person was described as one who has dealt and is dealing in a satisfactory manner with the conflicts inherent in each stage of human development. Inherent in this description is the implication that all persons have conflicts, problems, or stresses. In other words, life is not a bowl of cherries but a roller coaster with highs and lows. By acknowledging that all persons experience stress and crisis, the complicated task of the community health nurse is to determine when to intervene with individuals and families in need of assistance.

Stress is commonly associated with the rate of wear and tear on the body or the burden under which the individual is struggling. Rapoport referred to stress as the relation of the stressful stimulus, the individual's reaction to it, and the events to which it leads.[35] The state of crisis occurs when an imbalance between an important problem and the resources immediately available to deal with it are unsuccessful. In other words, the person in a state of crisis is unable to cope adequately with the immediate problem. The essence of crisis is struggle—a struggle to master an upsetting situation and to regain a state of balance.[36] For health professionals who utilize crisis theory, a crisis is an opportunity for respondents to try new actions or new coping mechanisms which will strengthen adaptive capacities and raise levels of emotional health.

In community health nursing the systems approach helps the nurse to view the family as an integral unit and as made up of individuals who are influenced by all occurrences within the family. She sees the family as a source of strength or a source of stress, dependent upon the constructive or destructive influences in operation within it. When a family is in crisis, they are at a turning point. They are faced with problems for which their coping mechanisms seem inadequate, they feel helpless and frustrated and are uncertain of how to act effectively to solve the problems.[37] It is at this point that the intervention of the community health nurse can be most effective. If her interaction occurs during the period of crisis, she has an optimum opportunity to guide the family toward improved coping mechanisms, which will successfully restore a state of balance within the family system and promote them toward a higher level of emotional health.

There are two types of crises which families undergo, developmental and situational. As described by Robischon, *developmental* or *maturational crises* are those which human beings experience in the process of their psychosocial growth. They are considered stages of the normal life cycle. For families, some examples of these crisis occur when a new baby is born, when the children reach adolescence, or when retirement occurs. *Situational* or *accidental crises* are external events or stresses. They are often more sudden, unexpected, and unfortunate.[38] For example, these crises

[35]Lydia Rapoport, "The State of Crisis: Some Theoretical Considerations," in Howard J. Parad (ed.), *Crisis Intervention: Selected Readings,* Family Service Association of America, New York, 1965, p. 23.
[36]Donald G. Langsley and David M. Kaplan, *The Treatment of Families in Crisis,* Grune & Stratton, Inc., New York, 1968, p. 3.
[37]Donna C. Aguilera, Janice M. Messick, and Marlene S. Farrell, *Crisis Intervention, Theory and Methodology,* The C. V. Mosby Company, St. Louis, 1970, p. 1.
[38]Paulette Robischon, "The Challenge of Crisis Theory for Nursing," *Nursing Outlook,* 15:7:28–32 (July) 1967.

occur when a member of the family dies, a handicapped child is born, a debilitating disease is diagnosed and seen as inevitable, or a serious accident maims a family member.

As stated by Leighton, there are three universal kinds of behavior with which individuals react to authority when subject to forces of stress that are disturbing to the emotions and thoughts of the individual. They are cooperation, withdrawal, and aggressiveness. When the nurse is watchful for these behaviors, she is better able to assess the dynamics involved in each family situation. Relief from excessive stress is assisted by the utilization of a sense of humor, observable facts, reasoned thinking, and new opportunities to achieve security and satisfactions.[39]

Some of the activities which the community health nurse can use in crisis intervention with an individual or family are:

**1.** Help the troubled to confront the crisis by helping him to verbalize and to comprehend the reality of the situation.

**2.** Help him to confront the crisis in doses he can manage. If the nurse uses cues that the individual reveals nonverbally, she may facilitate verbalization of feelings which the patient had considered to be taboo but were contributing to his state of tension.

**3.** Help him to find the facts of the situation and explore all possible ways of coping. Proceed at the patient's pace. When exploration is done mutually, the patient is helped to think and may devise solutions which are highly original and made possible because of the stimulus of another person engaging in the problem-solving process with him.

**4.** Help him by recognizing his strengths and encouraging the use of his capabilities.

**5.** Help him accept assistance from others as needed and as he is ready, until he has mobilized his own personal resources.[40]

By being available, patient, willing to listen, and supportive of strengths, the nurse can enable individuals or families in a state of crisis to move toward resolution of difficulties in an acceptable manner and promote their sense of responsibility and well-being at the same time.

### Homework

When working with individuals in the implementation phase of the nursing process, a simple activity or assignment is frequently accepted with keenness and ambivalence—eagerness to be doing something that may help

[39]Alexander H. Leighton, *The Governing of Men,* Princeton University Press, Princeton, N.J., 1945, pp. 252–286.
[40]Robischon, *op. cit.,* pp. 28–32

themselves and uncertainty about their ability to carry out the assignment. These tasks or activities are called "homework," a term used by David Kupfer, a transactional analyst who stated that people like to be given homework. The assignment given must be reasonable, fairly easily accomplished, and within the context of the goal toward which the patient is working. For example, for the person who has low self-esteem, an assignment can be given for that person to write down 100 strengths about himself and to show the list to the nurse on the next visit. Or the patient may be assigned a pamphlet to read and jot down questions for discussion on the nurse's return visit. Or the patient may be requested to tally on a chart the number of times he performed a prescribed set of exercises, and the nurse will anticipate examining the chart on the next visit. The performance of an assignment sometimes relieves tension, gives a sense of movement toward a desired goal, and a feeling of accomplishment that is satisfying. The achievement of the assignment, whether partial or complete, must always be recognized and reinforced positively by the nurse.

In a study reported by Geismar and Krisberg, it was found that families respond most favorably to communication which is focused on problem solving. The approach very frequently sought by families was the quick solution. However, when family members were encouraged to think through the problem-solving process and their strengths were reinforced, movement toward their goals was more apt to be realized.[41] The assignment of homework which is individualized to fit the situation and gives the family something to do can be one of the methods used to reinforce family members about their existing strengths and latent capacity for problem solving.

## The Nursing Bag
For the nurse who gives bedside care in the home, the nursing bag has always been a necessary accessory. Historically, its contents have included equipment which the nurse needed to perform her functions. The equipment has varied dependent upon the period of history that nursing care was given. In the early 1800s, the nurse carried a satchel which contained black currant jelly for the parched throat and racking cough, Irish moss to be made into a soothing drink, chicken jelly for a nourishing broth, and perhaps an orange or a lemon.[42] In the 1900s, the nurses in New York City carried heavy "telescope" bags containing more than a dozen bottles and porcelain jars.[43] From 1900 to the present era, the bags that have been used are

[41]Ludwig Geismar and Jane Krisberg, "The Family Life Improvement Project: An Experiment in Preventive Intervention," Parts I and II, *Social Casework*, 47:9 (November) 1966 and 48:10 (December) 1966.

[42]Alfred Worcester, *Nurses and Nursing*, Harvard University Press, Cambridge, Mass., 1927, p. 40.

[43]Mary M. Roberts, *American Nursing, History and Interpretation*, The Macmillan Company, New York, 1954, pp. 3-4

familiar to most nurses because of their shape and black color. The contents include equipment for handwashing, taking temperatures, giving injections, doing occasional dressings, and performing other nursing skills necessary to carry out a physician's orders. Frequently the equipment is disposable and entails a careful daily scrutiny of the bag to ensure that all needed articles for the services to be performed on that day are included, are sterile or clean, and intact.

The manner with which the nurse uses the supplies in the nursing bag communicates much nonverbal data to families about her behavior, attitude, and skill. If the family members like what they see, their respect, confidence, and acceptance of the nurse as a skilled practitioner are increased. They may adopt unconsciously some of her practices of asepsis and cleanliness. By routinely using nursing skills which include vital signs, the nurse conveys that she is truly a nurse and is genuinely concerned about the patient's welfare. Many opportunities for teaching patients can be realized through the use of the nursing bag—and the teaching is often not on a verbal or a demonstration basis. The most effective teaching may be accomplished purely on the nonverbal basis, during which the nurse is performing unconsciously as a role model.

A nursing student who did a mini-study on nurses' attitudes about the bag asked the question, "Is the nursing bag a symbol of the community health nurse?" From a very small sample of practicing community health nurses, four out of five answered, "no." The fifth nurse said that the bag was "whatever the nurse makes of it." Two nursing students out of a sample of three stated that the bag was a symbol of the community health nurse.

In view of the ongoing technological advancements in medical and nursing care, it is difficult to predict if nursing bags will continue to retain the shape, color, and size that they currently have. However, a means for carrying necessary equipment which aids in the administration of nursing care in the home will always be required.

### Case Finding
Inherent in every community health nursing visit are the possibilities for case finding and referral. These are important functions of each member of the community health team and are carried out in the home, the school, the clinic, and in places of employment. During the nurse's home visit, while she is providing nursing care and health counseling, she has unusual opportunities for case finding. In her discussions with the family, the nurse must be alert to and observant of early symptoms of such conditions as cancer, diabetes, communicable diseases, birth injuries, and mental and emotional disturbances. The nurse must be perceptive; she must be alert to what the

patient and other family members are saying or doing and to objective and subjective symptoms that may be revealed.

A nurse calling on a migratory farm worker's family noted that Judy, a three-year-old, had a definite limp as she walked across the bare floor. The nurse questioned the mother about it, and possible symptoms, suggestive of bone tuberculosis, came to light. A referral to a children's orthopedic clinic brought a diagnosis of bone tuberculosis. Further study of the family revealed that the father had active tuberculosis.

An ostensible purpose of community health nursing service is the early finding of pregnancy and the referral of prospective mothers for medical care. At this time, i.e., early in pregnancy, the nurse can place the mothers under nursing supervision also and teach them care of themselves and their babies. This teaching can often be related to the health needs, e.g., nutritional needs, of other members of the family.

## Referral

Closely allied to case finding during the home visit is referral, i.e., the referral of the patient or family to the community agency best suited or equipped to help meet the particular problems recognized by the nurse. These might be of a health, welfare, social, or recreational nature.

Often, the major task of the nurse is not referring a family to an appropriate community agency, but getting the family *ready* to accept the services of the community resource as needed and desired. The process involved in preparing a family includes the initiation of an effective relationship with the family, the recognition that problems are existing and must be resolved, and a time period during which an exploration of problems and possible solutions can be discussed with the family. The time during which the family is searching for appropriate solutions may be extended into weeks or months, dependent upon their readiness to act. In the meantime, the nurse can be utilizing methods or ideas which will reveal the discomfort the problems are causing for the family, will communicate indirectly the family's inability to resolve the problems without competent assistance, will give promise that ultimate solutions are possible and available, and that a referral to an appropriate community resource is indeed necessary to attain a desired goal. An interpretation of the services of a designated community resource and the manner in which the personnel will work with the family must be made. Also, when the family is ready to visit a selected community resource, they should be taught how best to present their desires and goals to the agency from whom they are requesting help. Sometimes the process of preparing a family for a referral to a community resource is a lengthy one and requires a patient and persistent nurse.

In making a referral, the nurse must be well aware of the services and contributions of the community's health and social agencies. Usually lists are available of recognized agencies and their services. Some agencies have developed interagency referral forms. The simplest is a card that includes the name of the agency, its address, telephone number, and the hours that the agency is open. This is signed with the name of the nurse's agency and given to the family. Other types of referral forms may include more details. In certain instances, the nurse may send the agency a notice that the patient or family have been referred, with some pertinent information relating to the situation. Some agencies arrange to return these forms to the nurse with the findings and recommendations that were made to the family. The nurse can utilize this information on future visits.

A workable referral system is basic to any community wide program of continuity of care of the patient. It is the initial step in the development of such a program.

## Closing the Visit

The community health nurse terminates her visit with a brief review of the important points she has tried to make. She stresses the positive aspects, emphasizing family strengths, and reiterates the plans the patient and family will carry out in her absence. Together the nurse and the family plan for the next visit, establishing a date and approximate time convenient for family and nurse. Summarizing the visit can be a learning experience for the patient and family and will give the nurse an opportunity to organize her thoughts in preparation for recording the visit.

## Recording the Visit

Community health agencies are continuously seeking ways to improve their family records by eliminating the writing of unnecessary detail or duplication and focusing on a succinct accounting of important information. Because the search for a satisfactory record form is elusive, community health nurses must be flexible and adapt to whatever record form is in use in the particular agency for whom they are working. By concentrating on writing only essential information, nurses can limit their recording of family situations to a few well-stated sentences, phrases, or brief paragraphs. This ability takes continuous effort and self-discipline. All records must be accurate and complete and must indicate that the treatments were justified by the diagnosis.

When a correction is necessary, the nurse lines out the erroneous statement, writing the correct statement below it and initialing it. The confidentiality of patient and family records must be maintained at all times. As in the hospital, the community health record is considered a legal document and, as such, is subject to court order. Elements of good record keeping include accuracy, conciseness, legibility, promptness, and the use of standard abbreviations only. The record must be dated and signed by the nurse.

The appropriate use of the patient and family record enables the nursing staff to provide continuity of nursing care. Because of vacation relief, emergencies, and staff absences, it is not always possible for the same nurse to visit the patient each time. However, a clear, concise, and accurate record, always complete to date, makes it possible for a different nurse to make an effective home call without disturbing the sense of security the patient had in the former nurse or interfering with the general relationship between the agency and family.

The community health nursing record is used frequently as a supervisory tool. It is helpful to both supervisor and staff nurse to review it from time to time in order to trace the nurse's growth and development and to determine where she may need additional help in her work with families. The agency also reviews the records as a basis for program planning and in consideration of budgetary needs.

Record forms for the recording of visits vary from agency to agency. Most agencies require that the information be organized into four general categories: a description of the situation; the activities carried out or the services rendered; the attitudes or responses of patient and family; and the plan to be followed for the next visit and the date of the visit.

In describing the situation, the nurse includes any changes that may have taken place since the last visit, such as illnesses in the family, changes in employment or income, or change in housing. Her account of the activity carried out or the service given is the most detailed part of the narrative, as it describes what was done by the nurse as well as by the family. In describing the activity, the nurse records what she did and her reasons for doing so.

Examples of activities include:

1. Demonstrated—how to read a thermometer or bathe the baby

2. Explained—services of the agency, reasons for calling physicians, or rules and regulations of the health department

3. Explored—family's knowledge of budget making, or their nutritional habits, or their ideas and attitudes regarding fluoridation

4. Reviewed—postpartum exercises, or patterns of growth and development of a six-month-old baby

5. Reassured—that good care was being given, or that progress was being made by patient and family

6. Supported—decision of family to seek help from a psychiatrist or mental health clinic

**7.** Listened—to mother as she clarified her own thinking and made her own decision

A negative example of recording is the following statement found on a record, "Discussed diet, anatomy, and physiology of pregnancy and immunizations." Do we really know what was discussed and with whom? Another nurse, preparing to visit the same family, might well raise the following questions:

**1.** Was the nutrition adequate or inadequate for each member of the family? Why was it discussed? What suggestions or instructions were given?

**2.** What did the mother know already about her pregnancy? Did the discussion start with the period of conception? Did it conclude with the six weeks' postpartum examination by the physician?

**3.** What diseases and their immunizations were discussed? What were the family's attitudes? Their responses? What action did the nurse think the family would take regarding immunizations?

In the narrative record, always written in the third person, the nurse carefully selects her wording, remembering that she does not diagnose. She describes clinical and behavioral manifestations in a way that gives clear meaning. Rather than stating, for example, that the parents were "overprotective" or "well adjusted," the nurse should describe briefly the symptom or behavior that would lead to the use of such adjectives. An assumption or impression on the part of the nurse should be stated as such, e.g., "Impression of this community health nurse is that the parents will secure immunizations for the children."

When visual aids have been used during the visit, the name of the pamphlet or guide should be given, either underlined or in quotes. This will help in the planning for future visits by the nurse or another staff member who assumes the responsibility for the case load. It is frustrating to a nurse who has selected a pamphlet for use in teaching to be told during the visit, "The other nurse brought me that last time."

The nurse records her assessment of the attitudes of the patient and family toward the long-term and short-term goals they have selected. At the same time she evaluates their abilities to meet these goals. Is the nurse aware of any changes in relation to these goals since previous visits?

In recording her plans for the next visit, the nurse notes what she believes the family will be ready to accept and carry out. She might plan to teach a family member to administer insulin to a diabetic, or help a patient to get up in a chair for a little while, or to teach an antepartum mother regarding the rest and exercise she needs at this point in her pregnancy. The plan should also include a memorandum to see how much and how well the patient and family learned from the teaching done at the previous visit and how they have been able to use what they learned. The plan may include calling the physician for additional orders and listing teaching aids that might be helpful.

There is a difference of opinion among agencies as to the most appropriate time for staff nurses to write their records. Some agencies wish the nurse to complete the records before leaving the home; others prefer to have this done immediately following the visit but not in the home; still others wish the recording to be done either at the end of the day or on the following morning before the nurse goes to her district. Some agencies, particularly in rural areas, provide tape recorders to be used by the nurse in her car following her visit.

In summary, skillfully written records to ensure continuity of agency contact and nursing service must be accurate, complete, concise, and promptly done. They should include a description of the service given and of the short- and long-term goals established, a description of the family's attitudes and relationships, the plan and date for the next visit, the signature of the nurse, and the current date. The same principles apply in writing referrals, memorandums, and letters to professional workers in other agencies.

## THE NURSING PROCESS: EVALUATING

Evaluating the intervention of a community health nurse with an individual or family requires careful appraisal of the nurse's performance and behavior and the individual's and family's responses in terms of a temporarily or permanently changed mode of behavior. The nurse constantly must be watchful for evidences of change in individual or family behavior as an index that her plan of nursing care is indeed of value and beneficial to the patient and family. If she decides that her implementation approach is not showing any desired effects based on her appraisal of the patient's response, she frequently will change her plan of care in hopes that a new approach will produce clues indicating a desired change of response or behavior on the part of the patient or family. If the nurse accepts the fact that evaluation is an ongoing activity that is constantly present in every phase of the nursing process, she realizes how crucial her evaluative skills must be in order to intervene effectively with a patient or family.

Evaluation involves measuring behavior and interpreting the results in terms of the desired behavior change—which is complicated by the fact that all such measurement contains error.[44]  Since the purpose of evaluation is

[44]Barbara Klug Redman, *The Process of Patient Teaching In Nursing,* The C. V. Mosby Company, St. Louis, 1968, p. 106.

to predict how the individual or family will behave in the future, it is necessary to use as many measurements of behavior as are feasible. Some current evaluative methods available for nurses in community health nursing include direct observation of patient behavior by means of tangible results or attainment of desired goals, questionnaires or rating scales designed to elicit opinions or attitudes of consumers regarding effectiveness of health services, anecdotal notes jotted down on a sequential basis by the nurse, process recording or tape recording of interactions on an intermittent basis, or written family analyses. By making use of combinations of several measuring tools, an evaluation of the results of the nursing intervention tends to be more reliable. As yet, there are too few measurement tools for determining the effectiveness of nursing intervention with patients and families. Many complex factors contribute to behavior change and the endeavor to evaluate the effect of nursing intervention alone is elusive.

### Observation of Behavior

Direct observation of the patient's change of behavior or attainment of desired goals is easy in some instances but not always possible for all situations. For example, when a patient loses twenty pounds and maintains the weight loss according to the plan of care, this result represents successful accomplishment of a desired goal and tangible evidence of a change. When a mother of a family accepts a suggestion by the nurse to perform a prescribed task consistently and several weeks later exhibits the change of behavior on a routine, casual basis, this observation may be taken as evidence of successful learning by the mother. Sometimes a sensitive observation of the patient's behavior, attitude, or action will reveal clues to the nurse alerting her to think about the effectiveness of her approach. An example is cited as written by a nursing student:

> At first I thought it very easy to see what were the needs of this family. As a community health nurse, I saw my roles to be very obvious. I saw myself helping the mother to get appointments for herself and the children for their medical care. I also saw my role to be one of a health teacher, especially to the mother concerning her condition. I began to do these things. My first two or three visits were dedicated to carrying out these objectives. Mrs. S. would listen very patiently to everything I said. She would promise to make appointments for herself and the children. However, after three visits, I evaluated my progress and found that I was really getting nowhere. I would encourage her to make appointments, which she would do, but I found that most of them she was unable to keep for a variety of reasons. Actually, other than a medical check-up for Sammy, I had accomplished nothing.
>
> It was at this point that I realized that my diagnosis and plan were all wrong.

I was looking at the family from my point of view, which was that of an inexperienced community health nurse. I also realized that I had placed my values on what should be done and what was not necessary. I saw that although we had developed somewhat of a good relationship, I was not meeting Mrs. S's needs as she saw them. So in my future visits, I decided to sit and listen to her and find out what her needs were. I knew it was vital that she realize my interest and concern not only in her health problems but also in the family and its relationships. Mrs. S saw her family's two main problems to be marital and financial. Health problems were secondary. She felt the need to talk with someone about these problems because she knew so few people in whom she could confide.

When the nurse feels that observation of behavior change in the individual or family is insufficient or intangible, she can make use of other measurement tools.

### Questionnaires or Rating Scales
Brief questionnaires or rating scales can be used occasionally or on an intermittent basis to elicit the opinions or attitudes of consumers about the health services they are receiving or would like to receive. The use of a questionnaire or rating scale differs from a face-to-face oral evaluation by allowing the consumer to respond to questions or statements when the nurse is not present and providing time to think about the questions before expressing an honest opinion. The consumer can be requested to mail the completed questionnaire or rating scale to the nurse or to her supervisor or teacher, whichever course of action is desired. Examples of information that the nurse may wish to obtain from the consumer may consist of statements such as the following:

---

1.  I always learn something new about health when the nurse comes to visit me. ☐ yes    ☐ no
2.  It helps me to be able to talk to the nurse about things that concern me.
    ☐ strongly disagree
    ☐ disagree
    ☐ uncertain
    ☐ agree
    ☐ strongly agree
3.  I would like to talk about the latest ideas in:
    ☐ low-cost buying
    ☐ birth control
    ☐ nutrition
    ☐ developmental problems of preschool children
    Other _____

---

By carefully constructing the statements or questions, the nurse can elicit and receive information and ideas from the consumer regarding attitudes about the health services already experienced or receptivity to more comprehensive health services.

## Anecdotal Notes

By jotting down casual notes in a notebook from time to time about observations of the patient or family, specific levels of patient or family activity, attitudes of the patient, family, or nurse, or goals of the patient, family, or nurse, an examination of the notes at prescribed time intervals will frequently reveal minute changes that have occurred over the course of time. All too often as the nurse works with absorbed interest in the patient or family, she forgets the initial assessment of the situation and consequently is unable to determine the changes that have taken place until she is reminded to compare the status of the patient and family with the anecdotal notes written on the first visit. To be able to evaluate changes that have occurred during a specific time period and to realize that she played a role in effecting the change is strengthening to the nurse. If she discusses the changes as demonstrating the patient's or family's progress as revealed through the use of the written anecdotal notes, the patient and family members are also strengthened and motivated positively to continue to work toward desired goals. Anecdotal notes can also be shown to instructors or supervisors as evidence of a patient's or family's progress.

## Process Recording

By doing a process recording or tape recording of an interaction during a home visit, the nurse is enabled to evaluate her interpersonal relationship with patients and families by gaining sensitivity to her interviewing skills, her follow-up of cues, her phrasing of questions and statements, and the family's responses. If she elects to do a tape recording of an interaction, she must obtain permission from the patient or family to do so. Frequently, a signed permission form which indicates the patient's or family's willingness for the use of the tape recorder and the purpose for which the interview will be reviewed simplifies the procedure. Many families respond affirmatively to the request to do a tape recording of a visit.

When the nurse chooses to do a process recording of a visit, she must be cognizant of the desirability of writing the content of the interaction as soon as possible. Its value lies in its prompt recording, and therefore it should be written immediately after the visit, as recall of the verbal and nonverbal behavior lessens as the time interval lengthens.

Process recording has been described as a verbatim recording of all recallable verbal and nonverbal communication between the nurse and the patient or family member. The record includes introductory statements describing the family constellation and the purpose of the visit; the verbatim recording of the verbal and nonverbal communication that took place between the nurse and the patient or family member; comments and analysis of feelings the nurse experienced and those she may have noticed on the part of the patient or family member; evaluation and analysis of the interaction that took place during the visit; a summary statement evaluating the visit and making plans and objectives for ensuing visits (see Case Record 12).

Process recording requires considerable time to write, analyze, and review. To become skillful in the method requires a great deal of effort, practice, and experience on the part of the nurse. Following is a form employed by one agency in the use of this method; other agencies use variations of this form.

---

Process Recording Form

Family
Address
Date of Visit
Purpose of Visit
Introduction


---

| Patient-Nurse Verbal and Nonverbal Exchange and Interaction | Nurse's Comments and Analysis |
| --- | --- |


---

Summary


---

## Family Analysis
The best description of a family analysis was written by a nursing student as follows:

> During a home visit the community health nurse is involved with the nurse-patient interaction to the extent that it is impossible to separate out the different components of the interaction. Often recording of the home visit back at the office does not provide the nurse with insight of the changes that are going on in the family. Webster's definition of *analysis* is an examination of a com-

plex, its elements, and their relations. Thus, a *family analysis* could be defined as an examination of the complex which is a family, the different elements (persons) that compose it, and the relations between the elements.

The value of a family analysis lies in its potential to improve patient care. Through doing a family analysis, the nurse is able to get a grasp on what changes are going on within the family and to see her role in relation to the initiation of support of these changes. It is exciting for the nurse to get this overview of the family to see in what areas she has been effective, how, and what further needs should be concentrated on.

An analysis gives a comprehensive view of the family under study and can be done whenever such a study seems expedient. It requires a thoughtful review of all components of the nursing process, a knowledge in depth of the family, and deliberate study of the effect and direction of the nursing intervention. A guide for writing a family analysis is suggested as follows:

I. Assessment
    A. Identify health factors.
        1. Physical factors.
            *a.* Chronological age and physical level of growth and development.
            *b.* Past and present physical problems.
            *c.* Special physical abilities.
            *d.* Utilization of medical resources.
            *e.* Nutritional status.
        2. Mental factors.
            *a.* Achievement in school.
            *b.* Ability to solve problems.
            *c.* Presence of sense of humor.
            *d.* Special mental abilities.
            *e.* Sense of self-esteem.
        3. Social-cultural factors.
            *a.* Nationality and cultural influences.
            *b.* Religious beliefs.
            *c.* Interaction with family members.
            *d.* Dominant attitudes toward health, education, and life.
            *e.* Child-rearing skills.
         4. Environmental factors.
            *a.* Characteristics and atmosphere of home, car, and neighborhood.
            *b.* Safety hazards.
            *c.* Attitude of community toward family.
            *d.* Beauty in environment.
        5. Socioeconomic factors.
            *a.* Annual income of breadwinner

           *b.* Occupation and employment of family members.

           *c.* Management of money.

    B. What are the interfamily relationships?

       1. What are the dynamics?

           *a.* Interactional style of communication of family.

           *b.* Decision-making skills.

           *c.* Relationship of family members in seriousness and in fun.

       2. What are the strengths?

  II. Nursing diagnosis

    A. Identify the needs of the patient or family which were focused upon. List them in order of priority. Were the family members in agreement with these needs?

    B. State the contract that the family and nurse made mutually.

  III. Nursing plan and implementation

    A. Describe your plan of action to fulfill the contract.

    B. What was your rationale for the plan? State nursing principles or reasons as justificstion for your actions.

  IV. Evaluation

    A. What demonstrated fulfillment of the contract? How has the family indicated that they have achieved a higher level of health?

## SUMMARY

The home visit is one of the principal means by which community health nurses interact with families. The components that must be considered in all home visits include activities such as preparation for the visit, meeting the family, setting up an agreeable contract with the family, assessing, planning, implementing, evaluating, and recording. The objective of the nurse is consistently directed toward assisting the family to advance toward wellness.

Assessing the needs of the patient or family is a continuous process, during which flexibility and willingness to redirect goals in keeping with the family's desires are essential. Use of assessment tools is important to confirm the accuracy of nurses' perceptions. Planning the nursing intervention includes the determination of methodology and techniques required to meet the assessed and distinctive needs of the patient and family. Some methods that can be used with families, dependent upon their needs, include the behavior modification approach, the family therapy approach, the transactional analysis approach, the epidemiologic approach, and the paradoxical communication approach. Implementing a plan of care consists of taking action to meet the assessed need. By taking action, the nurse must be aware of the elements influencing behavior during the change process and stress and crisis periods. She must be cognizant of factors affecting the referral process. Evaluating the implementation of a plan consists of determining outcomes in terms of success and family and nurse satisfaction.

Evaluation is an ongoing activity, which can be measured and judged by the use of various methods. Some suggested evaluative techniques include direct observation of patient and family behavior, utilization of questionnaires or rating scales, writing anecdotal notes, doing process recordings or tape recordings, and writing family analyses. Recording the nursing activities of the home visit succinctly on the appropriate record form completes and summarizes the nursing process.

## SUGGESTED READING

Ackerman, Nathan W., Frances L. Beatman, and Sanford N. Sherman: *Expanding Theory and Practice in Family Therapy*, Family Service Association of America, New York, 1967.

Aguilera, Donna C., Janice M. Messick, and Marlene S. Farrell: *Crisis Intervention, Theory and Methodology*, The C. V. Mosby Company, St. Louis, 1970.

Axline, Virginia M.: *Dibs, In Search of Self*, Houghton Mifflin Company, Boston, 1964.

Barnard, Kathryn: "Teaching the Retarded Child Is a Family Affair," *American Journal of Nursing*, 68:2:305–311 (February) 1968.

Bennis, Warren G., Kenneth D. Benne, and Robert Chin: *The Planning of Change*, Holt, Rinehart and Winston, Inc., New York, 1961.

Bensberg, Gerard J.: *Teaching the Mentally Retarded*, Southern Regional Education Board, Atlanta, 1965.

Berne, Eric: *Transactional Analysis in Psychotherapy*, Grove Press, Inc., New York, 1961.

———: *Games People Play*, Grove Press, Inc., New York, 1964.

———: *Principles of Group Treatment*, Grove Press, Inc., New York, 1966.

Brammer, Lawrence M., and Everett L. Shostrom: *Therapeutic Psychology, Fundamentals of Actualization Counseling and Psychotherapy*, Prentice-Hall, Inc., Englewood Cliffs, N.J., 1968.

Caplan, Gerald: *Concepts of Mental and Consultation*, Social Security Administration, Children's Bureau: U.S. Department of Health, Education and Welfare, 1959.

———: *Principles of Preventive Psychiatry*, Basic Books, Inc., Publishers, New York, 1964.

Carlson, Carolyn: *Behavioral Concepts of Nursing Intervention*, J. B. Lippincott Company, Philadelphia, 1970.

Cornelius, Dorothy A., and Helen Connors: "The United States Social Security System and Medicare and Medicaid," *International Nursing Review*, 17:3:206–223, 1970.

Dunn, Halbert L.: *High-Level Wellness*, R. W. Beatty Co., Arlington, Virginia, 1961.

Fivars, Grace, and Doris Cosnell: *Nursing Evaluation: The Problem and the Process— The Critical Incident Technique*, The Macmillan Company, New York, 1966.

Fox, John P., Carrie E. Hall, and Lila R. Elveback: *Epidemiology, Man and Disease*, The Macmillan Company, New York, 1970.

Frankl, Victor E.: *Man's Search For Meaning*, Washington Square Press, New York, 1963.

Ginott, Haim G.: *Between Parent and Child*, The Macmillan Company, New York, 1965.

————: *Between Parent and Teenager,* The Macmillan Company, New York, 1969.

Haley, Jay: *Strategies of Psychotherapy,* Grune & Stratton, Inc., New York, 1963.

Harris, Thomas A.: *I'm OK–You're OK,* Harper & Row, Publishers, New York, 1969.

Helvie, Carl O., Ann E. Hill, and Charlotte F. Bambino: "The Setting and Nursing Practice," Parts I and II, *Nursing Outlook,* 16:8:27–29 (August) 1968; 16:9:35–38 (September) 1968.

Langsley, Donald G., and Kaplan, David M.: *The Treatment of Families In Crisis,* Grune & Stratton, Inc., New York, 1968.

Levine, Myra E.: "The Pursuit of Wholeness," *American Journal of Nursing,* 69:1:93–98 (January) 1969.

Lippitt, Ronald, Jeanne Watson, and Bruce Westley: *The Dynamics of Planned Change,* Harcourt Brace Jovanovich, Inc., New York, 1958.

Mager, Robert F.: *Preparing Instructional Objectives,* Fearon Publishers, Inc., Palo Alto, Calif., 1962.

————: *Developing Attitudes Toward Learning,* Fearon Publishers, Inc., Palo Alto, Calif., 1968.

Maier, Henry W.: *Three Theories of Child Development,* Harper & Row, Publishers, Incorporated, New York, 1965.

Maltz, Maxwell: *Creative Living For Today,* Trident Press, a division of Simon & Schuster, Inc., New York, 1967.

Menninger, Karl: *The Vital Balance,* The Viking Press, Inc., New York, 1963.

Parad, Howard J. (ed.): *Crisis Intervention: Selected Readings,* Family Service Association of America, New York, 1965.

Patterson, Gerald R., and M. Elizabeth Gullion: *Living With Children,* Research Press, Champaign, Illinois, 1968.

Phaneuf, Maria C.: "A Nursing Audit Method," *Nursing Outlook,* 12:5:42–45 (May) 1964.

————: "The Nursing Audit For Evaluation of Patient Care," *Nursing Outlook,* 14:6:51–54 (June) 1966.

————: "Analysis Of a Nursing Audit," *Nursing Outlook,* 16:1:57–60 (January) 1968.

Redman, Barbara Klug: *The Process of Patient Teaching In Nursing,* The C. V. Mosby Company, St. Louis, 1968.

Satir, Virginia: *Conjoint Family Therapy,* Science and Behavior Books, Inc., Palo Alto, Calif., 1967.

Schutz, William C.: *Joy, Expanding Human Awareness,* Grove Press, Inc., New York, 1967.

Stein, Leonard I.: "The Doctor-Nurse Game," *American Journal of Nursing,* 68:1:101–105 (January) 1968.

Sussman, Marvin B.: *Sourcebook In Marriage and the Family,* Houghton Mifflin Company, Boston, 1963.

Woods, Mary F.: "Measuring A Patient's Needs and Progress," *Nursing Outlook,* 14:10:38–41 (October) 1966.

Wright, Beatrice A.: *Physical Disability—A Psychological Approach,* Harper & Row, Publishers, Incorporated, New York, 1960.

Yura, Helen, and Mary B. Walsh: *The Nursing Process: Assessing, Planning, Implementing, and Evaluating,* The Catholic University of America Press, Washington, 1967.

# 6
# The Community Health Nurse And Communication

## THE NURSE AND COMMUNICATION

The effectiveness of much of the community health nurse's work is dependent on her communication skills, not only those of speaking and writing, but also those of observation and listening—not just hearing, but *listening* with an open mind even if she is not in agreement with what is being said. In simple terms, *communication* means "effective transmission of information." The key word is "effective." Communication is a two-way process, including both the giving and receiving of knowledge, ideas, information, attitudes, and opinions.

A ready command of language, which was invented to facilitate communication, is requisite for developing communication skills. A discriminating knowledge of words and their specific meanings, plus the ability to use them with accuracy are essential in successfully presenting thoughts and ideas to patients and families, community members, and professional coworkers, either by writing or by speech. The importance of accuracy in spelling and in meaning can scarcely be overrated. An example is the two words "discreet" and "discrete," pronounced the same but with a difference in spelling and in meaning, yet at times used interchangeably by persons who do not understand the meanings. It has been said that linguistic differences are a perpetual source of international misunderstanding. This is equally true on a person-to-person basis. The nurse must be certain that words have the same meaning for her patients as they do for her. A classic example is the nurse who asked a pregnant mother to save a twenty-four-hour urine specimen. The mother withheld her urine for twenty-four hours at a cost of much discomfort and some pain.

Four specific skills are employed in communications, namely, reading, writing, listening, and speaking. "These four skills are unevenly distributed in human beings. Some of us are good writers; some are good talkers; some, good listeners; some, avid readers. All of these skills can be improved immeasurably if we want to improve them."[1]

Inherent in the use of communication skills is the social responsibility to strive for clarity, accuracy, and truth. In speech, it is a choice of words, use of voice tones and inflections; in writing, a choice of words, correct spelling, punctuation, sentence construction, and paragraphing. The listener and the reader have the responsibility for making an honest effort to grasp the meaning of the speaker or writer.

Successful communication may be carried on by nonverbal means also. The tone of voice, a smile (Lillian Wald said a nurse could smile in twenty-seven different languages), a gesture, such as a shrug of the shoulders, silence or inaction when action is indicated, all can communicate in an expressive way and merit attention. Children have long been recognized as masters of nonverbal communication.

Frequently problems arise from unconscious nonverbal communication, partly because the person is not aware of his nonverbal behavior and partly because he is unaware that it is evident. The nurse must watch for her own nonverbal communication when talking to the patient and family. It could either strengthen or weaken her teaching. Those watching her might misinterpret a facial expression or a shrug of the shoulders as impatience with them, not herself, or they might think it was a lack of interest in them on the nurse's part. The nurse who will listen calmly and with poise to the patient's or family's difficulties and problems without revealing her own inner feelings or attitudes will be more helpful than the nurse who shows her impatience and frustration with the general situation by her facial expressions or gestures. The nurse needs to listen for unexpressed hopes and fears. Listen to the young woman expecting her first baby. What is she really saying? What are her hopes? What are her fears? A person may communicate what he is thinking or feeling by body posture, movements, and facial expressions, so that the nurse needs to watch, listen for, and learn to recognize the significance of these nonverbally expressed feelings with a comprehending silence. What is *not* said with words may be as important as what *is* said.

While working with patients and families, and with coworkers, too, the nurse will note clues to unspoken feelings and ideas. Sometimes an unexplained pause or hesitancy in speech or a sudden change of subject may be a person's way of saying that he does not wish to continue with the conversation. On the other hand, the hesitancy or pause may indicate that the person is thinking and searching for the exact word or phrase to express his thought. The nurse should consider this and allow time as necessary.

[1]C. M. Siggins, "A Professor of English Looks at Communication Skills," *Nursing Outlook,* 9: 666–668 (November) 1961.

Many older persons and those for whom English is a second language are not always facile with words and need adequate time in which to phrase their thoughts and ideas. Sometimes this may apply to children as well. It is important, therefore, to be understanding and patient and not to misinterpret a sudden pause or change of topic. The nurse's skill in interpreting this comes with thoughtfulness, observation, practice, experience, and understanding. Occasionally, the patient or family will tell the nurse what they assume she wants to hear, and then her hope of being effective lies in listening carefully and searching for the nuances. During a home call, the nurse may gain insight into the family situation by close observation of surroundings. A painful neatness or an extreme untidiness may communicate the patient's or family's reaction to an unhappy situation. Such feelings may be expressed in other ways, as well. This requires the nurse to be alert and understanding at all times.

## TEACHING AND LEARNING
### Goals and Objectives
Teaching and learning are interlocked. In teaching, the nurse's underlying goal or objective is to help the patient and family to learn to meet and solve their own health problems. In addition to establishing her goals for teaching, the nurse also helps the patient and family to determine *their* goals and expectations for learning.

Before the nurse can teach effectively, she must know the learner. What are his goals and objectives in relation to health? or does he have any? Those who live close to the poverty line and move from one family crisis to another, frequently have no objectives. The nurse will sense the lack of motivation toward optimal health in many low-income families, where there is the constant threat and fear of unemployment with resulting inability to pay the rent or buy sufficient food and clothing. The lack of independence engendered by welfare may be another reason for low motivation.   These families are more concerned with their critical situations than with long-range problems of health. A practical approach is usually the wisest one in teaching low-income groups. Their financial difficulties are frequently coupled with a limited educational background and this, with their many family crises, makes it difficult to challenge interest. A realistic discussion of nutrition within their culture and means may provide a starting point. In families with some affluence, another approach might be more effective and relevant, as for example the B. family in Case Situation 9.

## TEACHING
Teaching employs many forms of communication, verbal and nonverbal. In planned teaching, the nurse applies, in one way or another, the four specific communication skills mentioned earlier: reading, writing, listening, and

speaking. She may implement these with demonstrations and other types of visual aids: care of the patient, equipment, charts, pictures, slides, films, and television. At the same time, she communicates or teaches, often unconsciously, by other means such as her own standards, attitudes, feelings, and interests, or by her appearance, manner, mode of dress, tone of voice, and acceptance of others.

Teaching sound health practices to patient and family was recognized early in its history as basic to all community health nursing. That it was an accepted part of the early public health nursing programs in the United States is shown in a daily report of a pioneer district nurse in Boston, when she wrote, "Almost every day I find some former patient carrying out many of the simple directions that have been given during some former sickness."[2]

In thinking of the family, the nurse must give realistic consideration to what a family is. Any definition would have to consider not only the so-called "normal family," but also the "broken family" or the "solo parent," families of varying racial, educational, and cultural backgrounds and families on all economic levels. The nurse encounters all these types in her work, and the needs, expectations, and health and medical goals will vary from family to family.

The teaching done by the nurse takes place in various locales, the home, health center, school, industrial plant, and at community gatherings, such as meetings of the parent-teacher associations and neighborhood clubs. Some junior and senior high schools depend on the nurse to teach one or more classes of a planned course in the curriculum in health education or the home nursing course in the home economics curriculum. If the nurse accepts such a responsibility, she should determine the subject matter that she will be expected to cover, the objectives for the entire course, and those which are to be met in her particular presentation.

At times the nurse is asked to speak at meetings of the parent-teacher association on health matters relating to school children, such as drug abuse, nutrition, safety measures, or communicable disease control. At the beginning of the school year, and at other times also, the nurse may be asked to attend a teachers' meeting to present some phase of her program and to discuss some of the health problems current in the school and community which the teachers will encounter, such as the possibility of an influenza outbreak, or problems that relate to an influx of a new population in the community.

The teacher-nurse conference in the school can be a planned teaching and learning experience for both teacher and nurse. By sharing their knowledge of the health problems of the children under their care and direction, they can work together with children and parents toward the solution of

[2]Isabel A. Hampton et al.: *Nursing of the Sick, 1893,* McGraw-Hill Book Company, New York, 1949, p. 123.

many of these problems (see Case Situation 11). Because of unexpected needs of a patient or family, some teaching has to be done without prior planning in order to meet a specific situation, e.g., visit 2 in Case Record 9 concerning alcoholism. The nurse must be alert to take advantage of these opportunities.

Time is always a factor in the nurse's teaching, for there is seldom enough, especially on a home call. This is frequently true also in a scheduled contact at the clinic or even in a formal class presentation. This lack of time enhances the need for the nurse to make a thorough preparation for her teaching.

In working toward her goals to help patient and family learn to meet and solve their health problems, the nurse may encounter some resistance to change, and this is normal. Change is unsettling to some people, particularly the elderly. It is difficult for most of us to give up established behaviors in which we are comfortable and in which we feel we have certain skills for something unfamiliar. When a patient or family does not fully understand the new situation or if they think they would be more uncomfortable than under present conditions, they will resist.

An example is that of a young man who unexpectedly learns he has diabetes, which will involve a new way of living for him such as learning self-administration of insulin, eating a different diet, and accepting a degree of control of certain activities, including athletics, camping, and travel. In such instances the nurse will encounter resistance that must be met with understanding and appreciation of the feelings of the young man and his family, recognizing that these changes will cause uncertainty, discomfort, and anxiety until he finds usefulness and satisfaction in his new way of living.

The nurse must watch for both the readiness and resistance factors involved in change. The best teaching may be done by careful, intelligent listening, allowing patient and family opportunities to think through the situation for themselves by talking it over and gaining a perspective. A situation such as that which faced the young diabetic is difficult to accept and the nurse must not let herself become so involved emotionally that she is not free to think objectively.

There are several components of success in teaching. Perhaps the three most important are: (1) the teacher's mastery of the subject. This entails continuous study for the nurse, in order not only to add to her general knowledge but also to add to her knowledge and understanding of nursing and of the natural and social sciences. The importance of this point has been emphasized by the "knowledge explosion" in many fields, particularly medicine, with the new drugs, new laboratory findings, and new approaches to long-established treatments. (2) The teacher's appreciation and enjoyment of her subject. Her enthusiasm for it and her interest in sharing her knowledge will help to stimulate learning on the part of the patient and family. (3) The teacher's genuine liking for people, all people of varying cultures, creeds, and backgrounds, and in particular the patient, the family, or the community group she is trying to teach.

Continuous evaluation of the achievement of the goals—her own as well as those of patient and family—will enable the nurse to make her teaching a learning experience for herself as well as for others. It will help her to assess her ability and skills to bring about behavioral changes for better health practices by patients and families under her care.

## Learning

Closely allied with teaching is learning. It covers a wide range of activities, from the acquisition of manual skills to the mental processes of problem solving. Learning is one of man's principal activities, but how it actually takes place is not known. There is comparatively little information regarding the mechanism of the transfer of knowledge from instructor to student, an instructor being any one of a number of things—a book, a picture, an observation, or a person. There is general agreement, however, that learning is evidenced by a change of behavior. These behavioral changes involve not only the individual's overt actions, but his covert actions as well in ways of thinking and feeling. Learning may be thought of also as a learner's development of ways of satisfying motives or attaining goals.

The individual has not really learned unless the changes in behavior persist. If learning is to become relatively permanent, it must be used either in mental activity or in physical practice. Many people in low-income groups tend to be action-oriented rather than word-oriented and find learning easier when the demonstration and return demonstration of teaching or of role-playing is used. This becomes an important way of teaching for the nurse in the home and the health center. Teaching a mother how to examine her baby is one example. Another example would be by a role-playing situation in which the mother would play the role of her preschool child who says "No," with the nurse playing the role of the mother as she perceives that role.

Curiosity is a vital factor in the psychology of learning of any age group. It should be stimulated but at the same time given direction. A child's effort to learn why and how a match makes a flame can be disastrous without supervision and guidance.

**Principles of learning**     Many principles of learning have been formulated by various schools of psychology. Some that apply to the work of the nurse are included here.

1.  Learning takes place more effectively when an individual is ready, both physically and mentally, to learn.

2.  Individual differences must be considered if effective learning is to take place.

3.  Motivation, either from within or without the individual, is essential for learning.

4.  What the individual learns in any given situation depends on his perception of the situation.

5.  An individual learns what he actually uses or what has relevance for him.

6.  Learning takes place more effectively when the individual has a sense of satisfaction and when he feels the learning is his.

7.  Evaluation by learner and teacher is essential in determining whether desirable changes in behavior are taking place.

These principles bear consideration as the nurse plans and conducts her teaching and develops accompanying learning experiences. None of these principles functions alone, but they are interdependent and interact with each other. A consideration of these principles follows.

*Learning takes place more effectively when an individual is ready to learn*
This principle of the readiness element in learning points out that what is to be taught must not only be relevant to the individual but must meet his needs and interests and be within the range of his mastery and achievement. This principle is basic to all teaching of patients. For example, most pregnant women are interested in and ready to learn about the anatomy and physiology of pregnancy and of the birth process. Many mothers seek information about good nutrition for their school age children, and ask for assistance with emotional problems of their teen-agers.

Much of the success in teaching the patient and his family depends on utilizing their interests and expressed needs. In the situation of an unwanted baby, the nurse may encounter an emotional block on the part of the mother or the family to learning about the baby's needs and care. When the readiness to learn is not present, what can the nurse do to stimulate it? A great deal depends on her initiative and insight. She can determine some interests of the patient and family, and try to capitalize on them. The well-planned use of visual aids will help. In addition to the birth atlas, there is available literature prepared by government agencies, insurance companies, commercial companies such as milk and baby food companies, and the voluntary agencies such as the American Heart Association or the American Cancer Society.

Timing is a factor in readiness to learn. A mother's interest in learning may lag if she is more concerned with putting her washing on the line or preparing dinner than with the information the nurse has to offer. Readiness to learn may be inhibited also by the presence of neighbors or children, and there is always the chance that the mother frankly may not be interested at the time. The nurse must be sensitive to these and other hidden causes that may underlie the lack of readiness, and she must evaluate the situation carefully. Often it is wiser, under the circumstances, to plan for a return call under more fortunate circumstances, and close the visit.

*Individual differences must be considered if effective learning is to take place* In her work, the community health nurse observes wide variations in the cultural, ethnic, religious, economic, and educational backgrounds of the families assigned to her. She also notes differences in the life experiences, ages, and interests of these families. The pregnant woman who lost her previous baby has certain needs and fears that are different from those of her young neighbor, a primipara. These individual differences occur among families living in the same neighborhood, and sometimes the nurse sees marked differences between members of one family. Alertness in the nurse and consideration of the background differences of individuals, families, and neighborhoods will enhance both teaching and learning.

*Motivation, either from within or without the individual, is essential for learning* Motivation is related to readiness, and without it, either from within or from without, little learning by the patient and his family, with resultant changes in behavior, can take place. Many patients and families are motivated on their own to learn because they appreciate that what the nurse has to teach will promote their comfort, safety, and security. In addition, many recognize the long-term values of health instruction and what it can mean to their permanent health, e.g., the nurse's instruction regarding dental health and hygiene. On occasion the nurse needs to challenge and to motivate the patient and family to learn. Praising and showing appreciation for what has been learned and put into use constitute one way. The nurse's effort to make the family independent of her in meeting their health needs can motivate them to learn more. Sometimes she may motivate them unconsciously by her enthusiasm for teaching, her evident knowledge of health matters, and her interest in the patient and family as persons.

Motivation by fear or threat leads to negative teaching and should be avoided. However, the teaching the nurse has done, without apparent effect at the time, regarding immunization may result in a marked change of behavior by a family or a community that is galvanized into action by the report of the health department that cases of communicable diseases, such as smallpox or poliomyelitis, are occurring in the community.

Motivation may come also from satisfactions gained in the use of previous learning, with a resultant desire to learn more in order to gain further satisfaction. Many young mothers, as they gain skills and competencies in the care of their new babies, are motivated to learn more about child care as their babies grow older. Sound interpersonal relationships between nurse and family will be a positive element in stimulating motivation and determining behavior—social, emotional, and intellectual—which develops from the learning situations.

*What the individual learns in any given situation depends on his perception of the situation*   Patients and families frequently will see things differently from the nurse because of their backgrounds and life experiences. What the individual sees, hears, understands, and knows affects his learning. In community health nursing, language difficulties and cultural and religious customs may interfere with the learning of the patient and family. Furthermore, misinterpretation can occur easily if members of the family think they understand what the nurse is saying and doing, when actually they do not. Periodic repetition of important points in the discussion by the nurse, and the use of pertinent questions from time to time on the material covered, will give her an idea of how much or how little has been understood. In certain instances, the nurse may need to change her approach in teaching and try other means in order to help the patient and family increase their perception and learning.

*An individual learns what he actually uses or what has relevance for him*   The effect of this principle is recognized by students in many fields. How easy it is to forget a foreign language when there is no opportunity to use it, either by speaking or reading. This principle emphasizes the value to the learner of the return demonstration in the demonstration method of teaching. When a technique such as the administration of insulin has been taught by the demonstration method to patient or family member in the hospital, health center, or home, the nurse should observe a return demonstration as soon as possible, to assure herself that the basic principles of the procedure have been comprehended and are being applied with an appreciation of their importance.

*Learning takes place more effectively when the individual has a sense of satisfaction and when he feels the learning is his*   This principle is related to the principle of readiness to learn, and it depends on the goals and interest of the individual learner. The wise selection of the learning experiences by instructor and student will bear on the implementation of this principle. The experiences must be within the range of accomplishment by the learner, not too difficult, but not too easy if satisfaction is to be derived in carrying them out. Teaching the necessary exercises to Mr. F., the elderly patient in Case Record 1 who had had a stroke, is an example. In any plan for teaching, the instructor needs to consider how to incorporate this principle. Basically it is the goal of all teaching, and can provide satisfactions for both student and instructor.

*Evaluation by learner and teacher is essential in determining whether desirable changes in behavior are taking place* Evaluation may be carried out in a variety of ways and is helpful to both the learner and the teacher. For example, the nurse may discuss with the mother the learning experiences she had that were associated with the care of her previous baby. Is she able to utilize the knowledge and carry out the skills she acquired in the care of that baby when caring for her new baby? What additional skills and knowledge does the mother feel she needs? What additional skills and knowledge does the mother appear to the nurse to need? Can a family meet new health needs and problems as they arise in daily living and solve them satisfactorily on the basis of their previous learning experiences? Both nurse and family need to ask themselves these and similar questions from time to time. The nurse applies this principle to her own work when she evaluates the progress made by family and patient in learning to meet their own health problems. Have they made sufficient progress in meeting their own needs so that she can close or discharge the case until such time as a new health crisis arises for which help is needed? In evaluating the learning that has taken place, the nurse should take the long view. Results of change in behavior leading to better health practices by patient, family, or community need time to be identified; the process may even take years.

The principles of learning selected for discussion here are guidelines or suggestions to help the nurse to attain a measure of success in an important part of her work, health teaching. As the nurse gains experience in her teaching and continues her observations, evaluation, and study, other principles which she can utilize will become apparent to her.

## Concomitant Learnings

In addition to the primary learnings that are the principal objectives of planned learning activities, there are concomitant learnings that also concern the instructor. These learnings include such intangibles as attitudes, ideals, appreciation, pride in accomplishment, and habits of conduct. They may have positive or negative values and will occur simultaneously with the primary learnings. Both types of learning may be derived from the same activities.

When the nurse carefully demonstrates formula making in the home, observing principles of cleanliness and accuracy, maintaining neatness of the work area, and making skillful use of the equipment, the mother will gain an appreciation of the importance of these factors, as well as of the actual techniques of formula making. If, on the other hand, the demonstration is conducted in a careless, slovenly, and haphazard manner, the converse may be true.

In all her work, the nurse should not lose sight of the concomitant learnings that are constantly taking place, sometimes without her thought or knowledge. In evaluating her teaching of patient and family, the nurse should look for evidences of concomitant learnings and should be objective in recognizing both the positive and negative aspects.

## TECHNIQUES OF TEACHING

The community health nurse will always have a responsibility for teaching the patient and his family in the home. However, the demand for group teaching is increasing as communities become more aware of and interested in health matters. Group teaching is more economical in time and effort than individual teaching, but it requires methods and approaches that differ from those used with the individual patient or family in their own environment.

### Teaching Plan

Preparation of a teaching plan, whether for a group or individual, is the first step in organized teaching. The instructor begins such a plan with a statement of goals and objectives for both the learner and herself, for teaching should be defined in terms not of content to be covered or techniques to be used but of goals and objectives of both instructor and learner in the ends to be achieved. For example, a mother might request the nurse to bring her information regarding means of birth control on her next visit. On that planned visit, the nurse's objective as teacher would be to acquaint the mother, by use of the family-planning kit, with the variety of existing birth control devices. On the other hand, the mother's objective as learner would be to determine for herself the most feasible means of birth control for her own use.

The nurse should not impose her own health standards or values on the learner without first studying or investigating the existing situation. She should determine, with the help of the learner, what needs are being met satisfactorily for those concerned and what needs are unmet to the degree that achievement of optimal health is seriously affected by the current situation. From there, she works out ways of filling the unmet needs. The means of implementing desired change should be explored with the learner.

In addition to setting objectives that can reasonably be attained by a group, the instructor needs some information about the class. For instance, is it an expectant parents' class? The nurse should have some pertinent information about their community or neighborhood, its health facilities, and health needs. What behavioral changes or learning are desired *by* and *for* this group? What content would facilitate achievement of the aims?

A story is told of the women in a certain North African village during World War II whose cooperation was required during the African invasion. They were alerted to the situation but requested to keep it secret, which they carefully did. Their cooperation contributed markedly to the success of the Allied Forces. The commanding officer wished to repay them for their loyalty. On learning that all water used in the homes had to be carried from the village well, he ordered water to be piped to each house. When this was done, the women were outraged. Going for the water each morning was a social activity in the village. At the well the women met their friends and neighbors and learned the local news, births, marriages, and deaths. When there was no reason for gathering at the well each morning, the local mores were disturbed and the need for human contact was no longer being met.

The teaching plan is a blueprint, a suggested guide. It should be so flexible that it can be adapted easily to the needs of patient, family, or community group. The teaching method best suited to the subject and circumstances should be selected. It might be a lecture, formal talk, discussion, demonstration, or any combination of these methods, or it might be the problem-solving approach. Visual aids to accompany the teaching plan should be selected carefully. They might include any of the following: demonstration of equipment and techniques, charts, posters, maps, graphs, books, slides, films, health literature, and reports. Aids to be used, and when and where, should be noted on the margin of the teaching plan. Not only visual aids but verbal illustrations may also be listed in the margin. A question or two is helpful if the instructor sees that interest is waning in some members of the class.

The nurse outlines the content of the lesson, keeping the stated goals for that lesson and the principles of learning clearly in mind. Clarity is essential. It has been said that if you cannot phrase your ideas in simple terms, you do not understand them fully yourself. Terminology should be used with discrimination; such words as "carcinoma" or "nephrectomy" should be avoided, as they carry little or no meaning for the laity. Finally, a lesson plan should provide space in which to record an evaluation of the class session. Noting questions that were raised during or at the end of the class is helpful in making the evaluation.

### Lecture Method

The lecture is usually selected if formal teaching seems appropriate to the situation, as in a large, organized class or a community gathering, a situation in which it is desirable to present certain information to many people. The real value of the lecture method lies in arousing the listener's curiosity so that he will develop an interest in seeking further information and knowledge. Therefore, thorough preparation is mandatory.

A careful but not detailed outline is required, based on current and accurate information. If statistics are to be used, they must be the most recent available and must be clearly interpreted. The outline is only a guide. No more than three main ideas should be developed, as an instructor cannot do justice to more in the forty-five- to fifty-minute period usually allotted. In general, the lecture has three divisions, an introduction that establishes the framework of what is to follow, the development of the theme, and the conclusion or summary, to which nothing new is added. There should be only enough facts and figures to illustrate the three ideas; more could be confusing. The instructor should have enthusiasm and interest for the subject, be knowledgeable, and be responsive to the group interest.

If visual aids, such as slides or films, are to be used, it is essential to check the equipment, e.g., the projector, before it leaves the office and again at the meeting place before the group assembles. Do all the electric connections work? In selecting visual aids the instructor should verify that they contain the desired information to support the theme of the lecture. Before visual aids are presented, the audience should be briefed on their content; at the conclusion of the showing, this content should be related to the overall subject of the meeting.

If the audience is not too large and if there is enough time, a discussion may follow. It provides the instructor with an opportunity to clarify any necessary points. In the discussion, the nurse should be on guard against that member of the group who wants to do all the talking, describing her personal experiences, often irrelevant, and preventing general discussion.

### Demonstration Method

The demonstration method is effective when teaching such nursing activities in the home as body exercises, body positioning, dressing a wound, or making a formula. It is difficult to learn to carry out a procedure by listening to a description of it. An anonymous patient once wrote:

I can soon learn to do it
    If you can let me see it done,

I can watch your hands in action
But your tongue too fast will run.

In planning the demonstration, the equipment used should be the same as that found in the home, the same as that the patient or family will be using. In other words, not the shining chrome sterilizer in the health center, but an ordinary saucepan found in any home kitchen should be used in teaching the sterilization of equipment.

The demonstration lesson plan should note where and when each step will occur. Even though she is familiar with the procedure, the nurse should review each step prior to performing it in the teaching or class situation. Before commencing the demonstration, it is important to check that everyone in the group is able to see the demonstration and to hear the instructor.

It is expedient to demonstrate only one method of carrying out a procedure; otherwise the learner may be confused. However, the instructor may mention that there is more than one method but that only one method is being demonstrated at this time. It is helpful to have a few questions ready in case attention appears to be waning and the group needs a little thought stimulation. Neatness of the work area, organization of equipment and materials, and the nurse's manual dexterity in carrying out the procedure will be observed closely by the class. Because she sets standards for accomplishment by the group, her skills are important. Consciously or unconsciously, they will try to emulate her. The nurse must be aware of the opportunities for concomitant learnings and must consider them in planning her demonstration. She must never be guilty of implying, "Do as I say, not as I do."

The demonstration method is expensive timewise and should therefore be used on a group basis whenever and wherever possible, e.g., for mothers waiting in a clinic or for a class in a housing project. There are times, however, when an individual demonstration in the home or clinic is necessary to meet a specific need or situation. Demonstration is especially helpful when there is a language barrier. In such a situation, extreme care should be taken to avoid errors and to proceed slowly and carefully, checking each step with the learner.

As stated previously, a return demonstration is an integral part of this method. It enables the nurse to see how well the underlying principles of the procedure were grasped, understood, and incorporated into the learner's thinking. It also permits the nurse to check on her teaching and to determine what concomitant learning, positive and negative, has taken place. The demonstration method, even though it is time-consuming, probably is used more frequently than any other type of teaching by most community health nurses. The nurse must constantly evaluate her skills in its use and the results obtained. She must continually ask herself how she can improve her skills.

### Problem Solving

Problem solving is an important technique in all public health work, including community health nursing. Epidemiology, a part of a nurse's daily work, is problem solving. The nurse uses the epidemiologic approach in relation to much of her work in homes, in schools, and in the community. From whom did the little two-year-old boy contract his tuberculous infection? How can a beginning outbreak of mumps in the third grade be controlled? What might be the source of the food poisoning that occurred following a school picnic?

Problem solving has been defined as a planned attack upon a difficulty or an obstacle for the purpose of finding a satisfactory solution. Clarity in the statement of the problem and critical thinking are essential in this method. It can be used as a teaching technique with patients, families, and community groups. One important goal in community health nursing is to teach the patient, family, and community to become independent of the nurse in meeting and solving their own health problems.

This is illustrated by Nancy Milio in her book *9226 Kercheval: The Storefront That Did Not Burn.* She points out that eventually she realized she could withdraw from the health center and its direction because those concerned no longer needed her help and guidance; furthermore, she came to see that they could only grow strong and secure without her.

Following the recognition that a problem exists, five steps are taken toward its solution: (1) Define and limit the problem. Until it has been clearly defined, and its limitations have been recognized, little can be done toward the next step. (2) Analyze the problem. This step involves a consideration of the factors present and their relationships. Every nurse has observed a physician in the problem-solving process of analyzing such data as x-rays, laboratory reports, physical examinations, and the outcome of interviews with the patient before arriving at his diagnosis. (3) Determine possible solutions to the problem, on the basis of a discriminating review of the problem and the facts involved. (4) Select the most likely solutions to the problem and test them. (5) Put the solution or plan into effect and evaluate the results.

When using the problem-solving approach with a patient and his family, the nurse may find that the steps are not always so clearly defined as they are presented here, and that they may not occur always in exactly the same sequence. However, there must be an understanding and definition of the problem, some critical thinking relating to possible solutions, and a plan for effecting the solutions and testing them.

A modified form of the problem-solving approach is used by the nurse in many home visits. An example is found in Case Record 7 concerning Mrs. U., who had cancer in its terminal stage. Her parents, Mr. and Mrs. K., told the nurse that they were not strong enough to take care of Mrs. U. any longer but that they did not want to send her to the county hospital for fear she would die there alone. This was the problem and its limitations. The nurse was aware of the factors surrounding the problem, such as the close family ties, the strong religious feeling, the imminence of death, the difficulty of family transportation to the hospital, and the frailty of Mr. and Mrs. K. A possible solution was for the family to ask the doctor to request the cancer society to provide private duty nursing service on a temporary basis. The family approached the doctor, his request to the cancer society was made and granted, and a private duty nurse was sent to the home. The arrival of the private duty nurse in the home was putting the plan into effect, or step 5. Although the nurse made the suggestion for a solution to the problem, recognized by the family, the family carried out the solution themselves by making their request to the doctor. It was a learning situation for them, and the solution was arrived at by their own action. No evaluation was made, but it would have been based on the mental comfort the family had in the presence of the private duty nurse on the last day.

## Group Discussion
As a method of facilitating teaching and learning, group discussion can be used by the nurse to arouse interest and provide information in health matters. The nurse prepares as carefully for this type of teaching as for any other. She reviews the subject selected for discussion and prepares herself to be the resource person. This method is more successful when members have a fairly common background or a similar interest, such as a group of parents with the common problem of drug abuse among their teen-aged children. These parents would face many similar problems, emotional, social, health, and economic. A satisfactory size for such a group is from about five to not more than fifteen members. Having fewer than five or more than fifteen members inhibits purposeful discussion within the group. With fewer than five, an insufficient number of viewpoints may be presented, and with more than fifteen, it is not possible to secure an expression of opinion from each group member and there is less opportunity to raise pertinent questions.

The physical setting for the group discussion is important, such as ventilation, adequate space, lighting, and elimination of outside noises as far as possible. Members should be able to see and hear each other at all times. Usually chairs are placed in a circle or around a table. The nurse is included in the group but does not have a position of authority, as in a formal classroom. Members are introduced and an effort is made to pronounce their names carefully and correctly. Usually the group selects its leader and recorder and the nurse acts as the resource person and facilitator.

The leader's role is important, for he is responsible for helping the group to feel as comfortable and at ease as possible and for following the discussion carefully to see that it is kept within the limits of the subject matter. From time to time the leader asks the recorder to report on what has been said or accomplished. The leader tries to secure the viewpoint of every member, tactfully preventing any one person from dominating the discussion and encouraging the shy members to contribute their ideas. On occasion, if a crisis arises in the discussion, the nurse may suggest that role-playing be tried in order to clarify the situation. A summary by the leader or recorder concludes the meeting. Usually a subject that lends itself to group discussion extends over several meetings, since not a great deal can be accomplished in one meeting alone. Until a sense of unity and cohesion has developed among group members, little progress in learning can take place.

At the end of each session, the nurse makes an evaluation for her use. Did all the members participate? If not, why? What important points of the subject were not covered? How might they be covered at the next session? Did she, the resource person and facilitator, talk too much? Was she prepared with the information needed by the group?

One nurse tried this method successfully in a suburban area with a group of parents of mentally retarded children. They represented a wide segment of the local community which had this one problem in common. The group included the custodian of the local grade school, a chemistry professor from a nearby college, a clergyman, several businessmen and women, and some housewives, about twelve in all. The custodian was selected to be the leader. As she observed the group interaction, the nurse realized how many facets of the problem they presented and discussed that would have been difficult for her to do on an individual, one-to-one basis; she also saw that these parents were coming to realize that they were not alone with their problem but were able to share it with others who had appreciation and understanding.

### The Interview
Another form of communication that is frequently used by the nurse in her work is the interview, a discussion between two or more persons in which information and ideas are exchanged. Kahn and Cannell define the inter-

view as ". . . a specialized pattern of verbal interaction initiated for a specific purpose, and focused on some specific content area with consequent elimination of extraneous material."[3] They point out that attitudes, values, feelings, and plans may be expressed in an interview.

In its simplest form, interviewing is a method of securing information, such as facts, opinions, or personal histories. When used on a professional level, interviewing, according to Abramovitz, involves ". . . a process of interaction and communication between people. Through this process individuals can mutually clarify feelings, attitudes, and meaningful information. In this way professional people can gain increased understanding of the behavior and personal reactions of individuals they serve."[4] Abramovitz points out further that the interview process can help individuals come to recognize and understand their own problems.

Various types of interviews are used by professional workers. For example, there is the therapeutic interview frequently used in psychiatry. Many nursing students have read records based on this type of interview or have observed such interviews in progress while on psychiatric nursing service. There is also the conference interview, the type most frequently employed by the community health nurse. Often it can be used to provide the framework for the teaching and learning situations she plans to initiate with a patient and/or his family.

Essentials for a successful interview of any type include a satisfactory environment, privacy, and the assurance of confidentiality. Usually the home is the most suitable place for the community health nurse's interview, especially if the interview is her first contact with the family. As the host, the patient (or family) will feel more secure and relaxed in his own environment. For the nurse, the intrafamily relationships and the atmosphere of the home will be more apparent and will provide clues on which to base her interview. Furthermore, the photographs, framed certificates of birth, confirmation, and marriage seen in many homes, and also the books, musical instruments, and arrangements of household living will provide silent answers to some of the nurse's questions and cues for others.

In specialized services, such as school nursing, it may be more satisfactory for the mother (or both parents) to meet the nurse at the school, particularly if the nurse wishes to include the teacher and/or principal, whose contributions are often most helpful, in the interview. In planning for the interview, though, the nurse needs to consider whether a home call to a particular family might not be more productive than a conference with parent or parents at school in understanding the child's health problems,

[3]Robert L. Kahn and Charles F. Cannell, *Dynamics of Interviewing,* John Wiley & Sons, Inc., New York, 1959, p. 16.
[4]Abraham B. Abramovitz (ed.), *Emotional Factors in Public Health Nursing,* University of Wisconsin Press, Madison, 1961, p. 72.

which might stem from his environment. When interviews take place in clinics or health centers, the nurse is the hostess, and the patient or family are guests. In her role as hostess, the nurse must take this into consideration, recognizing that they may not be as comfortable as in their own home. During an interview the patient and family need ample time to develop their point of view. It is as valuable for the nurse to listen as it is for her to talk, and knowing *when* to do each is a skill in itself. The nurse should determine how she herself is reacting to the expectations of the interviewee.

In her eagerness to help, the nurse should be careful not to impose on others her own attitudes and standards in matters as cleanliness, mode of dress, food, medical care, or social behavior. An understanding tolerance is important here. It has been said that the true meaning of tolerance is to be found in the Sioux Indians' definition: "If you wish for tolerance you must ask the Great Spirit to help you never to judge another until you have walked for two miles in his moccasins." This is especially true when patient and family are trying to meet their problems not only in the light of their own traditions, culture, and religious customs but also within the general patterns of American culture. The nurse must try to recognize what the patient and family really want, need, and are ready to accept from the professional services she has to offer.

The nurse needs to look for and consider causative factors in the patient's background that may be operating in his behavior. Her expressed appreciation for what the patient has accomplished and the difficulties he has encountered will help to establish rapport. A judicious use of sympathy and empathy enters the relationship. There will be times when the patient or interviewee needs help in differentiating between reality and confusion created by his own defenses. Setting limits to prevent the patient from wandering too far from problems under discussion will help.

In planning for the interview, the nurse considers and selects those questions that will elicit the information needed, questions that are concise, clear, and pertinent to the situation. These questions need to be phrased carefully, with no evidence of disapproval by the nurse of her personal value judgments. If an appointment has been broken, a mother will respond less defensively to a general question such as "We missed you at the health center last Friday, how are you getting along?" Questions that may be answered with a "Yes" or "No," e.g., "Does Mary eat the right kind of breakfast?" are usually of little help to the nurse. Such a question elicits little information about Mary's eating patterns. A more specific question, such as, "What did Mary eat for her breakfast this morning?" would provide a more helpful answer.

Sometimes a nurse new to the community health nursing field hesitates to ask certain necessary questions in an interview, fearing she may appear to be prying into family affairs. If she asks only for the information she needs in order to plan with the family, she is not prying. Some areas of family life are not the concern of the nurse. For example, usually the nurse would not need to ask *why* the husband was sent to prison. It is enough to know he is there. The nurse needs such information as will help in the current rehabilitation of the family and that of the husband and father on his return to the home.

The interview should close with a summary of the positive things that have been accomplished, some of the things yet to be done, and suggested plans for another conference or interview at a later date. However, the interview is not complete until the salient points have been recorded and placed in the folder of the family or patient. The planned date for the next interview and what is hoped to be accomplished at that time should be a part of the record.

One type of interview, that with the venereal disease patient, is on the increase because of the rapid rise in the nationwide incidence of syphilis and gonorrhea. Such interviews may take place in the home, the health center or clinic, the school, or place of employment. Because of the implications and the attitudes toward these diseases, this type of interview requires special skills in establishing confidence and developing rapport with the patient in order to gain his cooperation in undertaking a program of treatment promptly, which is not only important to the patient's health but is of equal importance also to his family, to future children, and to the community's health and protection.

This type of interview involves asking the patient all about his sex experience history and offers opportunities for developing, with sensitivity, a nurse-patient relationship based on the authority of knowledge. It includes teaching the patient to understand the nature of the diseases and their progress if left untreated, as well as their means of spread and of control in the community. It involves patient cooperation for responsibility for seeking, and continuing, treatment for himself and his sex partners, despite the inconveniences, until all laboratory reports are negative.

There should be an appreciation on the part of the nurse that this type of interview may be uncomfortable, embarrassing, or even painful for some patients. Others may be receptive to the health information the nurse offers and more cooperative. As in all interviews, the nurse should be sensitive to behavioral cues, be objective, understanding, nonjudgmental, and factual and help the patient to take the long view of his situation. Her goals are to help the patient and to protect the community.

As the nurse records an interview, she has an opportunity to evaluate it. Skills in interviewing do not come easily but require constant practice and evaluation, so she should ask herself the following questions:

1. Were the purposes and objectives of the interview met?

2. Did the interviewee have adequate time to participate in the interview and express his point of view?

3. Was the interview, as far as possible, kept with an "open end" and not too structured?

4. Was the interviewee permitted to talk freely and without interruption unless he rambled or became too repetitious?

5. Did she maintain a critical, objective, and impartial attitude while listening and talking?

By evaluating her interviews, the nurse gains an awareness of her progress in developing the necessary skills and techniques, for interviewing is a professional skill that can, for the most part, be developed only by constant study, practice, and self-evaluation.

Weissman has listed some concerns that community health nurses and other public health workers have expressed in relation to their skills and techniques in the interviewing process. Following are some of these concerns:

1. How to ask questions that will elicit meaningful responses.

2. How to secure information and understanding about some of the underlying emotional aspects of problem situations.

3. How does the interviewer deal with her own anxieties and tensions during an interview?

4. How can the interviewer comfortably meet silences on the part of the interviewee?

5. Can a silence be constructive?

6. How can the interviewee be encouraged to break the silence?

7. How can the patient's or the family's anger or unwillingness to talk be handled?

8. What does it mean to be supportive, and how is it done?[5]

Workers in the professional fields who use interviewing techniques will recognize many of these concerns as their own.

The mechanics of the interviewing process are important, but of equal importance are the goals, attitudes, and motives of the nurse and the patient or family. Abramovitz points out that skillful interviewing is a medium in

[5]Isabel G. Weissman, "Make Interviewing a Creative Process," *California's Health,* 22:22:201–203 (May 15) 1965.

which "an integrated understanding of people is combined with the knowledge of one's own professional field in order to enable the patient to help
himself."[6]

## BARRIERS TO COMMUNICATION

Since communication involves people, it is not unnatural that barriers occur.
Sometimes these barriers to communication arise between the nurse and
patient or family because of circumstances beyond the nurse's control.
When the nurse, because of a language difficulty, cannot understand the
mother or the mother cannot understand the nurse, it becomes necessary
to depend on neighbors and children for translation. This does not ensure
confidentiality, and it provides opportunities for misinterpretation by the
neighbor, child, mother, or nurse. It is a frustrating experience for both
mother and nurse. Today an increasing amount of health information is
being published in French and Spanish and made available by the World
Health Organization and similar health services. Such material will be of
help to nurse and family in overcoming the language barrier.

The nurse encounters some patients and families with cultures and
religions of which she has no knowledge or understanding, and then she is
faced with another barrier to communication. What may be acceptable to
the nurse in her own culture may be highly distasteful to persons of other
cultures, and vice versa. For example, the American custom of eating a
sandwich held with the fingers is unpleasant to members of certain cultures,
in which the use of a knife and fork would be essential. It is understandable
that members of such a culture might reject an American nurse's health
teaching, because her health habits are not acceptable to them.

In her work, the nurse should recognize that to be culturally different
is not to be devoid of culture, and that uneducated or homeless families,
such as agricultural migrants, are entities with a sense of belonging to their
wider group, although they may have different assumptions and concepts
from those of the nurse upon which to base their living. The nurse and other
members of the health team must learn to recognize that though these
families have cultural values and behavior that appear strange and different,
they and their children can be helped to live in this society. This does not
necessarily mean changing their ways, but rather helping them to gain
some knowledge and understanding, especially of health practices, that will
assist them to live with people in a culture other than their own.

Every nurse is obligated to develop a knowledge, understanding, and
appreciation of the religious practices of the families under her care, especially as they apply to birth, marriage, illness, and death. This is particularly

[6]Abramovitz, *loc. cit.*

true for the nurse in her work in the home, where patients can carry on their religious practices more freely than in a hospital. Such a knowledge and appreciation on the part of the nurse will help to overcome some of the barriers to communication. Priests, rabbis, and clergy are always willing to explain the meaning of the religious practices of their people and to be helpful to the community health nurse.

In general, the nurse should know and understand, to some degree, the main tenets or principles of the world's major religions as they affect family health practices such as the status of women and children in the family, diet patterns, and acceptance of medical care. An understanding and appreciation of these points by the nurse will make it easier for her to communicate with families of various religious backgrounds.

Frequently in her work the nurse finds herself moving from one extreme in the socioeconomic level to another. This requires a philosophy of living and an adjustment to and acceptance of the social values of other people. On occasion, the socioeconomic level and background of a family will present barriers to communication. Some families in her district may be on a higher socioeconomic level than others. Although their needs may be the same, the nurse's approach may have to differ from one family to another, and she may have to adapt her methods to meet particular situations.

To meet the needs of all groups for health information is often a challenge. The college-educated mother may need even more help in learning to care for her baby or in planning nutritious meals than the mother with less academic background but more practical experience. Each requires a different approach to problems. A nurse was startled one day to find a young woman physician as a member of her expectant mothers' class. The physician explained, "I don't know how to bathe, feed, or otherwise care for my baby, and I have to learn just like these other mothers."

A barrier to communication may occur because of the nurse's lack of teaching skills and preparation. Not everyone with a great deal of knowledge on a specific subject is able to teach it. Furthermore, if for some reason stimulation of learner interest, consideration of individual differences, and concern for the learner's difficulties are lacking or neglected, a barrier has been raised between learner and instructor. In group teaching, this may occur between the instructor and only one member of the group, because the instructor has not realized fully the needs of one individual learner. The probability of the occurrence of such a barrier enhances the importance of the constant evaluation by the instructor of her own teaching and the progress of each learner. The basic goal of all health education is to improve health practices, not just to acquire knowledge.

Incompatibility is another barrier to communication. Personal feelings and attitudes may block the interaction of the patient or family and the nurse. Every nurse encounters certain patients, families, and coworkers with whom she finds it difficult to work. She cannot reach them or understand them, nor can they understand her; they may even mistrust her. Deep-seated psychologic factors, such as national, ethnic, or other dislikes, or lack of appreciation for the religion and culture of the other, may be operating on both sides, and no one may be aware of them. In recognizing such a situation, the nurse accepts it and does the best she can under the circumstances. A frank discussion with the supervisor or consultant will help the nurse to gain some insight into this type of problem.

At times the patient or family may be under such stress, physical or emotional, that satisfactory interpersonal communications are prevented temporarily, but the barrier may be absent later. The nurse needs to appreciate and accept such situations and adapt to them, taking the long viewpoint.

Finally, in all health teaching, barriers of fear, habit, and ignorance are to be found in all families on all social and economic levels, and in all ethnic groups. Fear of the "needle" is apt to be found wherever the nurse is trying to teach the importance of immunization for the control of certain diseases, such as typhoid or tetanus. There is the patient who fears he may have cancer or tuberculosis and yet delays consulting the physician in dread of what the diagnosis may reveal. Therefore he refuses to listen to what the nurse is saying about the value of a physical examination by his doctor. Certain families have for generations followed customary diet habits; though they may appear to agree with the nurse when she is trying to teach the importance of adding other foods to their usual diet, they are too habit-bound to change their ways. Ignorance on the part of a family of the needs of an alcoholic member and of the difficulties he faces is baffling and hard to overcome. Because of tradition, illiteracy, habit, apathy, and living conditions, some patients, families, and neighborhoods are so wrapped in ignorance, superstition, and prejudice that they need considerable time to overcome barriers and to change their health practices. There were evidences of barriers to communication between the nurse and the husband of the tuberculous patient in Case Record 6. These barriers were probably due in part to the husband's ignorance and fear of the disease and to his cultural background.

The true measure of success in health teaching is not so much what people *know* as what they *do.* The community health nurse meets expectant mothers from many walks of life who still have not seen a physician at the end of their seventh month of pregnancy; they tell the nurse, "I know better, but I just haven't gotten around to seeing my doctor yet." Was their behavior due to fear? to ignorance? to habit? or to apathy?

## SUMMARY
The nurse does not always see the results of her own teaching as that Boston nurse did years ago, but frequently she sees the results of the teach-

ing of former nurses in her district or agency. Learning may take time to produce results, i.e., a change of behavior. Furthermore these changes in behavior may have taken place so subtly that the learner, whether patient, family, or community, may not have been aware of them.

Many of the concepts of teaching have changed in the past few years. To achieve her goals in teaching, the nurse, by building on strengths and interests, must make it as easy as possible for patient and family to learn efficiently and quickly. Learning does not necessarily take place just because of talking or telling. There must be motivation from within and without. Were patient and family taught or did they learn?

The nurse needs to begin where the learner—patient, family, or community—is, and by determining what is already known and accepted, proceed from the known to the unknown, developing relationships between the two. The content of her teaching must fit the needs of the learner with appropriate learning activities. Planned time for review, reconsideration, and evaluation at spaced intervals is necessary, depending on the ability of patient, family, and community to learn and to put into practice what they have gained from the nurse's teaching.

Perhaps the philosophy of the well-known Russian educator, A. D. Alexandrov, applies to the teaching done by the community health nurse as well as to that of the instructor in the formal classroom or laboratory: "A student is not a vessel to be filled, but a lamp to be lighted."[7] This philosophy should guide the nurse in planning and carrying out her health teaching in the home and in the community. She does not order or command, she instructs and leads, and by communication (effective transmission of information) enables patients, families, and communities to learn to make their lives more satisfactory, productive, and healthful.

## SUGGESTED READING

Aiken, Linda Harman: "Patient Problems are Problems in Learning," *American Journal of Nursing,* 70:1916–1918 (September) 1970.

Bermosk, Loretta Sue, and Mary Jane Mordan: *Interviewing in Nursing,* The Macmillan Company, New York, 1964.

Coulter, Pearl Parvin, and Margaret J. Brown: "Parallel Experience: An Interview Technique," *American Journal of Nursing,* 69:1028–1030 (May) 1969.

Freeman, Ruth B.: *Community Health Nursing Practice,* W. B. Saunders Company, Philadelphia, 1970, pp. 211–217; 371–373.

Giffen, Kim: "Interpersonal Trust in the Helping Professions," *American Journal of Nursing,* 69:1491–1492 (July) 1969.

Goldsborough, Judith D.: "On Becoming Nonjudgmental," *American Journal of Nursing,* 70:2340–2343 (November) 1970.

[7]A. D. Alexandrov, quoted by Priscilla Johnson, "New Heretics in Soviet Writing," *Saturday Review,* May 5, 1962, pp. 8–11.

Kadushin, Alfred: "The Racial Factor in the Interview," *Social Work,* 17:88–98 (May) 1972.

Muecke, Marjorie A.: "Overcoming the Language Barrier," *Nursing Outlook,* 18: 53–54 (April) 1970.

Pohl, Margaret: *Teaching Function of the Nursing Practitioner,* Wm. C. Brown Company Publishers, Dubuque, Iowa, 1968.

Rogers, Carl R.: *Freedom to Learn,* Charles E. Merrill Books, Inc., Columbus, Ohio, 1968, Chapters 6 and 7.

Rubin, Floreene, Janet D. Allan, and Allison Leak: "The Seminar Process—An Aid to Learning," *Nursing Outlook,* 19:37–39 (January) 1971.

# 7
# Family
# Nutrition

Nutrition, or the lack of it, has played an important part in the long history of man. It has been an instrument of government and politics and often a cause of war and conquest. It has led to exploration, discovery, and colonization and has participated in the fate of whole populations. In recent history it has been closely allied with industry through agriculture, transportation, and trade and plays a part in all aspects of modern living. The ultimate aim of nutrition is to provide for the health of the individual and the prevention and treatment of, and recovery from, diseases.

The community health nurse needs an appreciation and knowledge of the culture and background of the families she serves and to use this understanding in developing her nutrition teaching, utilizing the current diets of the families as far as possible, but urging changes as necessary. People and animals have always sought food to satisfy their hunger, but the science of nutrition has shown that not only quantity but *quality* is necessary for health and that an adequate diet is essential to strengthen the body's general resistance to disease.

The prevalence of malnutrition and hunger is a problem and concern of nearly every country, not just the so-called "developing countries." Hunger and malnutrition can only be attacked successfully by a combination of several means. Economics and money, education, food production and distribution, and the recognition of the nutritional value of certain foods are all necessary in meeting the problem. There is no single way of overcoming hunger and malnutrition, for its control is closely associated with the need for adequate shelter and clothing, for fresh water, sanitation, requisite cooking facilities and equipment, and on occasion, the overcoming of communication and language barriers. Home visits often take place in the kitchen, and the nurse can utilize the opportunity to observe the conditions under which the homemaker must prepare meals.

Many families, both rich and poor, lack adequate nutrition despite the availability of food. This is caused by lack of knowledge of nutrition, by faulty traditional food habits, by religious beliefs and taboos, food dislikes, and food fads based on pseudo-science.

Families as well as persons living alone need to learn more about foods that provide normal nutrition and how to spend their money wisely and economically. A report relating to the 1969 White House Conference on Food, Nutrition and Health in Washington, D.C., considered that previous efforts in nutrition education have been to a large degree ineffective and concluded:

> Most Americans today are abysmally ignorant about the most elementary principles of applied nutrition. This ignorance makes the middle and upper classes ideal targets for food faddists and the poor suffer because their limited food budget allows them no room for mistakes. Although food habits are difficult to change, a national nutritional policy will only become a working reality if we are able to find new effective ways to educate the population in the basics of food and nutrition.[1]

This evaluation of the situation offers a challenge to the nutritionist and the community health nurse working in the home, health center, school, and place of employment. Regardless of adequate money for food, knowledge and understanding of food values, and the availability of food, there can be little success in combatting hunger and malnutrition unless people are *motivated* to eat the nutritious foods their bodies need. This is partly a matter of nutrition teaching, although more than teaching is involved. Learning must take place and be implemented by change, motivation, and new patterns of food use. Acting as a nutrition counselor, the nurse needs to be flexible and develop ways to apply nutrition values to families' eating habits. She works to bring about needed change when necessary, but the motivation to change must be present for it to last. In seeking to bring about change, she must guard against imposing her own values, standards, and enthusiasm on others. She also needs to recognize that there is no standardized cultural patterns even among people of the same nationality. Although every family on the block may be of the same national origin, there will be wide variations in familial customs and values. They may come from different regions of a country, speak different dialects, and have different standards of living.

The purposes of adequate nutrition are to provide for body growth and development, to maintain general health and resistance to disease, to pro-

---

[1]"Message from the White House," Editorial, *The Journal of Nursing Education,* 8:4:5, McGraw-Hill Publications, New York, 1969. By permission of the publisher.

vide for activity, and to maintain a desirable weight. Margaret Mead has said, "Food affects not only man's dignity, but the capacity of children to reach their full potential, and the capacity of adults to act from day to day."[2]

Every nurse learns that a normal, adequate diet includes a balance of proteins, carbohydrates, and fats in combination with vitamins, especially A, B complex, C, and D, minerals, especially calcium and iron, and an adequate amount of fluids. The problem, and at the same time the challenge, in teaching is to interpret to the homemaker in the family or the person living alone what this means in terms of economics, availability of food, attractive food combinations, preferences of family members, and what contributes to growth and development and to general health and well-being.

Many changes in family organization and living patterns have taken place in recent years that affect family nutrition and eating habits. The movement of families from rural to urban areas, varying work shifts at factories and plants of different family members, the increase in the number of homemakers working outside the home, and the many interests and social activities that family members have, such as scouting, clubs, unions, and church meetings, make it increasingly difficult to plan and serve nutritious meals to the family as a group. The extensive advertising of foods and food supplements such as vitamins and iron compounds and some of the "fear" advertising regarding the value of low-calorie foods are responsible in part for a considerable lack of accurate knowledge and understanding of nutrition by many people. It has been said that more Americans are malnourished because of nutritional ignorance and misinformation than because of poverty. In teaching, the nurse should consider some barriers to learning she may encounter, such as apathy, ignorance, and lack of understanding of basic principles of nutrition, long-established family food habits, personal tastes, and lack of money.

Homemakers should be encouraged to include in their meal planning foods selected from the four major food groups: milk and milk products; meat, fish, poultry, eggs, nuts, and vegetables high in protein, e.g., dried beans and peas; fruits and vegetables, especially citrus fruits, tomatoes, and carrots; and enriched or whole grain bread and cereals.

Many homemakers do not always find it possible to provide a completely balanced diet in each meal, but the homemaker or person living alone might think of the meals eaten within a twenty-four-hour period as a unit of meal planning, since meals are affected by modes of modern living and individual needs and preferences. Usually the body has been at rest and has had little food intake for the ten to twelve hours preceding breakfast. For many persons breakfast is an important meal and requires more nutri-

[2]Margaret Mead, "Changing Significance of Food," *Journal of Nutrition,* 2:1:17–18 (Summer) 1970.

tive elements than are supplied by a sweet roll or doughnut and a cup of coffee. Consideration should be given particularly to children's growth and energy needs and also to those family members engaged in physical activity. Protein should be an important part of breakfast, such as milk, fish, meat, or eggs. In some European countries, cheese is frequently eaten for breakfast. Bread, toast, and cereals, hot and cold, help to provide energy for the coming day. Many families include fruit or fruit juices for breakfast. This may or may not help to provide the daily requirements for vitamins. It depends on the source of the fruit and the juices, how long the fruit has been in storage in the market and the home, and how it has been treated in preparation, for freshness is essential to the vitamin content. Some vitamins may be destroyed by prolonged cooking, also.

A carefully planned and prepared breakfast is a necessity in our urban society, as lunch is often a sketchy meal, eaten away from home and usually in a short time period. This is in contrast to many foreign countries, where the midday meal is an important family activity, with one to one-and-a-half hours allowed for the meal and a rest or relaxation period. When family members carry their lunch to work or school, it is wise to include some fresh fruit, such as oranges, bananas, or apples, and raw vegetables, such as carrot sticks. Mothers should be warned that if they send their children to school with carefully planned and balanced lunches, children have been observed exchanging their lunches for those that contain dill pickles and other interesting but nonnutritive foods.

The evening meal is important to the family's nutrition and should be carefully planned to include adequate servings of protein foods, such as meat, fish, cheese, eggs, or vegetable protein dishes with leafy and root vegetables, milk for children, and a simple dessert—fruit, fresh or cooked, gelatins, or various milk and egg puddings. The dinner should be eaten under as pleasant surroundings as possible.

These are some of the points to be considered in relation to normal diets of an average family without special food needs beyond that of growing, active children and active adults whose health maintenance must be met.

In nutrition teaching and working for change in dietary habits, the nurse should help the homemaker or person living alone to build whenever possible on the accustomed diet. A "meat and potato" diet meets many nutritional requirements and with the addition of such leafy vegetables as spinach, broccoli, or a salad and some fruit could be made a satisfactory one. Low-income families tend to use a diet high in "starchy" foods, because it is less expensive, is temporarily filling, and gives quick energy. However, it does not meet the body's requirements for growth and development of muscles, bones, and teeth or for general well-being.

There are many approaches to teaching nutrition for the alert nurse that will enable her to help the homemaker or the person living alone. There are times when a visit is made before the remains of breakfast or lunch have been cleared away and by observing unobtrusively, the nurse can learn something about the family's eating patterns. In discussing diet and foods, the nurse needs to ask questions that will provide more information than just a "yes" or "no" response.

A review of a record of the family's menus for two or three days will provide insight into some of the nutrition problems. In one instance, the sixth-grade daughter of a family had a severe problem of overweight. By reviewing the family menus, including the snacks the girl had at school, for three days, it was discovered that the snacks alone—candy bars, ice cream, and doughnuts—came to more than 600 calories a day. This brought out several psychological problems of which the family was not aware.

The nurse needs to be nonthreatening in her teaching, recognizing that the homemaker may be doing the best she can under the circumstances and in the face of such problems as meal preparation on a low income and meal planning with foods available from "surplus foods" and "food stamps." Some nurses have recipes they can share or exchange with home-makers for casseroles, the cooking of cheap cuts of meat, and simple desserts. On occasion, a productive way to teach is to accompany the homemaker to the market to give assistance in economy buying, showing her how to read the labels and compare sizes and prices of cans and packages.

Not only are the nutritionists in health centers, health departments, and hospitals available to the nurse for consultation, but also many private health organizations, such as the local heart association, employ nutritionists who can be most helpful. Nutritionists associated with some of the commercial businesses such as food processing plants and dairies often help. They are interested in the nutrition problems the nurse encounters in her work with families. In one "company" town suffering from a severe economic depression, the nutritionist from the local gas and electric company worked with the nurse to present some cooking demonstrations of low-cost menus and provided copies of the recipes demonstrated.

When certain dietary restrictions conform to religious beliefs or cultural practices regarding the eating of meat or other foods, substitutions can be worked out. Assistance for this can be secured from a local nutritionist.

## NUTRITIONAL NEEDS OF SPECIAL GROUPS
### Pregnant and Lactating Mothers
Every expectant mother needs dietary supervision throughout her pregnancy. When carefully planned, meals for *both* the mother and her family can provide for all those nutrients needed for growth and development,

energy, and general well-being. Many foods are sources for more than one nutritional requirement. In planning for her diet with the pregnant and lactating mother, consideration should be given to her age. Is she a teen-ager? or does she belong to a later age group? If she is a single teen-ager, she faces difficult problems—personal, emotional, familial, and health, with all their complications. Furthermore, these problems can have a direct effect on her baby (see Case Record 4).

Most teen-age pregnant mothers are still in their own growth period. Studies have shown that the nutritional status of many adolescents is unfavorable for an early pregnancy. The unfortunate outcome of many teen-age pregnancies, including maternal morbidity and mortality and infant morbidity and mortality, reflects this. Attention should be given to the nutritional status of this group, based on individual needs determined by careful physical examination to discover the presence of nutritional anemias and poor dietary habits. The pregnant woman who has passed through adolescence and who spaces her pregnancies so that her body has the opportunity to rebuild its nutritional well-being can expect a much more favorable outcome of her pregnancy and a healthier infant.

**Calcium**  With the growth of the fetus and accessory tissues during pregnancy, a significant need for calcium and iron occurs in the mother's body. This becomes more pronounced in the second and third trimesters and even more so during the lactation period. Pregnant women should understand the importance of calcium in their diet and its contribution to the growth and development of the infant's tooth and bone structure. Milk and milk products are good sources of calcium. Turnip and mustard greens, broccoli, and cooked dry beans are considered fair sources, and oranges are also a fair source.

**Iron**  Iron is an essential in the prenatal diet and in the second and third trimesters there is an increasing need to include it in the diet in order to:

1. Maintain the mother's hemoglobin level
2. Maintain her body stores of iron
3. Provide iron for fetal development
4. Furnish the infant with iron stores needed for blood formation during his neonatal period before iron-rich foods are added to his diet

It requires careful planning to include sufficient iron in the mother's daily diet. Good sources of iron include liver (both pork and beef), kidneys, oysters and clams, heart, lean pork and beef, raisins, cooked dried beans, canned peas, dried peaches, apricots, and prunes. Fair sources include spinach, mustard greens, eggs, and whole wheat bread and cereals.

**Vitamins**   The pregnant mother has an increased need for vitamins, especially in the last six months, and also during the lactating period.

*Vitamin A*   A fat-soluble vitamin, vitamin A is an essential factor in cell development, in normal bone formation and tooth development, and for a healthy skin. Good sources include liver, kidneys, egg yolk, whole milk, cream and butter, dark green and deep yellow vegetables such as broccoli and carrots, and such fruits as peaches, apricots, and cantaloupes. If buttermilk or nonfat milk is used in place of whole milk, being cheaper, other sources of vitamin A should be added to the diet. Such foods as salad dressing made with mineral oil are not advised because mineral oil interferes with the body's ability to absorb carotene (vitamin A) and other fat-soluble vitamins and also affects calcium and phosphorus absorption.

*Thiamine (B-1)*   This vitamin helps to keep both the appetite and digestion normal. It is necessary for completion of carbohydrate metabolism and is a factor in the maintenance of a healthy nervous system. It occurs widely, but in small amounts in many foods; thus, it points up the value of a varied diet. Again the second and third trimesters of pregnancy require additional intake of thiamine, as does the lactation period. Good sources include liver, heart and kidney, lean pork, dried beans and peas, whole grains, nuts, peanut butter, white potatoes, and oranges. Fair sources include fish, poultry, other meats, eggs, milk, and many fruits and vegetables.

*Riboflavin (B-2)*   Riboflavin assists in the metabolism of carbohydrates and amino acids. It has an increasing importance in the second and third trimesters of pregnancy. Milk is a good source, also liver, heart, and kidney. Fair sources include lean meat, poultry, cheese, eggs, dark green leafy vegetables and whole wheat bread and cereals.

*Niacin (B-3)*   This vitamin aids the body in translating sources of energy into usable form. When the protein in the diet is of good quality and of sufficient amount, the body's niacin intake will be adequate. Good sources include fish, heart, liver, kidney, poultry, and peanuts. Fair sources are found in milk, whole grain bread and cereals, and white potatoes.

*Ascorbic acid (vitamin C)*   Vitamin C is an essential element in the diet of the entire family, but especially for the pregnant mother. During the second and third trimesters and lactation period, it is recommended that her diet include a minimum of one serving a day from a good source and one from a fair source. Vitamin C increases the body's ability to absorb iron and is necessary for the development and maintenance for normal connective tissue in bones, cartilage, and muscle. Good sources are to be found in fresh fruits, including oranges, strawberries, cantaloupe, and grapefruit, and in such vegetables as cooked greens (turnip, mustard, and spinach), Brussels sprouts, and red and green peppers. Fair sources include fresh tomatoes, cooked cauliflower, sweet or white potatoes, raw cabbage, and liver. The body does not store vitamin C as it does vitamin A, so it should be included in the daily diet.

*Vitamin D* Sources of vitamin D, a fat-soluble vitamin, include not only certain foods, but also sunshine. The pregnant mother requires an additional amount of vitamin D in her diet during the second and third trimesters and in the lactation period. This vitamin promotes the absorption and retention of calcium and phosphorus in the body and is necessary during the fetal growth period for the formation of teeth and bones. Frequently the physician orders supplementary vitamin D for the pregnant woman, especially during dark winter months, when there is little sunshine. The mother should be warned against the dangers of overdosing of vitamin D. Food sources include fortified milk, butter, fish oils, egg yolk, and liver.

### Special health problems
Pregnant and nursing mothers with special diet problems for underweight or obesity should have continuous medical supervision throughout pregnancy and the lactation period. Efforts to reduce during pregnancy should not be made, except under physician's orders and close supervision. The weight of current medical opinion is to the effect that "severe caloric restriction is potentially harmful to the developing fetus and to the mother and almost inevitably restricts other nutrients essential for the growth process."[3] The need for this medical supervision applies also to mothers with chronic diseases of the heart, nephritis, or diabetes, all of which would require dietary restrictions of certain foods.

### Superstitions
Among the superstitions found in the culture and folklore of different ethnic groups are those relating to the pregnant woman and her food. These have been handed down for generations and are firmly grounded in the thinking and practices of the group; examples are: "dry labor" could result from eating cheese, or eating pork could cause the mother's death. It is possible there could have been a basis at one time for such ideas, prior to refrigeration or the safe cooking of meat. When the nurse meets these or similar superstitions in her work in the home and in the health center, she must approach the problem with care and understanding.

[3]National Academy of Sciences, *Maternal Nutrition and the Course of Pregnancy: Summary Report,* Washington, D.C., 1970, p. 13.

In their study of food taboos, Bartholomew and Poston concluded there was "a need for further investigation and study of the background, beliefs and customs of an individual before determining his nutritional status and giving constructive guidance. Every effort should be made to explore new avenues and approaches in motivation, education and guidance in this area."[4]

## NUTRITIONAL NEEDS OF INFANTS, PRESCHOOL, AND SCHOOL CHILDREN
### Infants
Breast feeding is the natural way to feed a new baby. Human breast milk is suited to the digestive system of the normal baby and provides the nourishment he needs in the first few months of life. When breast feeding is not feasible for the new baby for reasons such as the mother's health or allergies, unusual food needs of the baby, or because of social or economic conditions, the baby should be under close medical supervision and a suitable formula prescribed, with semisolid foods added gradually upon the doctor's recommendation.

Babies develop at different rates of speed even within the same family. Some have teeth at five or six months, while others get teeth months later. Some infants are walking by their first birthday, while others begin later. It is the same with foods; every child is different, but usually by his first birthday he should be having some soft foods, such as pureed fruits, vegetables, and meats, eggs, bread, rice, and other cereals. Children begin new foods slowly, and it is better not to urge them to eat foods which at first taste they appear to dislike, but rather to wait and reintroduce the food again a few weeks later with one they do like.

Until he is about three years old, the child is in a rapid growth period in relation to his size. If his mother has eaten wisely and carefully during her pregnancy, the child will have a good head start nutritionally. His diet for the first three years of life is important to future growth and development and for his general health. He needs protein body-building foods and calories for energy. His stomach is small and he will not be able to eat much at a time. Usually he will need food more often than the family's three-meals-a-day pattern.

### Preschool Child
At about three years of age, his rate of growth tends to slow down and his appetite may decrease. Parents should not be unduly concerned unless he

[4]Mary Jo Bartholomew and Frances E. Poston, "Effect of Food Taboos on Prenatal Nutrition," *Journal of Nutrition Education,* 2:1:15–17 (Summer) 1970.

has other symptoms. A basic menu pattern for the preschool child is suggested that can be adapted to meal planning for the entire family.

| BREAKFAST | LUNCH | DINNER |
|---|---|---|
| Fruit or juice | Meat or substitute | Meat or substitute |
| Meat or substitute | Vegetable or salad | Vegetable or salad |
| Bread and/or cereal | Bread or substitute | Bread or substitute |
| Butter and milk | Butter and milk | Butter and milk |
| | Dessert: fruit, | Dessert: fruit, |
| | jello, or ice cream | jello, or ice cream |

Children often need between-meal snacks. These can be fruit, fruit juices, milk, celery or carrot sticks, bread and peanut butter, or a *small* serving of a sweet—cookies or ice cream. The between-meal snack contributes to the child's total nutrition intake.

## School-age Child
The child who has formed good eating habits in early childhood will have few diet problems at this age period. As he grows older, his energy needs increase. He needs larger servings, and some sugar and other sweets added to his diet. It should be emphasized to parents that all growing children need *protein*—milk and milk products, fish, and eggs; *carbohydrates*—bread, cereals, fruits, vegetables, and simple desserts; *fats*—butter, peanut butter, cream; and *vitamins* and *minerals* from fruits and vegetables.

## Teen-agers
**Boys** In this age period, boys are in a time of rapid growth and energy needs. They need foods richer in nutrients than perhaps at any other time of their lives. Many need snacks that have nutrition value, not just a cola or a candy bar, but foods selected from the four major food groups.

**Girls** The teen years are an important period of physical and psychological development for girls. They also need more essential nutrients than at any other time of their lives, except perhaps during the later months of their pregnancy and lactation periods. Yet, according to dietary studies, teen-age girls often have the poorest eating practices of any age group. They tend to become figure conscious and inclined to cut down on amounts of food without respect to the quality and nutritive content.

Breakfast is often neglected in order to allow more time for sleeping or for dressing. In these times of fashion awareness, many girls of normal weight consider themselves to be too fat and try for a more slender figure by "crash" or "fad" diets of calorie counting at the expense of essential nutritious foods, especially those needed for tissue development and for body reserves. It should be stressed that in attempting to reduce weight it is the quantity of food that should be restricted and not the nutritive *quality.*

Iron intake is frequently lessened in these diets with resulting nutritional anemias and susceptibility to colds and other infections, even tuberculosis. Teen-age girls with anemias are inclined to be apathetic, irritable, or fatigued and to lose interest in school achievement. Motivating this group to eat the foods they need is often difficult, but the nurse must try to be original and innovative in making suggestions. A good breakfast decreases the hunger and energy needs at lunch time, when it is so easy to consume high-calorie foods, such as potato chips, pie, and candy bars. Participation in such physical activities as swimming, hiking, tennis, or skating should be encouraged. Finally, giving the girl some responsibility for the planning, purchasing, and preparation of family meals stimulates interest in nutrition. With the increasing number of teen-age marriages and pregnancies, the nutritional status of the teen-age girl has a high priority, not only for her family but for society as well, since many teen-agers will be mothers before they are twenty.

Teen-age girls and boys with serious overweight problems should be seen by their physician for several reasons before commencing a weight-reduction regime. To date, the etiology of adolescent obesity is not clearly defined, and certain physiologic factors may be operating that are not understood. Some cases of obesity might possibly be associated with certain diseases, such as diabetes or heart and kidney difficulties, and this should be ruled out before undertaking a reducing program. In some instances, the obesity might result from generic traits, which would involve several approaches to the problem. A large proportion of obesity cases, however, appear to result from physical inactivity coupled with the availability of the ample and varied food supplies in our society. A psychological approach may be the most effective one, an approach in which there is no nagging or teasing, but a sense of support, cooperation, and encouragement by other members of the family. The content of the diet should be carefully watched to ensure that the foods so necessary to the growing adolescent are included.

In some cultures, children and other family members are urged to overeat, with the idea that the resulting obesity indicates that the parents, especially the father, have sufficient money to feed his family "well." The nurse and the nutritionist need to approach such a situation with extreme caution and delicacy, as this is a matter of family pride, and careful teaching is involved or the results could be destructive.

Appearances for girls and physical prowess for boys are the activating forces for good nutrition and the underlying relationships of sound nutrition to these forces should be demonstrated to all teen-agers. Nutrition affects appearance and is related not only to weight but to posture, as good posture is determined by strong muscles and bones. Skin, hair, and eyes will also reflect the teen-ager's nutritional state. It is important to teach, but not to preach, nutrition to teen-agers. There is no magic formula that will persuade them to eat the foods they really need. The challenge lies in presenting nutrition information in such a way that it will motivate them to think and voluntarily to select wisely from the variety of available foods.

### The Middle-aged (over thirty-five years)
The need for protective foods remain as high for this age group as for young adults. Adequate nutrition will help to lengthen the period of maximum enjoyment and vitality as well as the life span. Milk, meat or substitutes, fruits and vegetables, and bread and cereals are as necessary as in earlier years to maintain general good health and replace tissue. Many people of this age group are not as active as they were in former years. They need to watch their food intake, cutting down on quantity but not on quality, for there is still the need for food of nutritive value. General outdoor exercise such as walking, golf, and swimming should be encouraged and "crash" or "fad" diets discouraged.

   In this age group, some of the chronic diseases may appear, such as diabetes or cardiac disturbances that require diet restrictions. This will provide opportunities for teaching nutrition to the patient and the homemaker. When obesity is a problem, reducing should be undertaken on the physician's advice and the nurse can offer assistance and support. Obesity might have a psychological basis, with compulsive eating resulting from feelings of frustration or of not having a sense of being necessary now that the children are grown and have assumed their own responsibilities. Helping the individual to build new interests and diversions might aid in overcoming the obesity. In general, middle-aged persons need a well-rounded diet, still high in quality, but lower in quantity, and with sufficient outdoor exercise and interests.

### The Elderly
During their working years, most people invest their money with the hope and anticipation of adequate financial resources upon retirement. During this time they should also be making an investment in good health for their retirement years through sound dietary practices. Difficulties can result when there are not habits of good nutrition for retirement, when living patterns will be different. Preparation for retirement is more than just financial, for sound nutrition patterns will be important.

Faulty diets in the aged are commonly results of loneliness and financial worry, which can lead to a malnutrition so severe that life cannot be enjoyed. Loneliness tends to increase poor eating habits, such as overeating of starchy, unbalanced meals and nibbling sweets, eating too little food at irregular times, or foods that contain slight nutritional value, at times a "tea and toast" diet. Some elderly people excuse themselves for this by a "what's the use?" attitude.

The nurse's challenge is to encourage an interest in all aspects of the meal; the planning, shopping, cooking, and eating. People should be encouraged to have their meals in as pleasant a situation as possible, to eat slowly and savor the food. For some, listening to the radio, watching television, or reading while eating can contribute to the pleasure of the meal.

Many retired men and women living alone have never learned to plan, buy, or cook a meal, and they need help to undertake such a program for themselves. There are some community resources to help them, such as senior citizens center classes and clubs. They particularly need help with shopping when the food budget is limited, for it may be a problem in relation to small buying and cooking. Emphasis should be on the importance of a varied diet selected from the four major food groups. A home economist has offered the following suggestions for planning and shopping under these situations for this group.

**1.** Keep up-to-date on food prices by watching advertisements.
**2.** Buy no more food at one time than can be used easily; a big economy-sized package is not a bargain if it grows stale or spoils or the person tires of it.
**3.** Buy dry mixes for breads, cakes, and puddings; a portion can be used and the remainder will keep in a cool place.
**4.** Cook small amounts when possible; half a cup of shelled peas or cut string beans makes a normal serving.

The elderly need one or more servings a day of meat, fish, eggs, or other protein foods, also milk and milk products, cereal or bread, fruit, or fruit juices, and vegetables. Some elderly people may be unable to tolerate certain foods, such as raw fruits and vegetables. Vitamins and minerals play an important part in the individual's health and can be supplied through careful selection of foods. Although these persons may not be as active as formerly, a varied diet with plenty of fluids is still essential for good health.

Chronic diseases requiring diet restrictions occur frequently in this age group, including diabetes and cardiac disturbances, also degenerative diseases such as cancer and paralysis agitans. The physician will prescribe diets for these conditions, but the nurse will need to explain—more than once—why it is important to avoid salt or sugar and why soft foods may sometimes be necessary. Salt and sugar substitutes are available at pharmacies and grocery stores; they can make meals more palatable. Often the patient must experiment with them to find the one he likes best, as their flavors differ.

When older persons live in a household with younger people their diet regime can be adapted to the regular family meal, with the omission of raw fruits and vegetables as necessary and the avoidance of certain foods that are too rich or highly seasoned.

It is important to point out to the elderly, especially those living alone, the close relationship of nourishing food to good health and a sense of well-being in order to enjoy life.

## DIET IN DISEASE

Nutrition is not only essential in maintaining good health, but it is also an important factor in restoring the patient to health or at least enabling him to function to as normal a degree as possible. A discussion of the implications of nutrition in diseases frequently encountered by the community health nurse in the home is included here.

### Diabetes

Known to man for centuries, diabetes is a disease of nutritional interest and is encountered frequently by the community health nurse in her work. It is widespread, found in every economic and age group, but most often in women above forty years of age. There are indications that it might have an inherited tendency, although there are other causes.

When diabetes occurs in children and young adults, it is of a more serious nature. These young patients usually require insulin treatment and a special diet planned for their nutritional needs by the physician. Usually the patient or a family member is taught insulin administration at the health center, the physician's office, or during a hospital stay. The nutritionist confers with the patient and family members regarding the prescribed diet and ways of following it. She teaches the use of scales and other measures as needed and advises on menu planning and meal preparation. The community health nurse's responsibility is to follow up the teaching in the home by: (1) supervising the insulin administration until she is satisfied that either the patient or a family member understands and can carry out the procedure satisfactorily; (2) advising and assisting with diet problems as they arise in the home; and (3) watching for any unusual condition.

When diabetes occurs in patients over forty years of age, it usually has a milder course and can frequently be controlled by diet, sometimes a strict one. Obesity aggravates diabetes and often is a complicating factor and must be considered in the patient's entire treatment program in relation to diet, calorie intake, and exercise.

**Diet**  Obviously, any form of sugar, such as candy, cake, jam, cookies, pie, syrup, or honey, must be omitted from the diabetic's diet, yet he must have adequate nutrition for energy, body-building tissues, maintenance of good health, and resistance to infection. His food should have a psychological appeal and be attractively served. When a patient is placed on a diabetic diet he usually will have some resistance to the restrictions, and this is normal. In introducing the patient to his new diet, the nurse's objective is to change or adjust his behavior and former patterns of eating. It is important to teach him about the new diet slowly, as the learner must progress from one new idea to the next until he understands the restrictions the disease has put on his choice of foods. At first, some patients will place too much reliance on the effect of the insulin and tend to cheat a little in eating. The nurse should direct her teaching to activating the patient to accept the diet for its positive outcomes, e.g., lessening the chances of cataracts or foot circulation difficulties. It is important to help the patient recognize and accept his disease as a way of life. Listen to his accounts of frustration with the prescribed diet, the food substitutes, elimination from the diet of favorite foods, and change of eating habits. The nurse needs to amplify and reinforce what he has learned and assist him in translating it into his own changed dietary behavior.

*The exchange*  Diabetics, like other people, must have some carbohydrates, protein, and fat each day in their diet. It is essential for all but those with a very mild diabetic condition to eat the exact amount of the foods planned for their daily intake—no more, no less—especially if they are taking insulin. To facilitate planning for the patient's dietary needs, foods necessary to the diabetic's health were classified and divided in to six "exchanges": (1) milk; (2) vegetables; (3) fruits; (4) bread and cereals; (5) meats; and (6) fats. These are considered to be "protective" foods.

Most diabetic lists are made out in definite terms, indicating carefully weighed or measured amounts of carbohydrate, protein, and fats by grams, such as one cup of whole milk is carbohydrate, 12 grams; protein, 8 grams; and fat, 10 grams. One slice of baker's bread is carbohydrate, 15 grams; protein, 2 grams; and fat, 0 grams. Three ounces of cooked ground beef contains carbohydrate, 0; protein, 21 grams; and fat, 15 grams. The diet list and menus are made out for a twenty-four-hour period. An "exchange" system provides for wider choice in the diet and at the same time keeps the diet within the limitations of the patient's required grams of carbohydrate, protein, and fat for the twenty-four-hour period. A simple example would be that if a patient wanted a soft boiled egg for dinner in place of a meat serving, the egg would be considered equivalent to a meat allowance of 1 ounce in an exchange. A more involved exchange would be an apricot, cottage cheese, and lettuce salad for lunch, which would provide exchanges for one fruit, one meat, and one vegetable from the "A" list.

Vegetables on the "A" list include those that contain 3 grams or less of carbohydrates per one-half-cup serving; examples are lettuce, broccoli, young string beans, or greens. Usually they are allowed "as desired." Group "B" vegetables contain 7 percent or more carbohydrates per 100 grams and must be considered in the carbohydrate allowance for the twenty-four hours. They include green peas, winter squash, and such root vegetables as carrots, onions, beets, and turnips.[5]

Until the diabetic has full appreciation of the need for strict compliance to his required diet and is completely motivated to follow it, he will need the support of family and close friends to protect him from well-meaning people who will say, "This cake is very simple, it can't possibly hurt you." Or "Just one little piece of candy isn't anything."

Many patients have a diabetic condition so mild that medication is not indicated and treatment is based on a low carbohydrate intake. High blood sugar or sugar in the urine usually appears in this group only after a high carbohydrate intake including such sugar-rich foods as candy or cake. These patients need to be highly motivated to keep on their diet. The nurse can be of assistance to both patient and family in teaching the value of the diet and by her understanding and appreciation of the frustrations at not being able to have some of the "favorite" foods and foods that others are eating.

Together the nurse and patient and/or the family can plan a nutritious, satisfying diet that will maintain health and well-being. This should be a normal diet, but low in carbohydrate, and include meat and meat substitutes, some fats, and adequate vitamins and minerals. Fresh fruits can be used for dessert. Some bread and cereals are needed as a source of vitamin B complex. Families are always looking for new flavoring products which will mitigate the feeling of restriction regarding the patient's diet. Sugar and salt substitutes are available, which will enable the patient to have some of his favorite dishes. The addition of lemon juice or herbs and spices will often increase the tastiness of food that was lacking with the use of sugar substitute alone. When recipes can be devised which will satisfy the patient's taste, he is happier and the cook's work is made easier.

The patient should be alerted to the recognition and care of diabetic symptoms and conditions. The nurse should help the patient to learn the importance of following his diet and maintaining his personal care, e.g.,

[5]Linnea Anderson and John H. Browe, *Nutrituion and Family Health Service,* W. B. Saunders Company, Philadelphia, 1961, pp. 47–58.

care of the feet and daily exercise, so that his health and well-being can be sustained.

Because of improved diagnostic techniques, this mild type of diabetes is being discovered more frequently than in the past and provides the nurse with many opportunities for health teaching to patient and family regarding the disease and its care (see Case Situation 3).

## Heart Disease and Stroke

There are multiple causes for a person's suffering a heart attack or a stroke. Among them are obesity and a faulty diet extending over a period of years, lack of sufficient physical activity, emotionally stressful situations at home or at work, environmental factors, family history of such attacks, habitual cigarette smoking, and certain diseases such as diabetes. Usually an attack follows a combination of two or more of these causes or situations.

Many Americans have a diet high in cholesterol and animal (saturated) fats, such as eggs and meat, and dairy products such as butter, cream, and whole milk. Other foods of high caloric value such as ice cream and rich cakes and pies are common in the American diet. These foods tend to increase the cholesterol in the blood of many individuals, which in turn contributes to the development of artherosclerosis, a disease that underlies most heart attacks and strokes.

**Diet**   The diet of a patient convalescing from a heart attack or a stroke is of major importance in his return to health. He should understand that in all likelihood he will follow it fairly closely for the remainder of his life. In most cases, the physician orders a low-sodium diet, based on 1,200 to 1,800 calories per day. It is important that the patient and homemaker understand the major objectives of this diet, which are to provide for low calories, low-sodium intake, and low roughage and yet at the same time to supply sufficient amounts of vital nutrients. The patient's food likes and dislikes should be determined and respected in diet planning as far as possible. Sodium is an essential mineral for all human beings, animals, and plant life and a diet too low in sodium could prove harmful, but since sodium appears in practically all foods and drinking water, this is not of unusual concern. It is believed that the average person ingests between 5,000 and 8,000 milligrams of sodium in his daily diet. One level teaspoon of table salt contains approximately 2,300 milligrams of sodium. There are many sources of sodium in the average diet that the patient and his family might overlook in diet planning. In addition to table salt, foods may contain baking soda, baking powder, and often monosodium glutinate, the latter used for flavor accent. It is important to read food labels carefully on packaged, canned, or frozen foods to determine the amount of sodium included. Many frozen vegetables are processed with table salt, such as frozen lima beans, so patients and families should be alerted to the salt content of these foods.

A low-sodium diet is often flat and uninteresting to the taste, but care must be exercised in the use of seasonings. Table salt is to be avoided, also prepared mustard, meat sauces, celery and parsley flakes, and garlic, onion, and celery salts. Other herbs and spices, such as pepper, oregano, and paprika, may be added in small amounts unless limited by the physician. Fresh lemon and lime juice may be used for enhancing flavors. These juices could add to the vitamin C content of the diet, as well. Here, too, the family often needs help in finding substitutes for salt which will satisfy the patient's taste and increase variety in the diet. The nurse should show the patient or family how to appraise the content of the salt substitute so that they are aware of the meaning of the symbols on the label. Often the doctor will recommend a specific substitute.

The physician's diet list will include the foods the patient may have. This will be influenced by the severity of the attack and the resulting condition. Foods most patients should avoid include baked beans, bacon and ham, canned meats, canned soups, bread, crackers, and some cereals. Exchanges can provide flexibility in the diet, and with the physician's approval can be used by the heart patient as they are by the diabetic patient.

In planning a low-sodium diet to meet the heart patient's dietary needs, the homemaker or the patient himself must bear in mind the requirements for protein, carbohydrate, and fat as well as vitamins and minerals needed for general good health. It is important not to lose sight of the patient's general nutritional needs, while at the same time meeting those special dietary needs required by his heart condition. In other words, do not overlook the forest for the trees.

**Prevention**   As a preventive measure, the community health nurse should be alert while working with families to situations or health problems in the home that could lead to heart attacks in later years, such as emotionally stressful situations, heavy cigarette smoking, obesity, and diets apparently high in those foods conducive to heart disease. Helping families to face these situations objectively and before they become too serious provides opportunities that could be productive for teaching prevention of faulty heart conditions that could result in invalidism in later years.

Helpful material may be secured from the American Heart Association, and its local or state associations that the nurse can use in her teaching and the patient and family can have for reference.

## Phenylketonuria

There are other diseases of a chronic nature that require strict adherence to a specific diet if the patient is to live a normal, productive life. Man's knowledge of biochemistry, genetics, and other sciences is increasing at a rapid rate. This knowledge has implications for the health and care of many people with diseases about which little is known currently. The disease phenylketonuria, frequently referred to as PKU, is an example. The only treatment to date is severe dietary restrictions of certain proteins and a substitute formula, beginning at birth if possible and probably continuing throughout life. The physician prescribes a special diet which provides little variation, although as more knowledge is acquired about the disease it may be possible to widen the content of the diet. Research in this disease is still in the experimental stages. The nurse's function is to work closely with the physician and the parents, teaching the parents the reasons for the diet and for carrying it out to the letter. Some recent studies have pointed to the value of the mother following the diet, if indicated, during her pregnancy.

Parents need considerable emotional support because of the rigorous food restrictions that must be imposed on the infant and child and the frequent blood samples to be taken. Many parents and grandparents have some guilt feelings also, since this is a disease linked with heredity. Some members of the medical profession estimate that control of this disease eventually could result in the reduction of patient population in mental hospitals if the disease is discovered immediately after birth and treatment is instituted.

## SUMMARY

There is a growing reliance by many physicians on the part that diet therapy can play in the care of diseases and their prevention. The nurse must make an effort to keep abreast of current findings that are being added to the field of nutrition, so that she may work closely with the physician and the nutritionist in teaching families and individuals how to select foods that will contribute to their health and general well-being.

Much of what is known about nutrition today is pragmatic, but with continued studies and diet evaluations, underlying principles of nutrition will develop. Knowledge, supported by scientific studies, is being added constantly to what is already known from centuries of human experience with foods and by present-day studies and their application.

In her teaching, the nurse needs to keep in mind that nutrition is a personal matter, closely tied to cultural background, religious practices, family customs, present family organization, and individual preferences or likes and dislikes. The nutritionist, with special preparation in her field, is a valuable resource for the nurse. She will have many excellent ideas for menu planning and food selection. It is, however, the nurse's concern in her teaching of family and patient in the home and the health center to implement the prescribed diet in a way that satisfies the patient and family physically and psychologically so that the adjustment in food habits and menu selection becomes a way of life that will prolong health.

## SUGGESTED READING

Anderson, Linnea, and John H. Browe: *Nutrition in Family Health Service,* W. B. Saunders Company, Philadelphia, 1961, Chapters 2 and 9.

Benrman, Deaconess Maude: "Fresh Fruits in Season," *Forecast,* 23:4:20–24 (May-June) 1970.

Briggs, George M.: "Hunger and Nutrition," *Journal of Nutrition Education,* 1:3:4–6 (Winter) 1970.

Callahan, Catherine L.: "The White House Conference on Food, Nutrition and Health," *Nursing Outlook,* 18:58–60 (January) 1970.

Crim, Sarah R.: "Nutritional Problems of the Poor," *Nursing Outlook,* 17:65–67 (September) 1969.

Filer, L. J.: "The U.S.A. Today—Is It Free of Public Health Nutrition Problems? Anemia," *Journal of the American Public Health Association,* 59:327–338 (February) 1969.

Franklin, Ruth E.: "Know-Why and Nutrition," *Forecast,* 21:2:14–18 (March-April) 1968.

Martin, E. A.: *Nutrition in Action,* 3d ed., Holt, Rinehart and Winston, Inc., New York, 1971.

"Message From the White House," Editorial, *Journal of Nursing Education,* 8:4:3–7 (November) 1969.

Mitchell, H. S., et al.: *Cooper's Nutrition in Health and Disease,* 15th ed., J. B. Lippincott Company, Philadelphia, 1968.

National Research Council Report: *Recommended Dietary Allowances,* 7th rev. ed., National Academy of Science, Washington, D.C., 1968.

O'Brien, Marian M.: *The Bible Cook Book,* Collier Books, The Macmillan Company, New York, 1961.

Rosenstock, Irwin M.: "Psychological Forces, Motivation and Nutrition Education," *Journal of the American Public Health Association,* 59:1992–1997 (November) 1969.

Stokes, Shirlee Ann: "Fasting for Obesity," *American Journal of Nursing,* 69:796–799 (April) 1969.

Watkins, Julia D., and Fay T. Moss: "Confusion in the Management of Diabetes," *American Journal of Nursing,* 69:521–524 (March) 1969.

# 8
# Selected Concerns For Community Health Nurses

Frequently in the present era the emergence of selected health problems is brought dramatically to the attention of citizens by means of the communication media such as radio, newspapers, and television. The intent of the communication media is to focus the attention of citizens on existing health situations that are in need of corrective action. By covering all aspects of a selected health problem descriptively and from various viewpoints, the media reveal the complexity of any health concern that affects the population and attempt to stimulate all citizens to become more knowledgeable about the controversial aspects of the problem. The world in which we live and the multiple things that happen in it have a bearing on the lives of all consumers, whether they are cognizant of it or not. In the past, criticism has been directed toward citizens who would not become involved when someone was in trouble. The emphasis today is exerted toward involving consumers to participate more in matters affecting their lives. Some health concerns about which citizens are receiving information are those that are or should be of interest or importance to them, such as drug abuse, human sexuality, and ecologic problems. Because the needs of our society are changing so rapidly and the traditional modes of performance are often no longer valid, new and innovative measures must be taken by all citizens to cope with today's health problems.

Community health nurses must accept the challenge also and be willing to try new measures for which they may not always feel adequately prepared. The health concerns that are receiving constant daily attention may be problems that have not been sufficiently emphasized in nurses' educational programs. The concerns for which nurses must become better prepared and the particular families who often feel an inadequacy in coping with these concerns are discussed in this chapter. By making use of professional consultants, professional literature, audiovisual media, and appropriate community facilities, the nurse who desires additional preparation or increased knowledge can facilitate her readiness to assist families who want help for the prevailing health problems which confuse and frustrate them. She can implement activities for which successful results will contribute to the practices of the nursing profession. For example, the nurse could institute a short-term, intensive training program for an aphasic adult by getting a firm commitment from all family members to participate in a behavior-modification program which requires the patient to verbalize or write his desires at all times before his needs are attended to by any one in the family.[1] By requiring written or verbal data from the family preceding and during the training period, the frequency of the patient's speech or written activity can be tabulated and evaluated by the nurse and all participating members of the family. The nurse can supervise the project although she is not directly participating or making frequent home visits, and yet she is aiding the family to effect a desirable change in the patient's status. By so doing, the nurse is instrumental in training the family to implement activities that are gaining successful results and giving the family a sense of responsibility and satisfaction. At the same time, she is enlarging her field of practice with an economy of personal time. The nurse can also expand her depth of knowledge and practice successfully in any selected field of health if she wishes to be innovative and create an essential position for nurses that has not always been seen as suitable for nurses. For example, the nurse could institute regular meeting sessions with small groups of young people in schools or community centers to give them the opportunity to talk freely about any subject that interests them in an unstructured environment. By so doing, the nurse may be able to determine the basis for the "generation gap" and gather data regarding the nature of the communication difficulties between young and old which are cited so frequently by young people as a problem. By endeavoring to meet some of the crucial lacks in health care and needs of selected citizens in the society, nurses can do their part to achieve higher levels of health in the nation's population. The following health problems represent only a few of the health concerns requiring further study and innovative efforts by nurses.

## HUMAN SEXUALITY

Human sexuality, sex education, and family planning have diverse meanings for many persons in Western society. It has been a subject little talked about by health professionals, including nurses, because of moral values, ignorance, avoidance, or embarrassment.

[1] For an elaboration of the behavior modification program, see Chap. 5.

A person's sex is determined genetically and influenced by the psychosocial environment of the society and family in which he lives and interacts. Like other maturational phases, the sexual phase has its highs and lows, its agonies and ecstasies. Man's sexuality is intrinsic to his being and colors his thoughts, ideas, social interactions, physical well-being, and his ability not only to reproduce but to nurture his offspring. However, the road to adulthood and maturity—including sexual maturity—is rocky and unchartered for many in the society.[2]

Human sexuality is more than the physical sex act, and nurses must be prepared to counsel about sexuality, contraception, abortions, and venereal diseases. Most nurses are familiar with family-planning kits which contain contraceptive devices. However, to be more effective in meeting the specific needs of patients, they must be more than informational resources. According to Cassidy, they must assume four roles during the interview: (1) the nurse *resource*, who has correct information about contraception, sex, abortion, and venereal disease; (2) the nurse *friend*, who helps the patient to trust and confide in her; (3) the nurse *authority*, who defines the limits of use of contraceptive devices and medical-care resources; and (4) the nurse *mother surrogate*, who acts as a responsible adult figure and who listens nonjudgmentally.[3] Elder recommends that sexual histories must be taken on all persons from puberty to old age. A sexual history is an integral part of the psychological-social-physical evaluation of the patient and forms the basis of sexual counseling. It provides information about a person's needs, expectations, and behavior in his sexual role.[4] It should be taken when patients are pregnant, are having marital problems, are unwed mothers or fathers, are seeking an abortion or family-planning information, have a venereal disease, or are complaining about sexual inadequacy.

Community health nurses must be aware of their own feelings of self-acceptance regarding their sexuality, their own values, their biases regarding sexual activity, and the extent of their knowledge of sexuality at each developmental stage of a person. They must be acquainted with contraceptive methods, the anatomy, physiology, and diseases of the sexual organs, and community agencies dealing with family planning, venereal diseases, abortions, and sexual counseling.

When nursing students are given an assignment to do a teaching project or engage in some type of community project, they frequently select the subject of human sexuality with which to deal. For example, they sometimes devise questionnaires which elicit the knowledge of respondents

[2]Jeanne D. Fonseca, "Sexuality—A Quality of Being Human," Editorial, *Nursing Outlook*, 18:11:25 (November) 1970.
[3]Jean Trotter Cassidy, "Teenagers In a Family Planning Clinic," *Nursing Outlook*, 18:11:30–31 (November) 1970.
[4]Mary-Scovill Elder, "Nurse Counseling on Sexuality," *Nursing Outlook*, 18:11:39 (November) 1970.

about venereal diseases, sex education, or contraceptive methods. Others elect to teach a small class of students about a selected aspect of sex education. Teachers in schools generally respond favorably to students' requests to conduct a teaching project on selected health subjects. Recently a nursing student was given permission to teach a brief series of sex education classes to eighth-grade girls in a junior high school. At the beginning of the class, the nursing student gave a short quiz with one of the questions asking, "What do you know about the menstrual cycle?" The answers of the students revealed a distribution of replies showing ignorance, misperceptions, and accurate knowledge about menstruation. One girl wrote, "I think menestration is something I don't know about! It's taken place in me but I don't understand exactly what it is. I have only a vague idea. Something to do with the pituitary gland in the brain, which sends hormones or something like that to the lower part of the body, which is secreted through the vagina." Another girl replied, "It is when a girl's body changes and she has too much blood and this is when she gets rid of the extra blood."

When counseling about sexuality, community health nurses must initiate the subject in as comfortable a manner as possible, utilizing all the relationship skills they possess. Frequently the patient gives cues of being troubled and responds to questions with discomfort. However, if the nurse persists in being concerned about the patient's nonverbal evidences of anxiety, the patient may eventually divulge the thoughts or activities that are troubling her. The nurse is then enabled to give physiological and psychological explanations, clarify misconceptions, and be supportive as needed.

The families who are particularly in need of counseling about human sexuality are the young adults, adolescents, and the parents of teen-agers. Through the communications media, all people, but particularly the young people in our society, are influenced almost daily to believe that sex is fun, is free, and must be tried. What is not given emphasis is that with sexual activity comes responsibility—perhaps for another human life.[5] Concurrent with the concept of responsibility is the acceptance of the consequences of one's actions. Not all persons are immediately ready to assume responsibility for the consequences of their activities. The helping professions, particularly nurses, must deal in a nonjudgmental and individualized way with counseling all people who demonstrate overt and covert needs in relation to human sexuality.

## ALCOHOLISM

Many families with an alcoholism problem are not immediately detected by community health nurses as having this particular problem, because all overt evidences of drinking are disguised in any number of interesting ways.

[5]Ethel H. Naugle, "Nurse, Make It Well," *Nursing Outlook,* 18:11:41 (November) 1970.

Sometimes a nurse will be aware that a family member drinks to excess but does not offer her services because of a feeling of inability to cope with the problem, a preset conviction that nothing constructive can be effected, or an attitude of disapproval based on her own feelings regarding the use of alcohol.

There have been a number of descriptions of alcoholism that include ideas stating that it is a disease, a condition, a physiologic and psychological disturbance, or that alcohol is an addictive, tranquilizing drug. However, any person who drinks alcoholic beverages to the extent that it interferes with his meaningful living and breaks down relationships with his mate, children, relatives, employer, and friends may be an alcoholic. Common characteristics of an alcoholic include: (1) loneliness; a sense of estrangement, of isolation from his fellow man; (2) dependency; a desire for others to care for him; (3) depression; a sense of worthlessness, hopelessness, and helplessness, which he tries to cover up by putting on the mask of happiness and gaiety; (4) aggression or hostility, which is often turned inward by self-punishing and self-destructive drinking habits; (5) confusion about sexual identification; and (6) anxiety, which manifests itself as a free-floating feeling of unrest and uneasiness.[6] When one member of a household is alcoholic, all other family members are affected and influenced in one way or another (see Case Situation 8 and Case Record 9).

Community health nurses are just beginning to participate more actively with the rehabilitation and counseling services given to alcoholics and their families. They are becoming aware of their particular value in counseling family members. The family must maintain an adequate living standard whether or not the alcoholic seeks help. However, the family needs support and guidance from a professional person who understands the various manifestations of the alcoholism problem. The *attitude* of the nurse is extremely important, as is her *assessment* of the *readiness* of the family to seek assistance from a wide variety of appropriate community facilities. The alcoholic and the family members need understanding, caring, strengthening, and hope that life can be better.

The nurse can acquire essential data about all facets of alcoholism from a proliferation of new books and informational pamphlets dealing with the problem and from visitation of alcoholism treatment and referral centers. It is also educational and often a rewarding experience to visit Alcoholics Anonymous, Al-Anon, and Al-Ateen groups. Alcoholics Anonymous (AA) is a loosely knit organization of alcoholics who meet regularly to help themselves and others to stay sober. AA gives emotional support to its members and relies on a "Power greater than ourselves" for strength in overcoming

[6]James A. Knight and Winborn E. Davis, *Comprehensive Community Mental Health Clinic,* Charles C Thomas, Publisher, Springfield, Illinois, 1964, p. 78.

their difficulties. Al-Anon and Al-Ateen groups are spouses or children of alcoholics. Their meetings are patterned similarly to AA meetings.

A nursing student who became interested in the problem of alcoholism reported her reactions as follows:

I have to admit that I was not particularly excited to attend an open AA meeting, but afterward realized my preconceived notions were mistaken about what took place and the kind of people who attended. Then going to an Al-Anon meeting was just about the most exciting experience I have gained this quarter. There was a group of about fifteen women who were very friendly, frank, and ready to discuss their troubles at home with an alcoholic husband.

It is quite evident to me that learning about the problem of alcoholism from a textbook cannot compare to the first-hand experience of seeing and learning about the problem being dealt with through community resources and the families and victims of alcoholism. Certainly I feel much better qualified now to refer those in need of such help to the appropriate resources and interpret the program of the resource, since I know what really takes place.

Since alcoholism is a major public health problem that affects many families, the nurse must become familiar with the role for which she is best suited to move the family in the direction of rehabilitation. This role may be active counseling and education of the alcoholic or family members, persuasive referral of the alcoholic or family to appropriate community facilities, or purely supportive listening functions, which are designed with subtleness to motivate the alcoholic and family members to seek treatment as soon as possible.

## DRUG ABUSE

A public health problem which is affecting all social classes in America is the increasing use of legal and illegal drugs. Television programs, newspaper accounts, books, magazines, and other communication media are focusing on the drug abuse of youth as youth seek new thrills and new experiences in the realm of "mind expansion."

The word "drug" has many meanings. The medical approach is commonly associated with the meaning that a drug is a medicine prescribed by the physician for specified and limited use in the treatment and prevention of disease, in the relief of pain, and in the restoration of a feeling of well-being.[7] In this capacity the nurse is well acquainted with the multiplicity of drugs that some patients take with complete conformity to the physician's instructions. However, many patients require proper interpretation of the drugs they take, the purposes of the drugs, the recognition of side-effects

[7]Helen H. Nowlis, *Drugs On the College Campus,* Doubleday & Company, Inc., Garden City, N.Y., 1969, p. 4.

that may occur, requiring prompt reporting of new symptoms. They also need a coordination of their time schedules in taking drugs at various times of the day since some people are not reliable in adhering to the schedule advised by the physician. When the nurse requests to see all the medications the patient is taking, she must be thorough in eliciting all information the patient knows about the drugs he is taking, the frequency with which he takes them, and the commitment he feels about taking the drugs. By writing all the identifying information about the drugs on notepaper, she can return to her office and look up all descriptive data in the most current *Physicians Desk Reference.* Sometimes when all the information is assembled, she may feel compelled to speak with the physician about the patient's drug-taking practices in order to clear up misperceptions, omissions, or complicity of the patient's drug intake.

The legal approach to a drug is that it is a habit-forming narcotic that is widely believed to be dangerous to the individual and society. A common acceptance of the word "drug" as used by the youth of today is that it is any chemical substance that alters mood, perception, or consciousness and is misused, to the apparent detriment of society.[8] There seems to be an increasing fascination with the use of drugs by the youth culture, which encourages experimentation and new experiences. The youth culture attributes the generation gap of old and young with the consequent breakdown in communication, the pressures for achievement, the depersonalization of society, and the purposelessness of life as reasons for taking drugs and youth state that misuse of drugs is no different from misuse of alcohol. They point out the inconsistency with which adults view drug use as compared to the way adults use legal drugs and alcohol. They dislike intensely any teaching, advice, or conversation that is predominantly moralizing.

As pointed out by Nowlis, the real problem is not drugs, but people who use drugs. These are people with personal, social, and intellectual problems who feel the need to try drugs for innumerable reasons.[9] Community health nurses who are working in community clinics, treatment centers, or free unofficial clinics for drug addicts or teen-agers are learning that some youth have an extremely sophisticated knowledge of drugs and like to experiment imaginatively with combinations of drugs just for the exhilarating, dramatic effect. They are learning about the importance of communication, of listening, of honesty, of strengthening self-worth in others, and allowing for independence in others within acceptable boundaries. The nurse must be up-to-date in knowledge about drugs in usage, about current youth philosophies, likes, and dislikes, and she must be skilled in relating with troubled persons. If she will initiate opportunities to work with youth in schools or community groups, serve as a coordinator for all interested

[8]*Ibid.,* pp. 4–5.
[9]Helen H. Nowlis, "Why Students Use Drugs," *American Journal of Nursing,* 68:8:1680–1685 (August) 1968.

community personnel, enlist the services of people who have overcome the habit and are willing to talk and work with those who are still addicts or drug users, she will be viewed increasingly as a necessary accomplice among professionals and nonprofessionals who are dealing with problems of drug abuse.

## MENTAL HEALTH

In community health nursing the mental and emotional health of individuals and families are seen in terms of their everyday coping abilities. If pathologic symptoms of a psychiatric nature are apparent in any way, the nurse works toward referring the person to an appropriate physician or community facility. She counsels the family and lends support if the identified patient is hospitalized. If consultation is needed from a mental health expert, she makes use of this resource. However, her expertise is primarily with families who are momentarily overcome with stressful life events and need only temporary assistance to reestablish their equilibrium and sense of confidence in their own coping abilities. For some families the intervention by the nurse may be needed for only a few weeks, whereas for other families, the service may be prolonged because of the slow process of building and strengthening beliefs within persons who are distrustful of constructive efforts in their behalf.

Many individuals and families of all social classes show evidences of low self-esteem as characterized in their behavior or verbal remarks about themselves. To be a minimally effective person, one must have at least minimal self-esteem. As described by Ryan, an individual must be able to perceive himself as having some power, capable of influencing his environment to his own benefit based on the actual experience and exercise of such power.[10] For families living in poverty, the building of self-esteem within individuals is an essential component of the nurse's work with them. The process of strengthening and building is time-consuming, requires patience and tolerance for frustrations, but it is rewarding in the long run. Another component of equal importance is the family's right of self-determination to participate and make decisions about the activities designed to benefit them.

The focus of attention on the mental health of persons in society is gaining momentum to counteract fears about the depersonalization and alienation trends that are appearing daily along with technological innovations. Many positive, constructive influences are operating in America, but

---

[10]Dr. William Ryan, "Preventive Services In the Social Context: Power, Pathology, and Prevention," Bernard L. Bloom and Dorothy P. Buck (eds.), *Preventive Services in Mental Health Programs,* Western Interstate Commission for Higher Education, Boulder, Colorado, December, 1967, p. 50.

greater momentum can be achieved if the potential forces of a great diversity of peoples can be seen as parts of a whole, working toward improved mental and emotional health of the citizens in the society. Community health nurses play their part in this endeavor by helping to build self-esteem in individuals and families who have need for it, participating with and teaching consumers in neighborhood or community health centers, and supporting social legislation designed to remove inequities in the delivery of health care.

A trend is beginning in which the institutionalization of people for long-term treatment is no longer considered desirable, and comprehensive community mental health facilities and clinics are being built or planned for by geographic regions. A comprehensive health program makes use of promotional, supportive, and therapeutic resources and includes personnel from many related fields, such as mental health, public welfare, education, probation, child welfare, community health, and recreation. A cooperative effort is expended to assist populations at risk such as juvenile delinquents, persons who have attempted suicide, abused children, dysfunctional families, families with handicapped or retarded children, and others.[11] Increasing use is made of trained paraprofessionals and community health aides. The role of the mental health professional in the field requires considerable versatility because of the varying backgrounds of his professional and nonprofessional associates, the need for a common, understandable language, and the increased active participation of consumers in health programs affecting them.[12] The community health nurse is an essential team member in a community health center because of her belief in wellness and prevention of disease, experience with consumers with different backgrounds, and expertise in coordinating personnel and community resources.

## SUICIDE

Often community health nurses inadvertently learn that persons to whom they are giving service have formerly threatened suicide or are giving it serious thought because of their feelings of despair and helplessness and a belief that nothing can be done about their lives. In order to be responsive to any "cry for help," the nurse must be cognizant of prevention or postvention phases of suicide. Prevention of suicide involves the identification of high-risk groups and/or individuals; the ready availability of responsive services such as crisis clinics; the dissemination of information, particularly about prodromal clues; the lowering of taboos so that citizens can more easily ask for help; and the sensitization of professionals and ordinary citi-

[11]Knight and Davis, *op. cit.,* p. 5.
[12]Howard E. Freeman and Rosalind Gertner, "The Changing Posture of the Mental Health Consortium," *American Journal of Orthopsychiatry,* 39:1:116–124 (January) 1969.

zens to the recognition of potential suicide. Postvention activities are those that occur after a suicidal event, such as (1) working with an individual after he has made a suicide attempt, or (2) working with survivor victims of a committed suicide to help them with their sense of anguish, guilt, anger, shame, and perplexity.[13] Life has two aspects, its duration—length or shortness—and its scope—richness or aridity.[14] Community health nurses have frequent opportunity to enable others to see life as having meaning and richness, provided they recognize early behavioral clues of ambivalence regarding the value of life in their patients.

McLean defined a suicidal crisis as a period of time during which a person experiences an extremely strong wish to die, which conflicts with the wish to live. The crucial element that makes suicide prevention possible is the ambivalence. The nurse must utilize all her knowledge and relationship skills to keep a potentially suicidal patient focusing on the desire to live. Crisis intervention in suicide prevention is outlined in detail by McLean, consisting essentially of the following elements:

1. Establishing a relationship, maintaining contact, and obtaining information
2. Identifying and clarifying the focal problem or problems
3. Evaluating the suicidal potential
4. Assessing strengths and resources of the patient
5. Formulating a therapeutic plan and mobilizing the resources of the patient and others[15]

When the nurse tells the patient contemplating suicide, "Don't do it," she is communicating that she cares. If she is able to extract a promise from the patient which is purposely designed to be fulfilled at a later time, she has probably assisted the patient in overcoming his existing ambivalence of the moment. Few persons contemplating suicide renege on a promise. By being aware of the nature of suicide, in either the prevention or postvention phase, the nurse adds another dimension to her intervention skills.

## CHRONIC DEGENERATIVE DISEASES AND DEATH

For those individuals and family members who must learn to adjust to the changes evoked by the symptoms of chronic and degenerative diseases, such as multiple sclerosis, arthritis, emphysema, terminal carcinoma, cerebral vascular accident (stroke), and similar debilitating diseases, special

[13]Edwin S. Shneidman, *On the Nature of Suicide*, Jossey-Bass, Inc., Publishers, San Francisco, 1969, pp. 20–21.
[14]*Ibid.*, p. 29.
[15]Lenora J. McLean, "Action and Reaction in Suicidal Crisis," *Nursing Forum*, 8:1:28–41, 1969.

attention must be given. Not only the patient but all family members are affected in some way or other by the required adaptation to the existence and concurrent dependencies produced by chronic diseases. All patients and families adjust in their own individualistic ways and many need assistance in learning to accommodate with essential changes necessitated by the disruption of roles and tasks in the home. Many professional references deal with the stages of adaptation or coping mechanisms undergone by patients when chronic diseases are diagnosed or terminal prognoses are given. However, few authors as yet take heed of the distinct adjustments expected of family members who are directly affected by the change of status of the patient, a family member with a one-time vital role in the family structure. Kubler-Ross discussed the physical and emotional adjustments undergone by family members of patients who were dying and recognized that family members also went through emotional stages of adjustment very similar to those described for dying patients. She pointed out the importance of someone to befriend family members, allow them to work through their rational or irrational feelings about a pending death, and ease the movement of feelings toward acceptance without guilt.[16] The family-centered community health nurse is the qualified person for the role of comforting and assisting family members when chronic degenerative diseases are diagnosed and terminal prognoses are anticipated (see Case Record 7).

The stages of adaptation or coping mechanisms undergone by patients and family members when they realize the necessity for accepting a change in their lives have been identified by various authors as sequential and progressive in nature for most people. According to Crate, who studied stages of adaptation for the diagnosis of multiple sclerosis, the first stage is one of *denial* and *disbelief,* which is manifested in a variety of ways, depending upon the individual's life style of coping with crisis or conflict. Denial can be exhibited for a short period or it can be long-lasting. The nurse should listen to all expressions of feeling noncritically and help the individual to articulate with clarity. By drawing out existing feelings of resentment and bitterness, she facilitates the adjustment process. The second stage consists of a *developing awareness,* which is commonly manifested as anger. By being empathic, the nurse can listen to arguments, criticisms, and attacks without responding as a singled-out target. She must be aware that anger is a realistic defense when a person's life is capriciously changed without his consent. The nurse must consciously not argue with the patient or moralize about any issue. The third stage is one of *recrganization,* in which relationships with family members are adjusted and accommodations are made in the activities of daily living. At this time the nurse must continue to listen to the expressions of feelings of the patient and family

[16]Elisabeth Kubler-Ross, *On Death and Dying,* The Macmillan Company, New York, 1969, pp. 157–180.

members, suggest suitable practical rehabilitative methods for readjusting their household routines, encourage the use of appropriate self-help devices, and give verbal support for accomplishments successfully attained by the persons assuming new roles and duties. The fourth stage consists of a *resolution* or *identity change,* in which the patient acknowledges the reality changes he sees in himself. He begins to identify that he is similar to other patients with the same diagnosis. Dependent upon the diagnosis and the home situation, the nurse at this point must consider releasing the patient, encouraging him to become self-directive within his limits, and to seek out relationships with others.[17] If the diagnosis is a terminal one, the early stages of denial and anger precede the latter stages of adaptation, which are aptly described by Kubler-Ross as those of bargaining, depression, and acceptance. *Bargaining* is a period when the patient makes a bargain with God in the hope that his death will be postponed. *Depression* is the natural state during which a patient is filled with sorrow that he will soon lose everything and everyone he loves. If he is allowed to express his sorrow, he becomes emotionally prepared for the final stage of acceptance. During the final stage, effective communications are predominantly nonverbal rather than verbal.[18]

The concept of hope was graphically described by Kubler-Ross as an essential ingredient in all people. They are nourished by it and appreciate any small fragment of hope that is offered on a realistic basis. The hope may not necessarily be directed toward total cure, but a remission of the illness or an anticipation about the next life.[19] The role and potency of hope in a person's life must always be remembered by nurses caring for patients and families who are experiencing any type of illness, whether cure is envisioned or death is pending.

## ECOLOGIC HEALTH PROBLEMS

Only recently has man become concerned with ecology, the study of the relationship of total man with his total environment. Such environmental hazards as pollution of air, water, and soil by biologic, chemical, and physical contaminants; the urban ghettos, with overcrowding of people, unsafe housing, inadequate disposal of wastes, malnutrition, and drug abuse; radiation, accidents, inequities of health care, and additional hazards are brought to the attention of citizens with increasing urgency. Neighborhoods or communities can be found in almost any section of the United States that reflect severe inadequacies of the present health-care delivery system and existence of ecological problems. Breslow reported that after touring several

[17]Marjorie Crate, "Nursing Functions In Adaptation to Chronic Illness," *American Journal of Nursing,* 65:72–76 (October) 1965.
[18]Kubler-Ross, *op. cit.,* pp. 82–136.
[19]*Ibid.,* pp. 138–156.

communities in the United States to investigate typical environmental and medical-care situations directly related to the rise of serious health problems, he came away "shocked and still reeling. Circumstances that only can be called health brutality pervade the lives of millions of American people who live in communities that seem designed to break the human spirit."[20]

Recommendations were advanced for all health professionals, including community health nurses, to engage in strategies for health progress which are based on improvement in the quality of life for all people and meeting human needs. Health professionals must join hands with organizations that are emerging in neighborhoods to fight for better health conditions. In addition, new forms of local community health services must be initiated and maintained, so that there is a close relationship between health professionals and neighborhood organizations. Professional technical competence, as provided by health professionals, is as necessary as the fostering of social forces activated by neighborhood organizations. Both play a part toward compelling action programs designed to care for urgent health needs.[21] For community health nurses the broadening scope of community health requires an ever-increasing knowledge about man, health, and the influences of the physical and social environment as never before seen in the history of mankind. The necessity of being concerned with total health on a comprehensive basis has never been so urgent.


## SELECTED CONSUMER GROUPS

In addition to selected health problems and concerns, selected groups of consumers must receive more emphasis than has been currently practiced by community health nurses. By working with groups, the nurse reaches many more people than on the traditional one-to-one basis and expands the opportunity to integrate desirable health practices to the target population through exploration and discussion of ideas. In group work, everyone learns when all are viewed as resource persons who draw from past and present personal experiences and perceptions of the subject being studied. Opportunities are unlimited for setting up discussion groups with people who would be responsive to a variety of common interests related to health. The task of the nurse is complex, because while she is visiting an individual on a one-to-one basis and ascertaining his health needs and interests, at the same time she can be mentally visualizing future common-interest discussion groups which would be beneficial for this person in expanding his horizons through intellectual and socialization means. Two populations in America with whom the nurse could work in exciting ways because of their

[20]Lester Breslow, "The Urgency of Social Action For Health," *American Journal of Public Health,* 60:1:10–16 (January) 1970.
[21]*Ibid.*

unique needs, concerns, and segregation are the elderly and the youth. They comprise a large segment of a special population that requires deeper understanding than is presently evident by the general public.

## Elderly Groups

In America, the man retiring at sixty-five has a fifty-fifty chance for living twelve more years.[22] In living longer, the elderly person must adapt to many demanding changes at a time when adaptation is difficult. Retirement from an active work life, the death of spouse and friends, and failing health are some of the necessary adaptations that must be made. The elderly generally are not highly valued in our society, since their productivity and social contributions have lessened or ceased.[23] A complaint of an actively independent eighty-four-year-old housewife, who perceived herself as not as old as her friends, was voiced resentfully, "People discriminate against us because we're old. They expect us to *act* old and they treat us as if we were ancient."

Some of the crises which must be met by the elderly include completion of the parental role, withdrawal from active community and organizational leadership, termination of marriage through death of one's mate, loss of an independent household, loss of interest in distant goals and plans, the necessity of depending on others or on society for support, advice, and management of funds, physical disabilities such as arthritis and cataracts, assumption of a subordinate position to adult persons, and taking up membership in groups made up largely of old people.[24] The manner in which the elderly person copes with and adjusts to these crises as they occur in his life depends on his personality, attitude, and past experiences, which may have been negative or positive. In order for aging to occur satisfactorily, it is essential that flexibility in adjustment to new situations be developed. Community health nurses can play an important role in assisting the elderly to strengthen their coping abilities, since the nurses have the opportunity to interact with the aged in nursing homes, retirement homes, senior activity centers, and private homes.

Retirement has a definite effect on the elderly, because it forces them to change many of their basic relationships and habits. A new framework of activity and new interests have to be developed. Since a basic psychological hunger of man is for time structure, the retired person must find new purposeful and satisfactory ways of structuring his day. A variety of tasks, activities, or hobbies can be undertaken, dependent upon the energy, en-

[22]Benjamin A. Kogan, *Health, Man In a Changing Environment,* Harcourt Brace Jovanovich, Inc., New York, 1970, p. 594.
[23]Paul L. Niebanck, *The Elderly In Older Urban Areas,* Institute For Environmental Studies, University of Pennsylvania, Philadelphia, 1965, pp. 91–92.
[24]*Ibid.,* pp. 96–97.

thusiasm, and interest of the person. Sometimes a reduction of income affects the manner in which the retired person lives. Or the income may be ample but a decline in health changes the living pattern so that some former activities can no longer be enjoyed. When widowhood occurs, this often means a severance of a fundamental relationship that has given stability and meaning to life. The process of readjustment is a lengthy one, and often important decisions have to be made during this critical period which affects the remainder of the person's life.[25]

**Working with the Elderly**
Some myths about the elderly which must be checked out in terms of the acquaintance of the nurse with any aged patient include: (1) the expected passive behavior pattern of the person in retirement. He has earned the right to "take it easy" and now can rest. Does the patient conform to this myth? Is he content? What is his philosophy of life? Is he satisfied with resting? (2) Dependence on others for advice and assistance is a natural and inevitable consequence of advancing age. Does the patient accept dependence graciously or is he fiercely independent? Who are the acceptable persons from whom he will take advice and assistance? (3) Custodial care in institutions is the answer to chronic illness, invalidity, and mental disturbances. How does the patient feel about institutional care? Has he personally visited any nursing or retirement homes? If he needs custodial care, what does this mean to him? (4) Withdrawal from social participation tends to accompany departure from employment. Is the patient active socially? Has he withdrawn from former social groups voluntarily? Is he lonely? Does he need encouragement to join new groups, such as a senior activity center? (5) No preparation for retirement is required or expected. How is the patient adjusting to retirement? Did he anticipate most of the changes? How would he advise others to prepare for retirement? (6) Older persons are unable to learn new skills.[26] Does the patient believe this myth? What new skills might he be interested in trying? Is he a *possibility* thinker—a person who perceptively probes every problem, proposal, and opportunity to discover the positive aspects present in almost every human situation? Or is he an *impossibility* thinker—a person who makes swift, sweeping passes over a proposed idea, scanning it with a sharp, negative eye, looking only for reasons why something won't work instead of visualizing ways in which it could work?[27]

[25] *Ibid.,* pp. 97–102.
[26] Ernest W. Burgess, *Aging In Western Societies,* The University of Chicago Press, 1960, p. 20.
[27] Robert H. Schuller, *Move Ahead With Possibility Thinking,* Doubleday & Company, Inc., Garden City, N.Y., 1967, pp. 2–3.

Since most elderly persons experience chronic illness to some degree, they must adjust in a way most conducive to their life style. Consequently, the nurse must work with them in terms of the goals which meet their most urgent needs. The goals may be rehabilitative measures, positive attitudes which promote preventive means, educational practices which maintain optimum health, or combinations of all three objectives. By assessing the patient as a *whole* person, his needs can be determined by talking with him and gaining an inclusive perspective of his physical, nutritional, psychological, social, recreational, economic, and environmental condition. Conti described several elderly persons who had individually adapted to life styles that were unsatisfactory because of their loneliness. She described how the community health nurse visited these persons who initially denied their loneliness, but consented to receiving the attention of a "caring" person and eventually made adjustments to more satisfactory coping patterns. For some, this meant attendance of senior citizen groups for socialization or participation in a range of activities. The work of the nurse with these elderly people meant communicating her value of them as human beings and showing acceptance, understanding, and patience with them before they were ready to reveal their feelings or willingness to make a change in adjustment.[28] Elderly persons sometimes move slowly and think slowly, but they are very responsive to the enthusiasm and warmth of young people and delight in any kind of exchange with young people. They also are very responsive to sensory stimulation and should be touched or stroked whenever a practical opportunity arises. For example, the nurse should always feel the pulse whether she needs to know it or not, comb the hair, press the ankle for edema, or give a reassuring body squeeze whenever she wants to communicate approval or acceptance. In many ways, elderly persons are like little children and don't mind being treated with warmth, fun, or simple games. If encouraged to attend small group discussions where a subject of interest is being explored, participants can find this to be a stimulating way for sharing ideas or receiving recognition, particularly when they have an able nurse leader or facilitator.

## Youth Groups

The youth of America have been the focus of much publicity and concern in recent years. The terms identity, generation gap, alienation, anomie, withdrawal, noninvolvement, nonconformity, apathy, indifference, dropout, dissent, violence, protest, hair—all reflect the basis of the concern and puzzlement directed toward youth by adults. In studying a cross section of youth, one finds common problems but different manifestations of behavior. Alienation is said to be the predominant problem and manifests itself as a

[28]Mary Louise Conti, "The Loneliness of Old Age," *Nursing Outlook,* 18:8:28–30 (August) 1970.

way of life which is an explicit rejection of the values and outlooks of American culture and our technological society.[29] Alienation is the response of individuals to dilemmas and problems that confront our entire society. Extraordinary demands are made on the members of the society, forcing them to adapt to chronic social change, achieve a sense of personal wholeness in a complex and fragmented society, resolve major discontinuities between childhood and adulthood, and locate positive values in an intellectual climate that consistently undermines such values.[30] The youth have been exposed most of their young lives to television and communication mass media, which project an image of a stereotype personality with values, practices, and desirability that is created by the media and not based on the real desires of people.[31] Youth have been raised in a period of rapid change and so have a different sense of time—for example, about the time it takes to get things done. Youth live for today, in a time when parents' advice, which is based on yesterday, is not relevant to the world that they encounter. They have multiple sources for information—school, radio, television, movies, newspapers, periodicals, books. They see authority as something changeable, relative, and questionable.[32] Youth have been raised by families who taught them the skills, outlooks, and motivations needed in our society and yet have seen much inconsistency between what is taught and what is practiced. As a consequence, youth look distrustfully at the adult world and feel a lack of enthusiasm or commitment. They join the youth culture, which requires a refusal of conventional adulthood and adult values and encourages experimentation, experiences, living in the present, being irresponsible and carefree, valuing and creating color and excitement, being daring and sexually attractive.[33] A classification of ways that youth react to the social and psychological manipulation of mass society is described by Gerzon as follows. (1) The *traditionalists*. This group supports the institutions and the character ideals of Western society, and its members orient their lives toward the pursuit of established social goals. They have adopted the framework of attitudes and values represented by the older generations and find that framework compatible with the world as they see it. They do not consider adult society to be one-dimensional and unfulfilling but consider *themselves* to be inadequately measuring up to the challenging image of mass society's ideal personality. (2) The *cynics*. This group is aware of the incompleteness of the accepted adult way of life and mistrusts mass society, but its members do not feel sufficiently removed

[29]Kenneth Keniston, *The Uncommitted,* Harcourt Brace Jovanovich, Inc., New York, 1965, p. 5.
[30]*Ibid.,* pp. 179–180.
[31]From *The Whole World Is Watching: A Young Man Looks At Youth's Dissent* by Mark Gerzon, p. 80, Copyright© 1969 by Mark Gerzon. All rights reserved. Reprinted by permission of the Viking Press, Inc., New York.
[32]*Ibid.,* pp. 271–273.
[33]Keniston, *op. cit.,* p. 349.

from the prevailing system to be impelled to find alternative goals. Cynical young people have accepted the unparalleled value of doubt. Their contact with adult society has taught them that a philosophy of disbelief is the safest way to live. (3) The *activists*. Members of this group have a variety of goals and ideologies they wish to further, their end being to infuse adult society with their convictions. Their dissent is political, but it is rooted in psychological criticisms of adult society's hypocrisy. These people are the ones who are intellectually motivated, for they are searching for viable alternatives to the system that warrants their criticisms. They are politically active as well as politically alienated. The most vociferous activists question the capacity of the American political and economic system to deal with the problems of the modern world and, in their own disorganized way, attempt to spread their ideas. The activists stay in society in order to gain the influence and power to change the existing order. (4) The *hippies*. This group is dissatisfied with adult society for psychological reasons in addition to the political. The hippies function outside of any socially recognized institution because they abhor organizations. They use drugs extensively for psychological purposes and have been influenced by Oriental philosophies and their character ideals. They are preoccupied with their minds, often to the point of passivity. Their lives are individualistic, and they feel that others will escape from the hassles of modern life when they realize that the depersonalizing forces in society are becoming still more pervasive. To sustain their self-image, the hippies interact frequently with straight people and enjoy contrasting themselves to people who have not broken away from the socially patterned frustrations. (5) The *other-culturists*. This group has rejected adult society completely and has adopted a way of life associated with other cultures. It believes the American way of life is on the way out and that Western character ideals have very little to offer.[34]

Wilkerson has his own system of classifying alienated youth based on his contact with street gangs and drug addicts. A few of his classifications include: (1) *hippies,* of which there are three kinds. The first kind are the teenagers between fifteen and eighteen who are "hope-to-be" hippies. They are attracted primarily by the glamor and mystique of the abandoned free life without the strictures of parents and the pressures of having to produce in the straight world. These teen-agers confess to being tied up in knots; fear of sex, the draft, the threat of global nuclear suicide—all problems forced on them by the establishment. The second group of hippies range in age from seventeen to twenty-five and are called "tribal" hippies. They have about them a sense of destiny and take drugs mostly for "kicks." This group includes those who simply want to try something new and experiment with life. In a tribal kind of togetherness, they seek to shake off their terrible feelings of emptiness and to satisfy an inner craving for love and under-

[34]Gerzon, *op. cit.,* pp. 290–292.

standing. The third group of hippies are the "synthetic" ones. Among them are the city hippies, the suburban hippies, poetical hippies, weekend hippies, musical hippies, Polynesian hippies, and tourist hippies. They want the world to think they're hippies, but in their hearts they don't have the courage or the foolhardiness to go all the way. Most in this group are about twenty-five years of age but some of them range in age from thirty to sixty years. (2) *Yippies* are hard-core, political activists who lead demonstrations around the world. Though many are Maoists, others are members of the New Left, determined to overthrow the establishment. (3) *Freebie gypsies* are groups of hippies who live in communes or temporary shelters in search of freedom of their bodies, freedom of their social selves, and love. They devote their time to writing, painting, and scrounging for food and other commodities. They use drugs for a sacramental experience and deprecate money as a tool of the establishment used to acquire power. Their philosophy is closely related to the mysticism of the Orient.[35]

### Working with Youth Groups
In the present health-care system, nurses meet the youth sporadically in several different settings, including the schools, community centers, youth camps, youth organizations, hospital emergency rooms, free community clinics, and private homes. Many opportunities to work with youth and get better acquainted with their needs and wants are available, but these kinds of activities must be initiated by the nurse if she desires the contact. By being skillful, patient, and ingenious, she can play an influential role in relating with youth and facilitating their growth toward maturity. She cannot do so if she follows the traditional pattern of professional behavior, which is predominantly physical health-oriented, "parent"-focused, and all-knowingly expert. In all probability she is a "square," but must be honest about it, must show genuine warmth and concern for youth, must know how to listen with sensitivity, must be patient and accepting, and must try to understand the viewpoint of youth so that a meaningful interchange can ensue that is not hindered by emotional reactions or stereotyped views. She must know that young people need a sense of support from and acceptance by adults and that as an adult she must be open to provocative ideas and up-to-date on new influences pervading society as a whole. Nurses can play a helping role with youth if they will consciously change their nurse image from one of rigid authoritarianism or disinterested passivism to one of warmth, empathy, responsibility, and willingness to listen, accept, and *care.* It is not easy to relate to alienated youth, but it can be accomplished if nurses desire to make the effort.

[35]David Wilkerson, *Purple Violet Squish,* Zondervan Publishing House, Grand Rapids, Michigan, 1969, pp. 13–46.

An example was cited in Chap. 3 of a group of senior baccalaureate nursing students whose ages ranged from twenty to twenty-two and who became interested in establishing a drop-in center for teen-agers for their community project, an assignment required in the community health nursing practice course. The idea was conceived after visiting a drop-in center for youth with drug problems in a nearby community. The nursing students were "turned on" by splashy colors on the walls and the casual, comfortable environment of the old house that was being used as a place for youth to go to talk among themselves and to talk to concerned, caring adults who wanted to listen and assist with unresolved frustrations. As stated by the nursing students, "We, in community health nursing and as representatives of the community, want to alleviate some of the unrest and anger felt by the youth and get involved in a community project, a drop-in center, which will serve as a neutral ground where teens can come to voice their discontent to individuals who will listen nonjudgmentally." The nursing students succeeded, as one segment of a community team representing many disciplines, in getting a drop-in center instituted, although it took several months, many meetings with key community people, financial backing from the community, and many additional complex arrangements. Of particular interest among the community workers was the fact that nursing students were playing a role in community health organization which did not quite fit the concept of nurses as they are viewed by the public. However, the community workers were delighted with the enthusiasm and dedication of the nursing students. Another facet of interest to the nursing students was that they themselves were regarded as *adults* by the teen-agers, a perception about themselves they did not share. Much unanticipated learning occurred in this experience for all participants in the project, including the teen-agers, the nursing students, and the responsible community leaders and workers.

## SUMMARY

Selected health problems come to the attention of all citizens with frequency, either through the communication media or personally. It is the intent of selected health professionals to make citizens actively aware and involve them in matters that affect their lives. Health concerns are those problems which are or should be of interest to citizens and *all* health professionals, including nurses. Community health nurses must be represented as participating members in a wide variety of health concerns. They must assume new, innovative roles and become better known to a diversity of people in need of health services. Some health concerns about which nurses can be more knowledgeable include human sexuality, alcoholism, drug abuse, mental health, suicide, chronic degenerative diseases and death, and ecological health problems. Two consumer groups in need of improved health services and understanding are the elderly and the youth. Nurses can play more facilitative roles with these groups and profit from the additional insights gained.

## SUGGESTED READING

Doster, Daphine D.: "Utilization Of Available 'Nurse Power' In Public Health," *American Journal of Public Health,* 60:1:25–37 (January) 1970.

Fromm, Erich: *The Art Of Loving,* Harper & Row, Publishers, Inc., New York, 1956.

Gabrielson, Ira W., Lorraine V. Klerman, John B. Currie, Natalie C. Tyler, and James F. Jekel: "Suicide Attempts In a Population Pregnant As Teen-agers," *American Journal of Public Health,* 60:12:2289–2301 (December) 1970.

Gerzon, Mark: *The Whole World Is Watching: A Young Man Looks at Youth's Dissent,* The Viking Press, Inc., New York, 1969.

Ginott, Dr. Haim G.: *Between Parent & Teenager,* The Macmillan Company, New York, 1969.

Griffith, Valerie Eaton: *A Stroke In the Family,* Random House, Inc., New York, 1970.

Hanlon, John J.: "An Ecologic View of Public Health," *American Journal of Public Health,* 59:1:4–11 (January) 1969.

Keniston, Kenneth: *The Uncommitted: Alienated Youth In American Society,* Harcourt Brace Jovanovich, Inc., New York, 1965.

Kogan, Benjamin A.: *Health, Man In a Changing Environment,* Harcourt Brace Jovanovich, Inc., New York, 1970.

Kubler-Ross, Elisabeth: *On Death and Dying,* The Macmillan Company, New York, 1969.

Lingeman, Richard R.: *Drugs From A to Z: A Dictionary,* McGraw-Hill Book Company, New York, 1969.

McLean, Lenora J.: "Action and Reaction in Suicidal Crisis," *Nursing Forum,* 8:1: 28–41, 1969.

Moustakas, Clark E.: *Loneliness,* Prentice-Hall, Inc., Englewood Cliffs, N.J., 1961.

Nowlis, Helen H.: *Drugs On the College Campus,* Doubleday & Company, Garden City, N.Y., 1969.

Pittman, David J.: *Alcoholism In America,* McGraw-Hill Book Company, New York, 1966.

Ponchin, Jean: *Without a Wedding Ring,* Schocken Books Inc., New York, 1969.

Shneidman, Edwin S.: *On the Nature of Suicide,* Jossey-Bass, Inc., Publishers, San Francisco, 1969.

Valentine, Alan C.: *Fathers to Sons: Advice Without Consent,* University of Oklahoma Press, Oklahoma City, 1963.

Valles, Jorge: *How To Live With an Alcoholic,* Simon & Schuster, New York, 1967.

Wilkerson, David: *The Cross and the Switchblade,* Bernard Geis Associates, New York, 1962.

Zderad, Loretta T., and Helen C. Belcher: *Developing Behavioral Concepts In Nursing,* Southern Regional Education Board, Atlanta, 1968.

The emphasis on clinical and laboratory research in the past decade dictates that the nurse have an understanding and appreciation of statistics. An understanding of statistics is necessary in order to apply precept 8 as stated in Chap. 1: Periodic and continuing appraisal and evaluation of the health situation of the community, family, and patient are basic to community health nursing. Also, the Public Health Nurses' Section of the American Nurses' Association requires the nurse to have knowledge of the research method within the broad categories of evaluating, studying, and research.

## STUDY AND RESEARCH

Searching for increased knowledge in a systematic way requires curiosity, self-discipline, and familiarity with research methods. Nursing students who wish to promote the advancement of improved patient care must have a beginning acquaintance with research methods in order to study any aspect of the health-illness continuum which concerns them. For the nurse who is sufficiently curious about an intriguing health problem, a beginning step into research activities can be initiated by doing a mini-study. By investigating the variety of methods for doing studies, getting an idea from readings whether any other nurse has done a similar study, and determining exactly what she wants to find out, the neophyte nurse can start investigative activities which may bring exciting discoveries to light. Some problems that might be interesting to study include identification of consumers' attitudes or opinions regarding specific health issues, the coexistence of special problems with specific diseases, investigation of factors that promote wellness in families, investigation of factors contributing to communication problems, comparison of nurse

9
The
Community
Health
Nurse
and
Statistics

235

goals and family goals with ultimate outcomes of health services, and many other related ideas. When the nurse desires to do a study about a specific problem, it is frequently advisable to consult an expert in research so that the identified problem can be whittled down to a dimension that will be stimulating to work with and the results may impel the student to want to learn more about research methodology. In order to do study and research, a knowledge of statistics is required.

The purpose of presenting an elementary discussion of statistical concepts is to enable the nurse to participate in or to conduct studies of her own. Familiarity with these concepts will be of value in presenting and analyzing quantitative data. Also, it will help the nurse to become more critical of the proliferation of new knowledge in the health sciences. Terms such as variation, population, sample, data, observations, and central tendency, which may be familiar to the nurse, are explained from the point of view of statistics. The authors present this limited discussion knowing that the material is too elementary for some readers, that it will be a review for others, and that it will be helpful for some; it is in no way intended to bring about mastery in the science of statistics.

The student is directed to references mentioned throughout the text and to the bibliography at the end of the chapter for a detailed discussion of statistical concepts and techniques.

## DEFINITIONS

The term *statistics* is defined in various ways. For the purpose of this presentation, statistics refers to a systematic approach for obtaining, organizing, and analyzing numerical facts so that conclusions may be drawn from them. Statistics allow for description and for making statistical inference. They present fact rather than an assumption or a hunch.

*Vital statistics* in the broad sense refers to births, deaths, populations, illnesses, marriages, and divorces. In the narrow sense the term refers to births, deaths, and population. Illnesses in the population are classified as morbidity statistics. Generally marriage and divorce statistics are used more frequently by social agencies than by health departments. Since the disciplines of public health and community health nursing are concerned with people, vital statistics are an important tool in the field of public health.

## SOURCES OF DATA

The family record is an excellent source for such statistical information as age, sex, ethnic background, and specific disease or condition. Information from the records facilitates program planning and is useful in evaluating the service given to the family. Roberts and Hudson developed a method of studying the patient's progress through his record. Their study method gives direction for collecting, presenting, and analyzing data concerning:

**1.** The scope of needs identified in patients and families by the public health nurse

**2.** The progress made by families in meeting their own needs for nursing care

**3.** The proportion of persons who obtain needed immunizations and diagnostic tests

**4.** The number and kinds of conditions which are brought to medical attention for diagnosis, periodic medical evaluation, and treatment

**5.** The extent to which patients with chronic illness and disability attain self-care[1]

Information from records is used in compiling monthly and annual reports required by the agency. Such information is used by the local community health agency as well as by state and Federal health agencies, grant-in-aid programs, voluntary and contracting agencies—e.g., insurance companies, schools, or industrial firms that pay for service—and by sponsoring or coordinating groups such as the Community Chest or the united funds. The information is used to make comparisons with previous years, to predict and to determine needs for ensuing years, and to interpret to the community in order to obtain better understanding and support for community health nursing services.

The staff nurse rarely is responsible for compiling the agency's monthly or annual reports, but she is responsible for knowing the information contained in them. Her responsibility includes knowledge and understanding of the major accomplishments of the year, such as quantitative and qualitative attainments, concerns and plans for change, trends in activities and service needs, and the relation of service given to the estimated needs for such services.

Staff nurses may be involved in compiling statistics for special investigations of such topics as well-child care, premature births, epidemiologic problems, home-care programs, school health, congenital defects, rehabilitation, mental retardation, and migratory workers. The individual nurse may be interested in conducting a study within her district. The opportunities are unlimited and will vary according to the nurse's interest and the policies of the agency.

## STATISTICAL CONCEPTS AND TECHNIQUES

To aid the nurse in developing a systematic approach in classifying and analyzing data, certain statistical concepts and techniques are necessary.

[1]Doris E. Roberts and Helen H. Hudson, *How to Study Patient Progress,* Public Health Service Publication 1169, April, 1964, p. 1.

Those to be described are variation, qualitative and quantitative data, population and sample in collecting data, tables and graphs in presenting data, and analyzing the data.

First and foremost is the concept that any particular subject or subject area is characterized by variation. The field of nursing is an example, since nurses may work in a hospital, office, community health agency, clinic, school, or industry. Another example is provided by people. Some people are young, others are old; some are thin, others are obese; some are males, others are females; some have a specific disease, others do not. Human behavior differs, for no two persons are alike and all respond to the environment in different ways. The variables or factors are the characteristics which have more than one value to be studied.

## TYPES OF DATA

There are two types of data: qualitative and quantitative. Qualitative data refer to those variables that describe a quality or attribute observed in the people or subject being studied. The variables in qualitative data are referred to as enumerations, classifications, and discrete or counting data. Qualitative data are developed by counting the number of persons who possess or do not possess a quality or attribute, e.g., the number of persons who are male or not male, who wear dentures or do not wear dentures, who have chickenpox or do not have chickenpox. The number of children in a family or the number in a group is a discrete value, as one does not have a proportion or one-half of a child or person. Qualitative attributes are easy to classify since there is only a definite number of possibilities, such as sex, race, presence or absence of a disease. Caution must be taken in categorizing subjective judgments of such matters as severity of a disease, appearance or behavior. Personal bias may affect the classification when it is made by other persons, even though specific criteria are set up. Also, counting data can be misleading when they are based on small numbers of cases.

Quantitative data or variables are those having measurable values, instead of counts or enumerations as in qualitative data. Quantitative variables allow for measurement by recording the amount of a variable possessed by each person (or thing) studied. Age in years is measured by subtracting the birth date from the present date. Incubation period for a disease is the time interval in hours or days between the infection of a susceptible person or animal and the appearance of signs or symptoms of the disease in question. Variables in quantitative data are called continuous data, in the sense that they are capable of assuming any value of measurement, as seen in measuring heights, weights, temperatures, and blood pressure.

Grouping of quantitative data in which the measurements are made on a continuous scale should be done with care to avoid loss of detail. For example, classifying 65 nursing students weighing from 100 to 150 lb would not tell how many students weighed 110, 120, 125, or up to 150 lb. Generally, to determine groupings, one divides the range into equal size intervals from 5 to 20 and makes each group nonoverlapping with the succeeding one. The range is the difference between the largest and smallest observations. For instance, if class intervals of five were used for weight, you would count the number of persons falling into the class interval from 100 to 104.99; 105 to 109.99; or 110 to 114.99; and so on through 149.99. The distribution is summarized in Table 9-1.

**TABLE 9-1**  Frequency distribution of weight in pounds of 65 senior nursing students at school X

| WEIGHT, lb | NO. OF STUDENTS |
|---|---|
| 100—104.99 | 1 |
| 105—109.99 | 1 |
| 110—114.99 | 5 |
| 115—119.99 | 11 |
| 120—124.99 | 12 |
| 125—129.99 | 19 |
| 130—134.99 | 10 |
| 135—139.99 | 4 |
| 140—144.99 | 1 |
| 145—149.99 | 1 |
| Total | 65 |

Such characteristics as heights, temperatures, pulse, blood pressures, or specific laboratory findings also could be shown in a frequency distribution table.

## COLLECTING THE DATA

The kind of data to be collected and the way in which they are collected depend on the hypothesis or purpose of the study. However, two important concepts are those of population and sample. Population, or universe, refers to the full group or collection of subjects under study. In practice, complete access to the total population may be difficult or impossible and therefore population refers to an aggregate of observations. The observations are measurements of characteristics, such as age, height, weight, income, and disease, of individuals in the population. The observations are made not of the persons themselves but only of some characteristic of the persons. Other examples might be the cholesterol level of persons in a certain group, the economic level of persons in a group, or a value held by members of a certain group.

A sample is a portion or a fraction of the population or universe which is to be investigated. Sampling is a method of collecting data on a small number of the total population under study and then generalizing the findings to the total population. There are many types of samples, of which the simple random sample is the only one mentioned here. A random sample is a sample from a population such that every sample of the same size has the same probability of being chosen. This eliminates bias. Another advantage of the random sample is that there are mathematic techniques which allow for drawing conclusions about the population on the basis of the sample.

When dealing with small numbers, a way of selecting a sample would be to copy the name or measurement on a piece of paper, place the pieces of paper in a hat or box, mix them up, and draw without looking into the hat or box, so that the sample is drawn by chance alone. For larger samples, a table of random numbers is helpful. Tables of random numbers are found in books of statistics such as those by Dunn, Hill, and Fisher and Yates listed at the end of the chapter. Sampling allows for generalizations about a population or universe in relation to averages and variations from the sample. Samples are used because it may be impossible to study the whole population, and because of the tremendous saving of time and money that is accomplished by studying only a small portion of the whole population. The reader is referred to texts which discuss sampling techniques in detail, such as those by McCollough and Van Atta or by Dunn, found in the bibliography at the end of the chapter.

Suppose, for example, that you are evaluating the effectiveness of immune globulin for prophylaxis of infectious hepatitis in an open community. Such an investigation requires information concerning the disease during a specified period of time from all persons who received the immune globulin. Decisions must be reached as to how the information is to be obtained. Is the history to be obtained by an interview, a home visit, a telephone call, or a mailed questionnaire? Decisions must be reached as to what information is needed. What variables are pertinent? Are household contacts a factor? Are age, sex, occupation, race, or economic level essential in contributing to the study?

The very nature of the question regarding the effectiveness of the globulin in the example dictates that similar information be obtained from the group receiving immune globulin and from the group who did not receive immune globulin. A controlled study of this type is essential; otherwise it would be impossible to evaluate whether the frequency of attack among the group receiving immune globulin was significant.

The method for collecting data depends on the hypothesis, the size of the sample, and the variables being studied. A few sources for data are records from the community health nursing agency, clinic, school, or industry; employment records, birth, and death certificates, United States census reports; morbidity and mortality reports from local, state, national, or international agencies.

There are many ways of developing a form for recording the variables. The form may be a simple listing of facts, such as age and sex; a complex form may contain age, sex, race, housing, income, occupation, education, immunizations, behavior, attitudes and beliefs. The form may be a checklist or a number of columns for entering information. A 3- by 5-in. card is often used for entering a few items, or a pre-punched card for many items, up to the limit of the card. Use of pre-punched or large cards with a number of items makes tabulation more difficult unless mechanical means are employed.

## TABULATING THE DATA

Tables are the most common way of presenting observations in a systematic arrangement, as they show the interrelationship among the variables. The simplest form of a table is a two-column frequency table which may be used for quantitative or qualitative data. The first column gives the classes into which data are grouped, and the second column lists the frequencies for each classification or group. Table 9-1 is an example of a two-column frequency table.

Since tables show the interrelationship between variables, the form may be arranged showing several variables. This type of table presents data in relation to a specific variable and in relation to any combination of the variables. For example, to determine the source of referrals to a district during a certain period of time, the data would be tabulated as shown in Table 9-2.

In this example the total number of referrals from all sources can be determined. In addition the table gives information concerning the interrelationship between the source of referral and the service given, as well as the combination of sources referring persons to a particular service.

## GRAPHICAL PRESENTATION OF DATA

A graph is a way of showing quantitative data. It allows for a rapid interpretation of the material presented. There are many types of graphs; a few of the most common, such as the bar graph, histogram, and polygon, will be presented. The bar graph is the simplest type, with bars of uniform width usually arranged according to magnitude (Fig. 9-1). It is useful in comparing quantitative data or qualitative data of discrete type.

**TABLE 9-2**  Source of referral for nursing service

| NURSING SERVICE | Source | | | | | | |
|---|---|---|---|---|---|---|---|
| | PRIVATE PHYSICIAN | PATIENT OR FAMILY | HOSPITAL OR OUT-PATIENT DEPARTMENT | HEALTH DEPARTMENT CLINIC | COMMU-NITY HEALTH NURSE | SCHOOL | TOTAL |
| Newborn ................... | | | | | | | |
| Infant ...................... | | | | | | | |
| Preschool.................. | | | | | | | |
| School ..................... | | | | | | | |
| Adult....................... | | | | | | | |
| Maternity.................. | | | | | | | |
| Tuberculosis............... | | | | | | | |
| Communicable disease...... | | | | | | | |
| Noncommunicable disease .. | | | | | | | |
| Chronic disease............ | | | | | | | |
| Orthopedic disease ......... | | | | | | | |
| Mental health.............. | | | | | | | |
| Total ..................... | | | | | | | |

The histogram is a bar chart showing frequency distributions of quantitative and continuous data. It is a series of adjacent rectangles of which the frequency is equal to the class if all intervals are of the same width. When intervals are not of the same width, the relative frequency may be used. This is an advantage in comparing class intervals of an unequal size. The relative frequency is expressed in percentage. It is calculated by taking

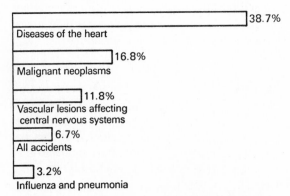

Fig. 9-1  Five leading causes of death in the state of Washington in 1969.

the frequency of a class, dividing by the total observations in the class, and multiplying by 100. The relative frequency of the weight in pounds of the example in Table 9-1 is shown in Table 9-3. The histogram for showing the frequency distribution is presented in Fig. 9-2.

The frequency polygon is essentially the same as the histogram; the data are computed in the same way. In the frequency polygon, the frequency is plotted at the midpoint of the class interval and each point is connected by a line. The rectangles of the histogram are replaced by the connecting lines at midpoint of the interval, resulting in a continuous line. Using the same data as in Fig. 9-2, a frequency polygon is plotted in Fig. 9-3. When the frequency polygon is superimposed on the histogram, it is evident that the frequency polygon is an approximation of the area of the histogram (see Fig. 9-4). The reader is referred to the volumes by Dunn, Hill, and Bancroft listed at the end of the chapter for a detailed presentation of different types of graphs, such as a spot map, shaded map, or pie diagram, and their construction.

## ANALYZING THE DATA

Analysis of data is a process for the purpose of drawing pertinent conclusions from them. The analysis of data is one of the most important parts of any study. The techniques used for drawing conclusions vary according to the hypothesis and the type and amount of data collected. This is why the

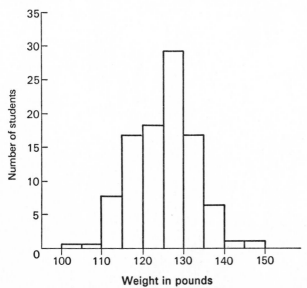

Fig. 9-2   Histogram of weight in pounds of sixty-five students.

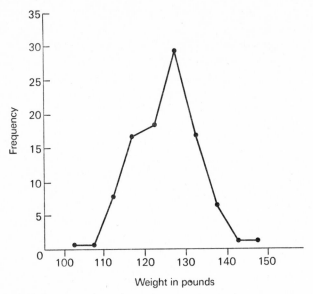

Fig. 9-3  Frequency polygon of weight in pounds of sixty-five students.

problem must be clearly defined and the data carefully obtained and well organized.

Vital statistics furnish data on quantity, quality, and composition with respect to a population. The data give a picture of the population and allow

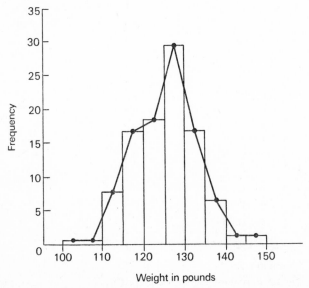

Fig. 9-4  Frequency polygon superimposed on histogram.

**TABLE 9-3** Relative frequency distribution of weight in pounds of 65 senior nursing students at school X

| WEIGHT, lb | FREQUENCY | RELATIVE FREQUENCY, % |
|---|---|---|
| 100—104.99 | 1 | 1.54 |
| 105—109.99 | 1 | 1.54 |
| 110—114.99 | 5 | 7.69 |
| 115—119.99 | 11 | 16.92 |
| 120—124.99 | 12 | 18.46 |
| 125—129.99 | 19 | 29.23 |
| 130—134.99 | 10 | 15.39 |
| 135—139.99 | 4 | 6.15 |
| 140—144.99 | 1 | 1.54 |
| 145—149.99 | 1 | 1.54 |
| Total | 65 | 100.00 |

for comparison; e.g., comparing the mortality of one group treated with a certain drug and that of another group not treated with the drug, or comparing the incidence or prevalence of disease in a given area with the incidence and prevalence in another area.

Data with qualitative characteristics usually are summarized in rates and ratios. A rate describes the proportion with which a given characteristic is occurring in a population. The ratio describes the proportion or relationship between two numerical quantities.

Many different kinds of rates are used in studying the various factors concerned in the formation and control of disease. Each rate serves a different purpose and is subject to a different interpretation. The general principles, however, that apply to any rate are numerator, denominator, population, base, and time element. In calculating a rate the numerator and denominator must be from the same population and they must relate to the same time period. The population at the middle of a time period under study is considered to be the population at risk. When the rate is an annual rate, the population as of July 1 of the specific year is used. The base for birth, death, or mortality generally is expressed as 1,000; for incidence as 100,000. In other words the birth, death, or mortality rate is expressed as number of cases per 1,000 population; and the incidence rate is expressed as number of cases per 100,000 population. Case fatality is expressed as number of cases per 100 population. The crude death rate illustrates the principles involved. The rate is calculated according to the following formula:

Crude death rate:

$$\frac{\text{Number of deaths reported in a given year}}{\text{Estimated population at middle of same year}} \times 1,000$$

The rate is easy to calculate. The numerator is found by adding up the number of deaths from all causes that occurred during a given period, usually one year. The denominator is the estimated population as of July 1 of same year, and the base usually is 1,000. The following example gives the calculation of the crude death rate for Seattle, Washington, in 1970:

$$\frac{\text{Total deaths in 1970}}{\text{Estimated population, 1970}} \text{ X } 1{,}000 = \frac{6{,}092}{524{,}263} \text{ X } 1{,}000 = 11.6$$

The findings are interpreted as indicating that, on the average, for every 1,000 persons in the population of Seattle in 1970 there were 11.6 deaths from all causes.

Specific rates for deaths, diseases, age, sex, race, or any combination of these factors may be found as long as the numerator can be related to the same population. The following example gives the formula for the specific death rate from neoplasms in the state of Washington, 1969:

$$\frac{\text{Number of deaths caused by a particular disease}}{\text{Estimated population, 1969}} \text{ X } 100{,}000$$

$$\frac{4{,}953 \text{ deaths from neoplasms}}{3{,}203{,}218 \text{ estimated population}} \text{ X } 100{,}000 = 154.6$$

The specific rate is interpreted as indicating that, on the average, 154.6 persons died from neoplasms per 100,000 population in the state of Washington in 1969.

Incidence and prevalence rates commonly are used to express the frequency of a disease in a population at a given point in time. Incidence rates are used when referring to new diseases which arise during a given year; prevalence rates refer to total rate of the disease in a population. For chronic disease the prevalence rate is high compared with incidence, but for acute or infectious disease, incidence is high compared with prevalence. The formulas for the two rates are as follows:

Incidence rate:

$$\frac{\text{No. of new cases of spec. disease occurring during given time period.}}{\text{Estimated population at risk during the same period of time}} \text{ X base}$$

Prevalence rate:

$$\frac{\text{No. of cases of spec. disease existing during given time period}}{\text{Estimated population at risk during the same period of time}} \times base$$

It is important to distinguish between these two rates, as can be seen when considering such diseases as arthritis, cancer, tuberculosis, and syphilis.

Adjusted rates are used in comparing rates and ratios of disease, age, sex, race, or specific characteristics between different geographic areas. The following hypothetical situation, summed up in Table 9-4, will illustrate the point.

**TABLE 9-4**   Morbidity from disease K in communities A and B

| SEX | COMMUNITY A | | | COMMUNITY B | | |
|---|---|---|---|---|---|---|
| | CASES | POPULATION | MORBIDITY RATE PER 10,000 | CASES | POPULATION | MORBIDITY RATE PER 10,000 |
| Males .............. | 50 | 10,000 | 25 | 50 | 15,000 | 25 |
| Females ........... | 10 | 10,000 | 05 | 10 | 5,000 | 05 |
| Total ............. | 60 | 20,000 | 30 | 60 | 20,000 | 30 |

In examining the crude rates for each community, the rate of 30 cases per 10,000 population appears to be the same. On further examination it appears that the sex rate is different, as there are more females with the disease in Community B than in Community A. Also, there are more males with the disease in Community A than in Community B. Therefore, to interpret information about the sex-specific rates of the two communities, the rates must be adjusted.

The simplest method of adjustment is to select a standard population and then apply the sex-specific rates of Communities A and B to this population. The method for calculating adjusted rates as shown in Table 9-4 is as follows:

1. Crude disease rate $= \dfrac{\text{cases of disease}}{\text{population}} \times base$

Community A:

$$\frac{60}{20,000} \times 10,000 = 30 \text{ cases per 10,000 population}$$

Community B:

$$\frac{60}{20,000} \times 10,000 = 30 \text{ cases per } 10,000 \text{ population}$$

**2.** Sex-specific case rate $= \dfrac{\text{no. of cases per sex group}}{\text{population of sex group}} \times \text{base}$

Community A (males):

$$\frac{50}{10,000} \times 10,000 = 50 \text{ males}$$

Community A (females):

$$\frac{10}{10,000} \times 10,000 = 10 \text{ females}$$

Community B (males):

$$\frac{50}{15,000} \times 10,000 = 33 \text{ males}$$

Community B (females):

$$\frac{10}{5,000} \times 10,000 = 20 \text{ females}$$

**3.** Specific sex population = Community A males
+ Community B males

Specific sex population = Community A females
+ Community B females

Community A + B males = 10,000 + 15,000 = 25,000 males

Community A + B females = 10,000 + 5,000 = 15,000 females

**4.** Expected cases $= \dfrac{\text{sex-specific rate}}{\text{base}} \times \text{specific sex population}$

Community A (males):

$$\frac{50}{10,000} \times 25,000 = 125$$

Community A (females):

$$\frac{10}{10,000} \text{ X } 15,000 = 15$$

Community B (males):

$$\frac{33}{10,000} \text{ X } 25,000 = 82$$

Community B (females):

$$\frac{20}{10,000} \text{ X } 15,000 = 30$$

5.  Sex-adjusted rate $= \dfrac{\text{total expected cases of each group}}{\text{total specific sex population}}$  X base

Community A:

$$\frac{140}{40,000} \text{ X } 10,000 = 35$$

Community B:

$$\frac{112}{40,000} \text{ X } 10,000 = 28$$

These sex-adjusted rates of 35 and 28 are now comparable. They reflect a higher rate for Community A than for Community B. For the sake of simplicity, race was considered to be similar in both communities. The age distribution for a disease or condition is often important, and it becomes necessary to adjust the rates according to age groups.

## Age Groups
The age groups frequently used for all causes of morbidity and mortality are:

Under 1 year—infant
1—4 years—preschool
5—15 years—school
15—24 years—adolescent
25—44 years—young adult
45—65 years—middle age
66 plus—old age

However, computing the age-specific rates of two populations from the above groupings is difficult; therefore ages may be regrouped into a greater span of years. The important principle is that the groupings must be the same for the two populations. The reader is referred to the books by Bancroft, Mainland, and Maxey listed at the end of the chapter for a further discussion on computing rates and ratios.

The following are some of the formulas for computing rates and ratios commonly used in public health:

Crude birth rate:

$$\frac{\text{No. of live births reported during a given year}}{\text{Estimated population as of July 1 of the same year}} \times 1{,}000$$

Age-specific birth rate:

$$\frac{\text{No. of live births to women of specific age reported during given year}}{\text{Est. female population of same age as of July 1 of same year}} \times 1{,}000$$

Crude death rate:

$$\frac{\text{No. of deaths reported during a given year}}{\text{Estimated population as of July 1 of the same year}} \times 1{,}000$$

Mortality rate for a specific disease:

$$\frac{\text{No. of deaths due to a specific disease during a given year}}{\text{Estimated population as of July 1 of the given year}} \times 100{,}000$$

Infant mortality rate:

$$\frac{\text{No. of deaths under 1 year reported during given year}}{\text{No. of live births reported during the same year}} \times 1{,}000$$

Neonatal mortality rate:

$$\frac{\text{No. of deaths under 28 days reported during given year}}{\text{No. of live births reported during the same year}} \times 1{,}000$$

Maternal mortality rate:

$$\frac{\text{No. of deaths from causes of pregnancy during a given year}}{\text{No. of live births reported during the same year}} \times 1{,}000$$

Fetal death ratio:

$$\frac{\text{No. of fetal deaths during a given year}}{\text{No. of live births reported during same year}} \times 1{,}000$$

Case fatality rate:

$$\frac{\text{No. of deaths from spec. disease during a given time period}}{\text{No. of cases of the disease during the same period of time}} \times 100$$

Proportional mortality rate:

$$\frac{\text{No. of deaths from a specific cause during a given year}}{\text{No. of deaths reported from all causes during the same year}} \times 100$$

Incidence rate:

$$\frac{\text{No. of new cases cf spec. disease during given time period}}{\text{Estimated population at risk during the same period of time}} \times \text{base}$$

Prevalence rate:

$$\frac{\text{No. of cases of spec. disease existing during given time period}}{\text{Estimated population at risk during the same period of time}} \times \text{base}$$

## Measurement Data

Data of all types, especially quantitative variables of age, weight, and time, are summarized in terms of their distribution. Measures of central tendency describe the center of the distribution, as frequency distributions tend to cluster where the frequency is the highest. The measures of central tendency are the mean, median, and mode.

The *mean* is the arithmetic average of a set of observations. It is calculated by adding up the value of each of the observations in a series and dividing by the total number of observations. Suppose that there is an outbreak of a waterborne disease in your district and you want to determine the mean age at onset. To find the average of the sum of the ages in years, add the ages as follows: 12 + 15 + 16 + 16 + 17 + 18 + 18 + 19 + 20 + 20 + 20 + 22 + 24 + 25 + 28 + 30 = 320; then divide the sum by the total number of observations (16), i.e., 320 divided by 16, which equals 20 years. Each of these numbers has had equal weight in determination of the mean. If the mean of all the observations is subtracted from each of the observations, the sum of the differences or deviations is equal to zero, which is the center of the distribution. An example of the deviation from the mean of 20 years is shown in Fig. 9-5. The distribution in this situation is fairly symmetric, as the frequencies on each side of the mean are similar.

The *median* is the middle observation of a series of observations when the observations are arranged in order of magnitude. If there is an even number of observations, the average of the two middle numbers is the

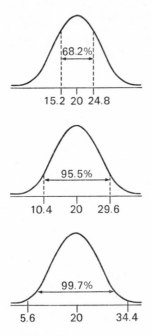

Fig. 9-5 Distribution of normal curve with standard deviation of
4.8 years.

median. For example, the median number for the age at onset of the waterborne disease is 19.5 years.

The *mode* is the observation occurring with the greatest frequency in
a set of observations. Thus in the example of age at onset of this waterborne
disease, the mode is equal to 20 years. A summary of these three measurements is shown in Table 9-5.

The mean is the central measure of choice except when the distribution is asymmetric or skewed. The median is used when the distribution is
asymmetric or when observations include occasional extreme values. For a
more detailed discussion of the use and of the calculation of the measures
of central tendency the reader is referred to the works of McCollough and
Van Atta, Dunn, Mainland, Hill, or Bancroft listed at the end of this chapter.

It is beyond the scope of this chapter to present the numerous statistical methods appropriate for analysis of different types of samples. It is
suggested that the reader consult a statistician within the agency or a
statistical consultant from the state health department for planning and
analyzing data.

Mention will be made of one measure of variation, the standard deviation, which is commonly used. The standard deviation is most useful with
reference to the normal frequency distribution. The measures of central

**TABLE 9-5**   Cases of waterborne disease

| AGE AT ONSET, YEARS | |
| --- | --- |
| | 12 |
| | 15 |
| | 16 |
| | 16 |
| | 17 |
| | 18 |
| *Range* = 18 years | 18 |
| | 19   *Median* = 19.5 years |
| | 20 |
| | 20 |
| | 20   *Mode* = 20 years |
| | 22 |
| | 24 |
| | 25 |
| | 28 |
| | 30 |

$320 \div 16 = 20.0$ years, *arithmetic mean*

*Arithmetic mean:* The sum of the observations in a series divided by the total number of observations.

*Median:* The middle observation when observations are arranged in order of magnitude. In an even number of observations, the average of the two middle observations is taken.

*Mode:* The observation occurring with the greatest frequency.

*Range:* The difference between the largest and smallest observations.

---

tendency will vary from sample to sample, giving a distribution of the sample mean. These will vary around the true mean of the population from which the samples were drawn. The standard deviation of the distribution of means gives the measure of the degree of chance variation or sampling within the population. The standard deviation is found by taking the square root of the sum of the squared deviations about the mean and dividing by the number in the sample or by the number of measurements. The formula, then, is:

$$S.D. = \sqrt{\frac{\text{sum of squared deviations}}{\text{no. of measurements}}}$$

or

$$S_x = \sqrt{\frac{\Sigma(x - \bar{x})^2}{n}}$$

When the standard deviation is calculated for a sample rather than for a population, the standard deviation is computed in the same way except that 1 is subtracted from the number of measurements, as a better estimate of the population is provided if the numbers are small. This would be the situation in the sample of age at onset of the waterborne disease. The formula would be:

$$\text{S.D.} = \sqrt{\frac{\text{sum of squared deviations}}{(\text{no. of measurements} - 1)}}$$

Even though the measures in the sample are discrete, the pattern is characteristic of the normal frequency distribution and is approximated by it. Substituting numbers from the same example, the formula is:

$$\text{S.D.} = \sqrt{\frac{\text{sum of squared deviations}}{(\text{no. of measurements} - 1)}} = \sqrt{\frac{348}{16 - 1}} = \sqrt{\frac{348}{15}} = 4.82$$

or 4.8 years

A summary of the distribution from the example is presented in Fig. 9-6. Since the sample is small and only approximates the frequency distribution, one is unable to generalize from the findings to large populations. The larger the sample, the closer is the approximation to normal frequency distribution.

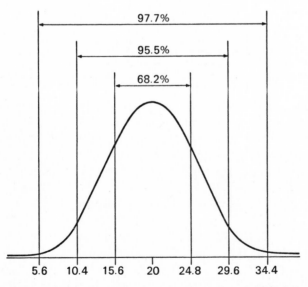

Fig. 9-6   Distribution of normal curve with standard deviation of 4.8 years.

If measurements are normally distributed, 68.26 percent of them will fall within 1 S.D. on either side of the mean, or approximately two-thirds of the measurements will not deviate from the mean by more than 1 S.D. In other words, in the same example, within 1 S.D., two-thirds of the observations will occur 4.8 years on either side of the mean of 20 years (Fig. 9-5).

Also, 95.5 percent of the measurements will fall within 2 S.D. on either

TABLE 9-6   Distribution of 16 cases of waterborne disease according to age in years

| AGE AT ONSET, YEARS | DEVIATION FROM MEAN OF 20 YEARS | SQUARED DEVIA- TION |
|---|---|---|
| 12 | −8 | 64 |
| 15 | −5 | 25 |
| 16 | −4 | 16 |
| 16 | −4 | 16 |
| 17 | −3 | 9 |
| 18 | −2 | 4 |
| 18 | −2 | 4 |
| 19 | −1 | 1 |
| 20 | 0 | 0 |
| 20 | 0 | 0 |
| 20 | 0 | 0 |
| 22 | +2 | 4 |
| 24 | +4 | 16 |
| 25 | +5 | 25 |
| 28 | +8 | 64 |
| 30 | +10 | 100 |
| | 0 | 348 |

*Range:* The difference between the largest and smallest measurements, e.g., 30 − 12 = 18 years.

*Standard deviation:* The square root of the average of the squared deviations of the measurements from the mean.

$$\sqrt{\frac{348}{16}} = \sqrt{21.75} = 4.66 = 4.7 \text{ years}$$

When the standard deviation is being computed for a sample, rather than for a population, it is computed as follows:

$$\sqrt{\frac{348}{16-1}} = \sqrt{\frac{348}{15}} = \sqrt{23.2} = 4.82 = 4.8 \text{ years}$$

side of the mean, or approximately 95 percent of the measurements will not deviate from the mean by more than 2 S.D. Therefore, continuing with the same example, 9.6 years on either side of the mean equals 2 S.D.

Last, 99.7 percent of the measurements will fall within 3 S.D. on either side of the mean. Applying this principle to the example, almost all the measurements will be within 14.4 years of the mean. Figure 9-6 summarizes the measurements of normal distribution.

## SUMMARY

A brief discussion with illustrations of some statistical concepts useful to the nurse in conducting studies is presented. Variation in people, behavior, and environment allows for study of special characteristics within the population. The purpose, or hypothesis, of a study determines the type of data, quantitative or qualitative, to be collected. When collecting the data, emphasis is given to the population and the sample. After collecting the data, the findings are systematically organized or tabulated to show the interrelationships among the variables under study. Analysis of data is the process of drawing conclusions so that intelligent judgments may be made. Rates and ratios allow for comparison of data with qualitative characteristics. Measurement data of all types, especially quantitative data, are summarized in terms of their distribution, e.g., measures of central tendency. Use of the data as a basis for generalization to the population requires statistical methods appropriate to different samples. The standard deviation is the most useful in normal frequency distribution.

It is suggested that the nurse interested in conducting a study of her own consult with a statistician or specialist in the field of statistics. This chapter provides an elementary discussion in the science of statistics.

## SUGGESTED READING

Bancroft, Huldah: *Introduction to Biostatistics,* Paul B. Hoeber, Inc., New York, medical book department of Harper & Row, Publishers, Incorporated, 1960.

Downie, N. M., and R. W. Heath: *Basic Statistical Methods,* 2d ed., Harper & Row, Publishers, Incorporated, New York, 1965.

Dunn, Olive Jean: *Basic Statistics: A Primer for the Biomedical Sciences,* John Wiley & Sons, Inc., New York, 1964.

Fisher, R. A., and F. Yates: *Statistical Tables for Biological, Agricultural, and Medical Research,* Hafner Publishing Company, Inc., New York, 1957.

Fox, John P., Carrie E. Hall, and Leila R. Elveback: *Epidemiology—Man and Disease,* Macmillan & Company, Ltd., London, 1970.

Hill, Bradford: *Principles of Medical Statistics,* 7th ed., Oxford University Press, New York, 1961.

Kenney, J. K.: *Mathematics of Statistics,* D. Van Nostrand Company, Inc., Princeton, N.J., 1939.

Levine, Eugene: "The ABC's of Statistics," *American Journal of Nursing,* 59:71–75 (January) 1959; and 59:230–233 (February) 1959.

McCollough, Celeste, and Loche Van Atta: *Statistical Concepts: A Program for Self-Instruction,* McGraw-Hill Book Company, New York, 1963.

Mainland, Donald: *Elementary Medical Statistics,* 2d ed., W. B. Saunders Company, Philadelphia, 1963.

Maxey, Kenneth F.: *Rosenau Preventive Medicine and Public Health,* 8th ed., Appleton-Century-Crofts, Inc., New York, 1956.

Roberts, Doris E., and Helen H. Hudson: *How to Study Patient Progress,* Public Health Service Publication 1169, U. S. Department of Health, Education and Welfare, Washington, D.C., 1964.

Seattle-King County Health Department, *Annual Report, 1970,* Seattle, Wash., 1971.

Washington State Department of Health, *Vital Statistics Summary 1969,* Olympia, Wash., 1969.

# 10
## History, Trends, and Philosophy of Community Health Nursing

## HISTORY OF COMMUNITY HEALTH NURSING
### Early History

"Concern with matters of personal and community health appears to have been widely reflected in the records of every major civilization and the majority of cultures known to man."[1]

Similar references are to be found in the general literature and in the Bible. The Old Testament cites the efforts of Moses to prevent the spread of disease among his people by curbing their use of shellfish and pork as food. He did not know specifically why the ingestion of certain shellfish caused dysentery (probably typhoid) and death, or why the ingestion of pork caused illness and disability (probably trichinosis), but he did observe that when he prohibited the use of these foods, the incidence of these diseases declined among his people.

Community health nursing is also an outgrowth and a development of an ancient practice, that of visiting the sick. About 60 A.D. St. Paul mentions in his writings Phebe, a deaconess in the early Christian church, whose duties included a combination of parish work, friendly visiting, and district nursing. She has often been called the first visiting nurse; "from her day the work of visiting nursing has never been unknown."[2]

### Nursing in Europe

For more than a thousand years after the time of Phebe, most of the nursing was done by men and women motivated by their religious faith. During the Crusades, illness and death

[1] Edward S. Rogers, *Human Ecology and Health,* The Macmillan Company, New York, 1960, p. 155.
[2] M. Adelaide Nutting and Lavinia L. Dock, *History of Nursing,* G. P. Putnam's Sons, New York, 1907, vol. 1, p. 102.

were the fate of many pilgrims on their way to the Holy Land. Monasteries were established on some routes to provide care for these sick and travel-worn pilgrims. Here was the beginning of hospitals and nursing.

Following the Crusades, a spirit of great unrest dominated Western Europe. Many who had visited eastern Mediterranean countries while on their pilgrimages, returned with a knowledge of new and easier modes of living, with stories of the luxuries of the East, its spices, jewels, and unfamiliar ideas about art and architecture. Important aftermaths of the Crusades were the improvement of economic conditions in many Western European countries; for example, the rise of the great maritime powers, Britain, France, Spain, and Italy, with their wealthy merchant class, and an eagerness for knowledge, especially in the sciences, in the universities.

Marked social reforms came with the end of the sixteenth century and the beginning of the seventeenth. This was also a period of creativity, resulting in an increased production in literature and the other arts, a broadening of the horizons of science, and, even more important to community health, a notable increase in social understanding, with a growing recognition of social responsibilities by those on different levels of power. The concept of the brotherhood of man and other such revolutionary ideas, for those times, as that men are born free and equal and entitled to equal chances, were gaining acceptance. Improvement in living conditions continued, resulting in better housing, improved sanitation, and more nutritious food. In some instances these gains were the results of the English Poor Laws of 1601 during the reign of Elizabeth I.

The sense of social responsibility for the welfare of others was demonstrated also by the sporadic attempts to provide nursing care for the sick, both in their homes and in hospitals. In 1610, in the little town of Annecy in eastern France, St. Francis de Sales (1567–1622) with the aid of Madame de Chantal, organized a nursing service for the care of the sick in their homes, the care to be given by a recently founded order of nuns drawn from women of the upper classes in the surrounding countryside. Unfortunately after five years, this order of nuns became cloistered and their home care of the sick was discontinued. Even though their project failed in such a short time, the work of St. Francis de Sales and Madame de Chantal created an interest in the venture, for in 1617 St. Vincent de Paul (1576–1660) founded a religious order of French women near Chatillon, France, to care for the sick on a home visiting nurse basis. St. Vincent de Paul had given much thought and study to the founding of this new organization while a university student in Paris. He introduced modern principles of social work and placed visiting nursing on a plane not reached in previous experiments of this nature. His order of nuns served local communities for many years, but after his death, it, too, became cloistered and could carry out its original purpose no longer.

Much of St. Vincent de Paul's philosophy of service to others is to be found in his writings, among which is the following, quoted from Nutting and Dock, which has significance and meaning for community health nurses today. "Lay off your jewels and fine clothing to visit the poor," said Vincent, "and treat them openly, respectfully and as persons of quality, avoiding all familiarity or stiffness. To send money is good, but we have not really begun to serve the poor until we visit them."[3]

In the centuries that followed, three movements or forces that stimulated interest in community health nursing were developing, slowly and unevenly, throughout Western Europe and were being carried to the New World.

These were (1) a sense of humanity, a deepening consciousness of the social problems affecting the lives of many people, such as poverty, inadequate housing, evils of the industrial revolution, child labor, deplorable prison conditions, and lack of opportunities for education; (2) the growth of medical science, which was developing from the curing of disease to the prevention of disease and the promotion of health; and (3) the development of nursing as a profession and a discipline.

Social conditions in England showed definite improvement in the late eighteenth and early nineteenth centuries because of the work of both John Howard and Octavia Hill. John Howard (1726–1790), a sheriff of Bedfordshire, brought about, through his observations and writings, outstanding prison reforms, not only in his native England but in many countries in Europe as well. He has been called an "inspiration to the whole Humanitarian Movement." Octavia Hill (1838–1912), a social worker and contemporary of Florence Nightingale, instigated practical housing reforms in the Liverpool and London slums, bringing comfort, safety, and health to thousands of poor families.

Another evidence of a growing sense of social justice was the founding of the International Red Cross in Switzerland in 1863, through the efforts of Henri Dunant, a young man interested in promoting the welfare of others. As the Red Cross societies developed in each country, their emphasis on humanity and their efforts to prevent and to alleviate human suffering wherever it existed widened opportunities for providing nursing care in hospitals and in the community, particularly in many European countries.

The concept of present-day nonreligious community health nursing service was introduced in 1859 under the aegis of William Rathbone of Liverpool, England, who saw visiting nursing as a service that encompassed the new perception of humanity, the knowledge of modern medical science, and the "renewed art of nursing." He was actively supported in his work by Miss Nightingale.

[3] *Ibid.,* p. 414.

Brainard has summarized the development of the three movements as follows:

> ... the "new humanity" had taught that universal brotherhood is but a name, unless it seeks to remove the causes of one's brother's degradation; and the new science had taught that disease and suffering are not a visitation from an angered God, but are the direct results of our own carelessness in not following the right principles of hygiene, sanitation and healthful living; and finally, the care of the sick had been raised from the despised occupation of unskilled, untrustworthy women, and placed in the hands of women of refinement and character, who looked upon it as a vocation, and were trained, not only to the gentle ways of the early nuns and deaconesses, but to the scientific care and treatment of the patient as well.[4]

## Community Health Nursing in the United States

Nursing care of the sick in their own homes by a graduate nurse was commenced in New York City in 1877, sponsored by the Women's Board of the New York City Mission. The nurse was Frances Root, a graduate of the newly established Bellvue Training School for Nurses. The visiting nurse program, though modest, was a success and similar ones were initiated on a sporadic basis in a few other American cities. Even in those early years, while providing bedside nursing care in city slums, these pioneer nurses recognized that many illnesses were caused by faulty economic and social conditions under which their patients and families lived, such as inadequate housing, lack of sanitation, insufficient food, and unfair, often vicious, labor conditions, and that measures for the prevention of these abuses were a necessity.

Nine years later the first district nursing associations were started, one in Boston and one in Philadelphia. They reflected a knowledge and understanding of the experience of the visiting nurse programs commenced previously in England. This was the period of prosperity in the reconstruction era following the Civil War. Standards of living were rising, and opportunities for education and travel, both in the United States and abroad, were becoming available to many people. Communication of ideas by post, telegraph, newspapers, and magazines was becoming a part of daily living. The idea of an organized district or visiting nurse service for the city poor spread rapidly west and south, and by 1900, twenty such agencies had been established in the major cities.

Robert Koch, director of the Imperial Health Bureau in Berlin, in 1882 reported on his studies and those of his confreres, which demonstrated that tuberculosis was a transmissible disease, caused by a specific organism. This new concept of the cause of tuberculosis, with its bearing on the care

[4]Annie M. Brainard, *The Evolution of Public Health Nursing,* W. B. Saunders Company, Philadelphia, 1922, pp. 102–103.

and control of the disease, was quickly accepted by a large part of the medical profession, both in Europe and in the United States. Koch's discovery brought a new approach to the control of tuberculosis, that of public health measures, e.g., epidemiology and health education. The contribution that community health nurses could make to the control of this disease was recognized soon by the medical profession and the community. Community health nurses became responsible for much of the case finding and case holding, for teaching patients and their families, and for providing both pre- and postsanatorium home nursing care. Nurses soon discovered that the families of their tuberculous patients, many of them in the upper socioeconomic brackets in the community, had other health problems, too. This widened the scope of the community health nursing program at the beginning of the twentieth century. This new aspect in the care and control of a specific disease by community health measures was important in the early development of community health nursing.

The leadership of Lillian Wald (1867–1940), both a nurse and social worker, at the beginning of this century was responsible for many developments in community health nursing. Miss Wald brought to her work a basic love of and faith in mankind, a brilliant mind trained in the sciences, a sense of the practical, and a vision of what community health nursing and social work could do for communities and their people. In 1893, she and Mary Brewster established a visiting nurse service as a part of their Henry Street Settlement in New York City. This became a model for similar organizations and a training center to which community health nurses were sent for many years, both on an apprenticeship basis and for advanced work in supervision and administration.

Miss Wald, in 1909, persuaded the Metropolitan Life Insurance Company to begin, at first on an experimental basis, a home nursing service for its policy holders through a working arrangement with the Henry Street Settlement. Twelve years later, a study and review of the project showed that the program had been highly successful and had been adopted by community health nursing agencies in many communities. When the number of policy holders warranted it and no community health nursing agency existed in the area, the company set up its own visiting nurse service to care for its policy holders. This program, with some variations, was adopted by other insurance companies in succeeding years.

With the assured income from the provision of nursing services to policy holders for which the insurance companies paid full cost, community health nursing agencies had a firm basis on which to build their overall budget. The remainder of the budget could then be raised in the community by charging full or part fees for visits to non-policy holders who could afford to pay, by gifts, and by allotments from community funds. This contributed to a healthy and steady growth of privately supported visiting nurse agencies throughout the country. With a group of persons (the insurance company policy holders) who were fairly secure economically and who were receiving home nursing service in times of illness from the visiting nurse, the feeling that nursing services were only for the sick poor began to change in many communities. Community health nursing organizations began to note an increase in requests for nursing services from families able and willing to pay for them.

The programs of caring for insurance companies' policy holders continued on a nationwide basis until several years after World War II, when changing social, economic, and health conditions made them no longer feasible. Many communities, however, had learned the value of community nursing services and had come to realize their responsibilities for supporting, by both public and private means, this health service to the community.

Lillian Wald, while on a visit to London, had an opportunity to observe a school nursing program that had been functioning in the London schools for nearly ten years. She was impressed to see that the nurses' work showed an improvement in school attendance and a reduction in the spread of communicable diseases among the children, especially skin diseases such as scabies and impetigo.

Through the efforts of Miss Wald, school nursing as a full-time program for a community health nurse was demonstrated and adopted in the New York City schools in 1902. This had followed by a few years the beginning of an industrial or occupational health nursing program in 1895 and was succeeded later by the development, on a specialty basis, of tuberculosis nursing in 1904, following the founding of the National Tuberculosis Association, and of venereal disease nursing as a specialty in 1909, when improved laboratory methods of diagnosis and treatment for syphilis and gonorrhea were developed through the work of Ehrlich.

Maternal and child health had its beginning as a specialty following the first White House Conference on Children called in 1909 through the interest and support of President Theodore Roosevelt. The program received an impetus in its development with the founding of the Children's Bureau by the Federal government in 1912 and 1913. Outstanding landmarks in the development of maternal and child health followed rapidly. The New York City Health Department had established a Division of Child Hygiene in 1908, and the New York State Health Department followed in 1914. In 1922, Congress passed the Sheppard-Towner Act for Federal aid for local infant welfare work. This money was distributed nationwide, generally through the state departments of health. The Social Security Act of 1935 and its amendments in succeeding years included, among other measures, provisions for public assistance, social services, and means of strengthening family life. These all had an important bearing on maternal and child health work in all parts of the country, rural and urban.

During the 1960s, additional health and welfare programs were initiated by Congress and state legislatures, such as the provisions for Medicare, Medicaid, and similar programs sponsored by individual states. All this social legislation has increased the opportunities for the community health nurse to provide nursing care and health teaching to patients and families in all age groups.

In the years immediately preceding World War I, certain social, economic, and humanitarian forces, implemented by such leaders as Annie W. Goodrich, Lillian Wald, and Edith Abbott of the Children's Bureau brought about several events that were important in the development of community health nursing. In 1910, Mrs. Helen Hartley Jenkins, a friend of Miss Wald's, gave funds to Teachers' College Columbia University to establish an academic program of study in community health nursing. Thus a little more than thirty years after Frances Root began her work in district nursing, college preparation in that field became available to nurses. Prior to this, whatever preparation nurses had been able to secure had been provided on an apprenticeship basis by some of the big city nursing agencies, such as the Henry Street Settlement and the Instructive District Nursing Association of Boston.

Following World War I, many colleges and universities initiated study programs in community health nursing for graduate nurses. These were discontinued as community health nursing preparation became recognized as an integral part of the preparation for *all* nurses in the collegiate programs for nursing.

The National Organization for Public Health Nursing was founded in Chicago in 1912. Miss Wald was its first president. The new organization had three types of membership: nurse members, lay members, and corporate members. The key word in the name of the organization was "for." Lay members were active participants and were considered important to the new organization. They worked closely with community health nurses for forty years to improve the standards of nursing service and education. In 1952, the organization became a part of the National League for Nursing at the reorganization of the nursing organizations.

At the time of its founding, the National Organization for Public Health Nursing received a small but successful quarterly publication from the Cleveland, Ohio, Visiting Nurse Association. This became the official national magazine of the young organization, and was best known as *Public Health Nursing*. It devoted its contents to the interests of those in the public health field. In 1953 it was absorbed by a new publication, *Nursing Outlook*, founded to meet, on a broader basis, the needs of an expanding profession.

The American Red Cross pioneered in rural community health nursing when, in 1912, it provided demonstrations of community health nursing care to people in the villages and on the farms. Much of the work was done by "itinerant nurses," who were sent to an area for a period of several months to demonstrate home care of the sick, school nursing, and well-baby conferences. These nurses also conducted mothers' classes and home nursing classes. It was hoped that the communities would recognize the need to employ full-time community health nurses to carry on the program.

Following the introduction of the Red Cross program, rural nursing developed rapidly. County health departments, particularly in the Southern and Western states, were established. Nearly every county health department had a full-time nurse on its staff, though often she was the only full-time professional member of the department. Rural nursing was facilitated further by the production and marketing of the first inexpensive automobile, which made it possible for many nurses to reach patients and families on distant farms and ranches. Putting nurses "on wheels" opened up many new opportunities for nursing services in both rural and urban areas.

The organization of the Children's Bureau by the Federal government was completed in 1913. The Bureau stimulated programs of mother and child care by preparing and distributing health literature, e.g., *Prenatal Care*, by investigating unsatisfactory conditions relating to mothers and children, and by assisting with community health studies. The Children's Bureau programs expanded rapidly following the Social Security Act of 1935. The Bureau is now a division of the Department of Health, Education and Welfare.

Following World War I, a trend from specialization toward generalization occurred, with the staff nurse being responsible for all types of community health nursing services in her district, and the agency providing her with consultant service. This shift from specialization to generalization, and an increasing demand for community health nursing services, contributed to the rapid expansion of community health nursing programs of study for graduate nurses, as previously mentioned, in colleges and universities. The National Organization for Public Health Nursing offered consultant service in the development of such programs, and helped to promote standards by an accreditation service and by studies and surveys.

For many years Annie W. Goodrich had pointed out that although nursing had a place in the institutions of the sick, it could not render its full service to the community until it had found a place also in colleges and universities. In 1923 Miss Goodrich founded the Yale School of Nursing as a collegiate school, and for the first time adequate preparation for community health nursing was included in the basic curriculum. This was an innovation closely watched by other collegiate schools of nursing. Slowly they adopted the program, but it was not until after World War II that community health nursing preparation became an integral part of the basic collegiate curriculum and a requirement for national accreditation for a collegiate school of nursing.

During and after World War II, the increased demand for nursing services by the military and by the civilian population made mandatory many improvements in the utilization of nursing services, both in hospitals and in community health agencies, including a discriminating use of the professional nurse's knowledge, abilities, and time. Wider use of the team concept and more carefully planned services by auxiliary personnel were instituted in many hospitals and community health agencies.

Across the country, there was a growing effort to prevent duplication of services offered by the official and nonofficial agencies in any one community. One means was to combine such agencies wherever possible, thereby conserving the nurses' time and efforts and reducing such overhead costs as those of rent, administration, and travel. Knowledge regarding health practices acquired by the laity during and since World War II and the new public health and community health nursing practices that developed from the nation's war experiences facilitated the movement for the combining of community health nursing agencies.

Some nursing studies had been made in the period between World War I and World War II, such as *Nursing and Nursing Education in the United States, Nurses, Patients and Pocketbooks,* and the *Survey of Public Health Nursing.* In order to determine how to meet adequately the country's needs for nursing in the period following World War II, and how to provide the kind of professional education and preparation required by nurses, it was recognized that more studies and research regarding nursing and nursing education were needed. Such additional studies, e.g., *Nursing for the Future, Collegiate Education for Nurses, Twenty Thousand Nurses Tell Their Story,* and *Toward Quality in Nursing,* have been published. Many other studies relating to curriculum needs and development have been made; these have pointed out the need for deepening the content of the preparation for nursing, for supporting nursing knowledge with contributions from other disciplines in the natural and social sciences and the humanities, for developing skills and abilities in the problem-solving approach, and for preparing students in collegiate programs in basic nursing for beginning positions in both hospitals and community health agencies. Current developments in nursing education attempt to meet these needs on both basic and graduate levels of study.

The nursing profession recognized the need also for continued research in other aspects of nursing, nursing practice, and research methodology as well as education, thus the founding in 1952 of the periodical *Nursing Research Report,* sponsored by the National League for Nursing and later by the American Nurses' Association also. Through its pages, *Nursing Research* has made the results of many studies in the various fields of nursing available to the profession as a whole and to allied disciplines. In 1955, the American Nurses' Association created the American Nurses'

Foundation to meet the needs for a permanent nonprofit organization devoted to research in nursing.[5] Research programs to determine community needs for nursing in all its aspects and ways for meeting these needs will continue for years to come.

## TRENDS IN COMMUNITY HEALTH NURSING
### General Trends
Trends in community health nursing are part of the overall trends in general nursing and reflect those evidenced in current medicine. Furthermore they are closely allied to the social, economic, and political trends of the times. A distinction should be made between a tendency and a trend. A trend is a turn toward a specific direction; a tendency is an aptness to move or act in a particular way. A tendency should be watched, as it could be the beginning of a trend. An alert nurse might note a tendency in a family or a neighborhood which could become a trend, e.g., if two or three families with school-aged children move from the neighborhood, the nurse might wonder if this tendency could become a trend, producing a change in the average age of those living in the neighborhood and requiring a different type of nursing service, with more emphasis on geriatrics and less on preschool and school-age child health programs.

## TRENDS IN NURSING SERVICES AND FUNCTIONS
Community health nursing practice is a changing and evolutionary concept of our time and nurses must prepare and adapt to the needs of a dynamic society, which itself is in a continuous state of change and new order. Community health nurses are expected to assume many new duties and functions in America's move toward comprehensive health care, not only for the poor, but for the entire community.

The outstanding trend in community health programs is that of establishing the delivery of a comprehensive, effective system of health care for every citizen. This trend is in response to demands that have been made in the past few decades by leaders in community health and other groups of society. Such a trend is developing and will eventually be accepted and become a part of American life. National health insurance programs, health maintenance organizations, and health education foundations for expanded citizen health education are all proposals under study. Every nurse, especially the community health nurse, will play a large part in the delivery of this comprehensive health program. Nurses need to study the development of

[5]Susan D. Taylor, "American Nurses' Foundation, 1955–1970," *Nursing Research Report,* 5:4:1-6 (December) 1970.

these plans so that the nursing profession can actively participate and contribute to the planning and execution of such a health service.

According to The Carnegie Commission on Higher Education,[6] the trends that will affect the nation's health and the nature of health-care delivery include:

**1.** An increase in prepaid professional group practice plans, with emphasis on preventive services

**2.** Greater concern for achieving effective functioning of health-care teams, which would include professional and allied health personnel

**3.** Greater emphasis on care outside the hospital in a wider variety of health-care facilities, such as neighborhood health centers, facilities for ambulatory care of convalescing patients, and homemaker services to facilitate care in the home

**4.** Increased acceptance of health care as a public utility with government backing

**5.** Acquisition of new knowledge and technology on a continuing basis, with more extensive use of computers and automation techniques, which will lead to new therapeutic techniques requiring in turn new technologies, new kinds of trained personnel, and cooperation of many persons working closely together toward prevention of physical diseases and mental illnesses

**6.** A shift of education, service, and research functions into an organized, integrated system of health-care delivery for the consumer

The above trends will have a direct or indirect impact on the functioning of all nurses and will greatly influence the practices and the emphases of community health nurses as practitioners, coordinators, teachers, supervisors, counselors, and health educators. As practitioners, nurses will be giving specialized services in community health centers, which focus on comprehensive health problems such as mental health, chronic and degenerative diseases, child spacing and abortion counseling, drug abuse, support of those attempting to rid themselves of the drug habit, social and medical conditions arising from environmental health problems, and other conditions meriting nursing specialization. As coordinators, nurses will initiate multidisciplinary team conferences, act as liaison agents between per-

---

[6]The Carnegie Commission on Higher Education, *Higher Education and the Nation's Health,* McGraw-Hill Book Company, New York, 1970, pp. 31–33.

sonnel of allied professional fields, and encourage greater team effort in health activities in behalf of consumers.

As teachers and supervisors, nurses will have an increasing responsibility for instructing, guiding, and supervising nonprofessional personnel, such as community health aides, to perform duties in homes and health centers. The nurse also will direct attention toward achieving an interpersonal cohesion between professional and nonprofessional personnel to facilitate team functioning. As counselors, nurses will interact with consumers to give assistance with health needs as desired and will encourage consumer participation, responsibility, and self-direction in community health activities. As health educators, nurses will need to be knowledgeable regarding current social problems in the community, pending health legislation and policies, community organization processes, existing health planning committees, and ways of implementing desirable community health activities.

Nurses will also need to maintain their preparation by additional study, research, and writing for both professional and lay publications and will be expected to speak to public groups about their work and community health needs.

It will be many years before this long-term trend reaches completion nationwide, but some aspects are currently under way. Other less comprehensive trends appearing today are discussed here.

**Maternal and child health care.**   Maternal and child health programs have always been an integral part of community health nursing. New trends in this field are evident. Changing sexual mores are bringing about a wider acceptance and use of birth control methods. Society is becoming more permissive toward the practice of abortions, and there is a growing acceptance of the unmarried or single mother as a member of the community. Some states have liberalized their abortion laws, providing that the abortion takes place prior to the twentieth week of pregnancy and that it is performed by a licensed, practicing physician in a licensed hospital. In most states with such laws, the decision to have the abortion lies with the mother and her physician. In this changing trend in American culture, some nurses will have emotional difficulties in being accepting of this situation if it is counter to their own religious background and family culture. Nurses must be nonjudgmental in such matters, however, and not force their personal values on others.

Nurse midwifery has an expanding role in the maternal child health program, especially in crowded urban areas. The nurse midwife must be an experienced community health nurse who sees the family as a unit and has additional preparation in midwifery. Such preparation is offered currently by a few university schools of nursing on a master's level of study. The nurse midwife functions within a medically directed health service as a part of the hospital obstetrical team and not independently, as in some European countries.

The nurse midwife follows the mother in her pregnancy, conducts the normal delivery in the hospital, provides care and counseling in the postpartum period in the health center or outpatient department, and makes follow-up home calls to observe the progress of the mother and infant. It is expected that this trend will develop to help meet the need for safe obstetrical care.

**Increased life expectancy.** This social and health trend places added responsibility on community health nursing to provide more services to persons who have chronic diseases, such as cardiovascular disease or cancer, and crippling diseases due in part to arthritis and accidents, as well as to those who are mentally retarded or have mental illnesses. This will require an added number of nurses who not only will have had additional preparation in these fields, but who also will participate in continuing education programs.

With increasing hospital care costs and the many new medications and treatments now available to patients, there will be more movement by patients from home to hospital to home. Community health nurses will play a larger role in the care of these patients, who may have brief periods of hospitalization interspersed with home care. This will require an increasing identification of the community health nurse with the hospital staff, including nurses, doctors, dietitians, social workers, and the various therapists, and will depend on practical methods of patient referral for success.

**Rehabilitation.** Basic to the care of patients in all age groups with physical, emotional, and mental diseases, acute or chronic, is rehabilitation. It is of vital importance for the child born deaf, the victim of an industrial accident, the patient with an emotional or mental disorder, or the elderly victim of stroke. In order to secure the best results, rehabilitation of the patient must begin as early as possible after the diagnosis is established. In the past few years, the growing number of older persons in the general population, the higher incidence of accidents, with resulting incapacities, and war casualties have stimulated a marked interest in rehabilitation on the part of many groups in the community. This appreciation by the general public and by the health professions of the possibilities and importance of the patient's rehabilitation emphasizes this trend in community health nursing. Community health nursing agencies are assuming increasing responsibility for developing and promoting rehabilitation programs in the home, school, industry, and community, and for assisting families in the care and rehabilitation of patients in their own homes (see Case Record 1).

### Trends in Health Center Development

Nurses will have greater professional responsibilities in the health centers now undergoing rapid changes resulting from the insufficient health care that many communities provided the poor, the isolated, and members of minority groups in the past. A new phenomenon has appeared in many large cities, "the people's health center" offering free health services to the socially "disenfranchized," especially those ethnic and social groups living in slum areas. This new type of neighborhood health center is planned, developed, and operated by those neighborhood groups who use it, usually with no charge and functioning in a nonjudgmental atmosphere. The program is comprehensive. The nurse emphasizes the prevention of disease by her teaching and participates in disease care, cure, and control.

Some rural areas with critical medical-care shortages are beginning to have the services of specially prepared community health nurses having the knowledge and abilities to provide for diagnosis and therapeutic care of patient and family as well as for the prevention of disease. This trend is similar to that of the developing trend in midwifery. These increases in the community health nurse's duties and responsibilities adds to the need for additional services of the health aide group in health centers and the home.

**Evaluation and appraisal.** The use of evaluation and appraisal procedures is essential in all fields of public health, and especially in community health nursing. This field of nursing depends on a continuous evaluation and appraisal process in order to meet the needs of family and patient in the face of the rapid changes taking place in current society. Not only their needs should be assessed, but also the goals of the patient and family, for they may change rapidly with new family situations: a birth, a death, a new job, or a move to a different neighborhood.

Community health nursing methods of teaching and assisting families to meet their health problems need continuous evaluation. Frequent appraisal of the performance of the family and patient in meeting successfully their own problems, without constant supervision by the nurse, provides essential information for agency and community planning. Both the agency and the nurse need to know the ability of patients and families who have had community health nursing supervision to react satisfactorily to a new health crisis.

**Community health nursing and international health.** International health is a new responsibility on the world scene and one of today's major health problems. Community health nurses in all parts of the world share the concerns of their governments for improving the health of their own people. It is well known in public health that health or the lack of it in *one* country can affect directly the health of people in *other* countries. One country's communicable disease incidence can quickly become a serious matter to other nations, because of modern transportation, international commerce, and increased global travel (see Case Record 8).

It is necessary for all nations and their health professions to work together to protect the health of the world. Many governments and their leading health personnel do this through participation in the specialized agencies of the United Nations, e.g., the World Health Organization and the Food and Agricultural Organization.

The International Council of Nurses provides channels for nurses of many countries to work together and to share their knowledge and skills. The basic desire to help others, which is a part of nursing, provides a common bond between nurses of every country. Since the days of Miss Goodrich, Miss Wald, and Miss Nutting, American nurses have taken a deep interest in the responsibilities they share with nurses of other countries, such as care and teaching of the patient, nursing service administration, nursing education, and community health nursing. They participate in the study and development of these subjects on an international basis through the International Council of Nurses, the World Health Organization, and other agencies of the United Nations.

Helen Nussbaum, the former general secretary of the International Council of Nurses, spoke on this point at a conference at the University of Edinburgh, Scotland, in the summer of 1964. She pointed out the barrier of language in achieving understanding of problems in nursing education and nursing service in various countries, citing the word "welfare" as being difficult to translate into certain languages.

She believed that understanding between nurses of different countries could be reached by developing insight into the cultural background of others, by being tolerant, by having patience in trying to understand the philosophy and beliefs of others, particularly as they pertain to health matters, illness, and death, and finally, by gaining *wisdom*. The latter she considered to be the supreme quality in the definition of understanding.


### Trends in Public Health

Emerging trends in public health that will affect community health nursing include solutions to some of the newer problems to be found in connection with environment, such as control of air, sound, and smog, and radiation activity. There are problems of accident prevention, especially in the home, rehabilitation, care and rehabilitation of the alcoholic and drug abuser, and care of the mentally ill and the mentally retarded, including new approaches to the care of the mental patient by the community, such as day hospitals and increased provisions for out-patient department services.

With the shifts in social, economic, political, and health situations, additional trends in public health and community health nursing will emerge to meet new and different needs of the patient, family, and community. These trends will lead to more satisfying and productive ways of reaching the goals of public health and of nursing.

### The Continuing Education of the Nurse

The above trends all point to another need, that of the community health nurse for continuous and on-going preparation, both in nursing and in allied disciplines, in order to interpret and utilize new methods in medicine, social work, and nursing practices. Nursing shares this challenge with all professions today. The changes rapidly taking place in the care of the mentally retarded provide one example of the nurse's responsibility for continuous study. Recent developments in assisting the alcoholic patient or the drug abuser and his family point to another area in which the nurse must have a growing awareness. The traditional patterns of psychiatric care of the patient in institutions are no longer considered by many psychiatrists to be compatible with current medical thinking and practice. There is growing evidence that care and treatment in the patient's home community are more efficacious. This involves the concept of "family therapy." For such a program the family needs professional assistance and support from doctors and nurses in learning to understand and solve their problems. The community health nurse must be prepared to help and teach both patient and family.

These new trends in community health nursing require both agencies and nurses to plan and to carry out education programs that will increase the knowledge and skills of the nurse. Although many agencies have had such programs in the past, new and revitalized ones are necessary, for as the Red Queen said to Alice, ". . . it takes all the running you can do to keep in the same place."

### PHILOSOPHY OF COMMUNITY HEALTH NURSING

The philosophy of community health nursing, like that of all nursing, has always been based on the concept of the "worth and dignity of the individual." A hundred years ago, Octavia Hill, a social worker active in slum housing reform, expressed the same idea:

> It is essential to remember that each man has his own view of his life, and must be free to fulfill it; that in many ways he is a far better judge of it than we, as

he has lived through and felt what we have only seen. Our work is rather to bring him to the point of considering, and to the spirit of judging rightly, than to consider or judge for him.[7]

Basic to the belief of all nurses is the acceptance that all persons have the capacity and the potential to develop better physical health and improve psychosocial well-being, dependent upon their desires, willingness to change, and adaptability to prescribed therapies. Nursing practice assists individuals and families in adjusting their health needs and wants, resolving health problems in the social, emotional, and physical environments, and facilitating coping abilities to achieve higher levels of health maintenance satisfactory to all persons.

Each community health nurse develops her own personal philosophy of nursing, tempered by her background, preparation, experience, and personality. Her philosophy will grow and deepen as she acquires experience in working with others—patients, families, communities, and coworkers—and as she adds to her preparation and understanding by continuous study, reading, and thinking. It has been said that "the community health nurse has lots to learn, to teach and to do."

The philosophy that community health nursing is based on "the worth and dignity of the individual" is identified closely with the age-old purpose of nursing, which Marion Sheahan so ably stated to be, "... caring for, giving comfort and ease, helping persons with health problems to become healed in body and mind or helping them to live with their infirmities with grace."[8] The nurse who can successfully teach others to "live with their infirmities with grace" has that same ability deep within herself and has achieved a philosophy in accord with that of community health nursing.

## SUGGESTED READING

Bierman, Jessie M.: "Some Things Learned," *American Journal of Public Health,* 59:930–935 (June) 1969.

Breslow, Lester: "Standards for Changing Practice in Abortion," Editorial, *American Journal of Public Health,* 61:215–217 (February) 1971.

Christy, Teresa E.: "Portrait of a Leader: M. Adelaide Nutting," *Nursing Outlook,* 17:20–22 (June) 1969.

———: "Portrait of a Leader: Annie Warburton Goodrich," *Nursing Outlook,* 18: 46–50 (August) 1970.

[7]Octavia Hill, *Through the Ages,* Family Welfare Association of America, New York (no date of publication), p. 42.

[8]Marion W. Sheahan, "This I Believe About Nursing," *Nursing Outlook,* 11:641 (September) 1963.

————: "Portrait of a Leader: Lillian D. Wald," *Nursing Outlook,* 18:50–54 (March) 1970.

Hanlon, John J.: "An Ecologic View of Public Health," *American Journal of Public Health,* 59:4–11 (January) 1969.

Harris, David, et al.: "Nurse-Midwifery in New York City," *American Journal of Public Health,* 61:64–77 (January) 1971.

Leppert, Phyllis G.: "A Proposal for Educating More Nurse Midwives," *Nursing Outlook,* 18:42–43 (September) 1970.

Levine, Eugene: "Nurse Manpower: Yesterday, Today, and Tomorrow," *American Journal of Nursing,* 69:290–296 (February) 1969.

Lewis, M. D.: "Health Care for Denver's Poor," *American Journal of Nursing,* 69: 1469–1471 (July) 1969.

McNerney, Walter J.: "Health Care Reforms—The Myths and Realities," *American Journal of Public Health,* 61:222–232 (February) 1971.

Mussallem, Helen K.: "The Changing Role of the Nurse," *American Journal of Nursing,* 69:514–517 (March) 1969.

National Commission for the Study of Nursing and Nursing Education, *An Abstract for Action,* vol. 1, McGraw-Hill Book Company, New York, 1970.

Paynich, Mary Louise, et al.: "Is There a Role for Nurse Clinician in Public Health?" *Nursing Outlook,* 17:32–36 (July) 1969.

Roberts, Mary M.: *American Nursing: History and Interpretation,* The Macmillan Company, New York, 1954.

Rothberg, June S.: "Challenges for Rehabilitative Nursing," *Nursing Outlook,* 17: 37–39 (November) 1969.

Smith, Richard A., and James E. Banta: "Global Community Health—A New Health Direction," *American Journal of Public Health,* 59:1713–1719 (September) 1969.

Walker, A. Elizabeth: "Primex—The Family Nurse Practitioner Program," *Nursing Outlook,* 20:1:28–31 (January) 1972.

# PART TWO

Part Two offers some case situations and case records. The first are brief descriptions of actual situations experienced and problems encountered by community health nurses in their work in urban and rural areas. Topics and questions are presented for class discussion at the end of each situation.

A series of case records follows. These are not case studies; rather, they describe the community health nurse's plans and work with individual patients and families. Topics and questions for class discussion are included at the end of each record. Many precepts of community health nursing and principles of learning presented in Part One are illustrated in these case situations and case records.

What knowledge drawn from nursing and its associated disciplines did the nurse need in order to help the patient, the family, and the community? What understanding, appreciation, and awareness did the nurse need as she worked in the situations described? For example, Mrs. G., the tuberculous patient, and Mr. G. demonstrated many needs based on their physical and emotional problems. What knowledge, understanding, and skills did the nurse utilize in attempting to meet their needs?

It is hoped that these descriptions of what community health nursing is and what community health nurses do will provide some insight into this phase of nursing and add depth to the student's understanding that she can apply in her own experience with patients and families in homes and community situations.

# 1 CASE SITUATION

# A Failure in Communication

A mother, with a Spanish-speaking background and a limited knowledge of English and whose husband had recently been hospitalized for tuberculosis, was urged by the community health nurse to secure x-rays for herself and her five children at the county clinic. A neighbor agreed to drive them to the clinic. The nurse made appointments for the following morning and notified the mother, but the appointments were not kept.

A few days later, the nurse made a home visit to learn why the family did not go to the clinic. During the visit, the mother said with some hostility, "I like Miss A. (a local church worker) better than you, she 'presents' me." The nurse, startled, realized she had failed in her teaching and that little learning or change of behavior had taken place with this mother, who was waiting to be paid for going to the clinic with gifts, such as clothes, which she received from the church worker. It became obvious to the nurse that the mother had agreed to go for the x-rays to satisfy the nurse, not for any value she could see for herself and her family and therefore wished to be recompensed for her trouble.

## DISCUSSION

1. What precepts of community health nursing had the nurse overlooked?

2. What principles of learning had she failed to apply?

Three times a week for the past several weeks the community health nurse had been visiting the Q. family to assist Mrs. Q. in the care of her mother, who had cancer in its terminal stage. Mrs. Q. was deeply devoted to her mother.

In addition to the patient, the family included Mr. and Mrs. Q. and their five-year-old son, Peter. The family lived in a comfortable home in a pleasant neighborhood. Mr. Q. was a divisional manager of a large firm and was away from home on business much of the time.

This particular morning, the nurse arrived about ten o'clock. Peter answered the doorbell and greeted the nurse.

"Good morning," responded the nurse, "how are you this morning, and how is Grandmother?" At the word "Grandmother," Peter scowled darkly at the nurse and kicked the door vehemently.

"I wish I could put grandmother in a black, black closet." And he added for emphasis, "I'd like to lock her up tight." At that moment, Mrs. Q. appeared, gravely concerned with her mother's failing condition.

# Family Stress

## DISCUSSION

**1.** Should the nurse discuss Peter's reaction with his mother? If so, what should be her approach?

**2.** Should the nurse talk to Peter about his grandmother? Or should she ignore his attitude?

**3.** If she ignores Peter's reaction, how do you think the situation might resolve itself?

# Planning the Teaching for a Mild Diabetic

**Mrs. Rachel R., age fifty-four; diagnosis: mild diabetes.**

Mrs. R., a childless widow, lived alone in a small apartment. During a recent general physical examination, she was found to have a mild diabetic condition. Her physician told her that medication was not indicated and that her condition could be controlled by diet. He advised her to avoid all foods containing sugar, saying, "no candy, jam, cake, cookies, ice cream, or similar foods."

A neighbor thought Mrs. R. needed help in planning her meals, especially as she was on a low-income food budget, and requested a visit from the local visiting nurse agency to help Mrs. R. with diet planning. The nurse called the next day about 11 A.M. Mrs. R. was resting after a morning of general house cleaning. She was a slender, attractive woman, not robust. She said she had grown up on a farm in the Midwest, the youngest of a large family. Her mother and sisters were all considered to be good cooks and her mother had been noted for the good meals she provided for her family.

Mrs. R. was not aware of any incidence of diabetes in her family and knew nothing about the disease—its symptoms, effects, or treatment. She said she was always tired, often very thirsty, had frequent urination, especially at night, and chronic constipation. The doctor had told her she had high blood sugar, but that no sugar appeared in her urine.

When asked about her current diet, Mrs. R. replied that for breakfast she usually had a bran cereal with one-half cup of low-fat milk and a handful of raisins, a small piece of buttered whole wheat bread and a hard-boiled egg. She did not like egg yolk, so threw most of it away. She also had a cup of black coffee. Usually her lunch consisted of a cup of low-fat cottage cheese, two apples, and one slice of whole wheat bread with butter. For dinner, she had meat, potatoes or rice, a vegetable, frequently frozen carrots or peas, and fresh fruit. She added that she craved a piece of cake, but was afraid to bake one for fear she would eat it all at one sitting. She was disturbed by all she had read and heard about cyclamates and had discontinued the use of sugarless ice cream and desserts.

The nurse recognized that Mrs. R. needed help in understanding the implications and nature of her diabetic condition, such as: (1) within the limits of her budget, how to plan a nutritious and satisfying diet, including an understanding of "exchanges" on a twenty-four-hour basis; (2) some mental health aspects relating to her situation; (3) the need for personal care she must take of herself, such as skin care, care of cuts and scratches, care of her feet, the need for regular exercise because of the problems of arteriosclerosis in the large blood vessels in her legs, eating at stated hours, and the care and protection of her eyes.

## DISCUSSION

Outline the teaching content for the nurse's next two visits to Mrs. R. Suggest some teaching aids the nurse might use.

# 4 CASE SITUATION

# A Hospital Extension Program Patient

Mr. and Mrs. Z., a childless couple, lived in a small house, which they owned, in a quiet neighborhood. Mr. Z., age eighty, and Mrs. Z., age seventy-five, attended their nearby church regularly and participated in church affairs. Mr. Z. looked after their small garden. Nearly every day, he walked to an adjacent park where he met and talked with other elderly, retired men. The couple had a small pension that was adequate for their needs. Friends and neighbors visited them regularly and helped with the shopping when necessary.

Mr. Z. began to complain of stiffness and pain in both hips. Following consultation, surgery was proposed, and bilateral arthroplasty was done. An infection developed in the left hip, and several castings were necessary, requiring the patient to remain in the hospital for several months.

Mrs. Z. grew eager to have her husband return home. She assured the medical service at the hospital that with the help of a visiting nurse, she was sure she could care for him at home.

The patient was placed on the hospital extension program. The orthopedic resident, the ward head nurse, the physiotherapist, and the social worker met with the community health nurse who would help Mrs. Z., and a program of care for Mr. Z. was outlined. The services of the hospital staff and other clinical resources were made available to Mrs. Z. if necessary.

After Mr. Z.'s return home, the nurse visited him every day, and then gradually reduced her visits to once a week. She reported regularly to the hospital team regarding Mr. Z.'s progress. Soon after returning home, Mr. Z. had a urinary infection. The hospital team was notified; a staff doctor made three home calls, and medications were left.

After that, Mr. Z. improved steadily, and slowly he was able to resume his former pattern of living.

## DISCUSSION

**1.** What community health nursing precepts functioned in relation to the home care of Mr. Z?

**2.** In providing care for this family, what responsibilities did the community health nurse have for Mr. Z? for Mrs. Z?

**3.** There are several types of hospital extension programs. Describe one program with which you are familiar, either from your own experience in the field or from your reading.

## 5 CASE SITUATION

## Need—A Factor in Learning

The director of a home for single pregnant mothers asked a community health nurse to discuss venereal diseases with the young women in the home. The group ranged from thirteen to thirty years in age, with a median age of sixteen. The nurse, recognizing that this was a difficult assignment, prepared her outline with much care.

On the evening of the meeting, the group filed into the dayroom, looking bored and uninterested. They listened politely but with little change of expression. After about ten minutes, the nurse seeing that they were not interested in what she was saying, brought the talk to a close and asked for questions. There was silence; then the thirteen-year-old girl raised her hand timidly and asked, "What kind of diapers do you think are best, the three-cornered ones or the long ones?" Realizing that the question indicated what the young women were interested in, the nurse hastened to answer the question. Before she had finished, other questions on baby care and growth and development came so fast that there was not time to answer them all, and she promised to return another evening.

### DISCUSSION

**1.** What principles of learning were operating here?

**2.** What principles were not operating?

**3.** Since these young women had been exposed to venereal disease, would you have accepted the director's request for such a talk? Give reasons for your answer.

**4.** Outline the content of a talk to young people on venereal diseases.

A nurse, new to the district, was visiting schools in a remote mountainous area of the county for the first time. She watched the children playing at the recess period and noticed two unhappy little girls in long cotton dresses, standing apart from their schoolmates. On questioning the teacher, the nurse learned that each autumn their mother sent to a mail-order house for their school clothes but always lengthened the skirts to their ankles. This naturally caused comment and laughter from the other children.

"What is this mother trying to communicate?" the nurse thought later. Was it some form of prudery? If so, what was the underlying cause? What could be done to lessen the burden of ridicule these little girls were suffering?

The next day the nurse conferred with the county social worker, who immediately recognized the situation and explained that the children's mother, who had limited mental ability, had been an unwed mother in her early teens and that several years later she had married an older man in the district. The two little girls had been born to the marriage. By hiding their legs with the long dresses, did the mother think she was protecting them from the unhappy experience of her own girlhood? A home call to the mother showed that this was the case.

**6** CASE SITUATION

# Recognition of a Nonverbal Communication

## DISCUSSION

**1.** What social and psychologic forces were operating here?

**2.** What plans for helping mother and daughters would you suggest?

**3.** Would you involve the schoolteacher in your plans? If so, how would you do it? If not, what are your reasons?

**4.** If this situation had occurred in your district, what community organizations or agencies could you and the social worker have used?

# Syphilis in an Itinerant Family

An itinerant construction worker, with his pregnant wife and two children, was en route from one job to another in a car and trailer. Late in the evening, while they were traveling on a lonely mountain road, the mother commenced her labor. The father ran to a nearby ranch house to inquire for the nearest hospital and was told that it was 30 miles down the valley but that there was a doctor in a small town 2 miles away. The rancher offered to call him.

The doctor arrived in time to deliver the patient by candlelight in the trailer. The delivery was quick and easy. He recommended that the family not move on for a few days and promised to ask the community health nurse to call in the morning.

The next morning the doctor called the local health department to request a nursing visit to the family, for the purpose of bathing mother and baby and checking their conditions. The nurse found them without difficulty. She bathed the baby. His physical condition aroused suspicions in the nurse. Then, while bathing the mother, the nurse noted some signs and symptoms which she thought might be caused by secondary syphilis. (Later, laboratory findings confirmed the nurse's suspicions.)

## DISCUSSION

**1.** What steps should the nurse take at this point? List them in order of importance.

**2.** What precepts of community health nursing were important to observe in this case?

**3.** Name some possible signs and symptoms of secondary syphilis that the nurse might have observed while bathing this mother.

**4.** What symptoms might the nurse have observed in bathing the baby?

# 8 CASE SITUATION

## A Family with an Alcoholic Member

During a teacher-nurse conference one afternoon, the teacher mentioned Jean N.'s periodic absences from school for no apparent reason and said that she was falling behind in her schoolwork.

"I used to have her brother, Jimmie, in my class last year," the teacher commented, "and he was absent this way, too. Usually the mother telephones that the children will not be in school that day, but gives no reason. They come on the school bus, and I've asked the driver if he knows anything about them. He said the mother told him if the children were not at the bus stop in the morning not to wait for them. I'm sure it's not a matter of money, they are always nicely dressed. Do you think a home call would be in order?"

The nurse agreed that it would be; she, too, had wondered about the children lately, as neither of them looked well and both seemed unhappy. She planned for a home call that afternoon.

The nurse found the home, a large well-kept farmhouse, about 15 miles from the school. Mrs. N., a neat-looking somewhat tense woman, answered the nurse's knock. The two children were with her. The nurse introduced herself and was invited into a pleasant living room. The mother was courteous but unresponsive. She gave some vague excuses for the children's absences. After about ten minutes, the nurse, realizing that nothing was being accomplished, took her leave, baffled by the situation. She made another home call en route to her office. It was nearly five o'clock when she reached her desk, to find a note to call Mrs. N. as soon as she came in. Somewhat puzzled, the nurse returned the call. Mrs. N. was almost sobbing as she said, "I didn't know what to say to you this afternoon. My children and I are in great trouble. My husband is really a very good man, but often he drinks too much, and then I have to keep the children home on those days to help me with the chores. Could you come back in the morning to see me?"

The nurse promised to do so, and made an appointment for about ten-thirty the next day.

## DISCUSSION

**1.** What should the nurse include in her preparation for the next day's visit?

**2.** How should the nurse approach the situation?

**3.** In reporting back to the teacher, what information should be shared with her regarding the family?

**4.** What can a nurse contribute to a family faced with problems due to alcoholism?

**5.** List the official and nonofficial resource agencies available in your community for helping a family with this sort of problem.

# 9 CASE SITUATION

# A Family's Reaction to Death

In May, Mrs. B. brought Mark to a preschool registration conference. While talking to the community health nurse, Mrs. B. said she expected a new baby early in October. When the nurse offered to call to help her plan for the baby, Mrs. B. eagerly accepted.

The nurse found the family living in an attractive duplex in a pleasant area, one block from the school. They had lived in this home about a year. Mr. B., age thirty, had been a Federal government employee for the past nine years. He had been attending night school classes at a nearby college. The nurse did not meet him, but from his wife's comments, he appeared to be conscientious, stable, and intelligent. He helped at home when he could, took the children to the park to play, and seemed to understand the importance of physical and emotional health.

Mrs. B., twenty-eight, was a bright, energetic young woman with a variety of interests, her main ones being her family and their welfare. The children, Eileen, seven, and Mark, five, appeared to be normal, healthy, and active.

Although Mrs. B. had seen her physician several times, she had questions relating to her pregnancy and was interested in having help. Her other pregnancies had been normal, and she had breast-fed her babies. With this pregnancy, she experienced great fatigue and was completely exhausted by evening. This concerned her. As she was talking, she suddenly interrupted herself and said, "I should tell you why we are having this baby, and why it is so important to us."

She explained that five months previously, their fourteen-month-old daughter had suffocated to death on a rattle while asleep in her crib. She said that she and her husband did not talk about the tragedy, but that both of them got up at repeated intervals during the night to check and recheck that Eileen and

Mark were all right. Since the accident, Eileen had refused to mention her baby sister, had frequent nightmares and unexplained severe crying spells, once at school. The doctor had ordered sedatives for her. The neighbors were supportive and included the family in their social activities.

The physician had advised the parents, shortly after the accident, to consider having another baby as soon as possible.

## DISCUSSION

**1.** How can Mr. and Mrs. B. be helped to accept the loss of their little daughter, and accept the new baby? *Talk about it*

**2.** Is the frequent checking on the children during the night by the parents a normal reaction five months after the accident? *Extremism*

**3.** What could be done to help Eileen overcome her sense of grief and loss? *Explanations*

**4.** Assume the role of the nurse. What is your reaction to this family's problems?

# 10 CASE SITUATION

## A Family with a Mentally Ill Member

Mr. J., age forty-seven, father, laborer.
Mrs. J., age forty-five, mother, patient.
Jane J., age fifteen, high school student.

The girls' advisor at Central High School called the visiting nurse association to ask if a visit could be made to the J. home. Jane J. had dropped out of school two weeks previously, and it was reported that her mother was ill. The family had lived in the community less than a year. Jane was considered an outstanding student by her teachers.

It was two o'clock that afternoon when the community health nurse made the home call. The address was a small frame house somewhat in need of repair. The tiny flower garden in front showed neglect. There were vacant lots, overgrown with weeds, on each side of the house. The nurse noted that all the window shades were tightly drawn and the place had a deserted air.

There was no door bell, and the nurse knocked several times, but there was no response. It appeared that no one was home, but as she turned to leave, she saw a slight movement of the window shade nearest the door, so she knocked once more. This time Jane opened the door a crack. She was relieved when she saw the nurse, and she invited her into a small, sparsely furnished living room.

The nurse inquired about Mrs. J. and Jane began to cry. The nurse waited quietly, and finally Jane was able to talk. She explained that her mother was sent to the state mental hospital (about 60 miles away) ten days ago. Her father considered her mother's illness to be such a terrible disgrace that he told Jane she could no longer go to school and that they could not have anything to do with the neighbors because of this shame. Jane remained alone in the house all day, with the shades drawn. The nurse saw little evidence of any amenities in the home—no books, pictures, radio, or television.

In response to the nurse's question about what she did with her time, Jane said she did the housework and the laundry, which she hung in the basement, and read her school books. She had read them all several times and did not know what she would do now. Her father left for work at seven in the morning and returned about four-thirty in the afternoon. Three evenings a week, she and her father went to a corner grocery store about a block away to buy their food. Jane said they had formerly lived in an isolated farming area of the state, where her father was a tenant farmer, but had moved to the city because her father thought he could get medical care for her mother. However, the mother had grown steadily worse, and about two weeks ago it had been necessary to take her by ambulance to the city-county hospital; a few days later she was transferred to the state mental hospital.

The nurse asked if Jane thought she might come to see her father that afternoon at about five. Hesitantly, Jane agreed, saying her father seemed so overwhelmed with grief and with the shame and disgrace of her mother's condition that he had not talked to anyone, but she thought he might talk with the nurse. The nurse left, promising to return at five o'clock.

## DISCUSSION

**1.** Assume the role of the nurse. How would you plan for this late-afternoon visit?

**2.** What assessment would you make of Mr. J.'s needs?

**3.** What do you see to be Jane's needs? Do you think her reaction to this family situation was a normal one? Why?

**4.** How would you work with Mr. J. to help him see the need for Jane to return to school and have friends of her own age?

**5.** What would you report to the girls' advisor regarding this situation? On the basis of your assessment of Jane's needs, what recommendations would you make to her regarding Jane's return to school?

**6.** If this family lived in your district, what community resources would be available for the prevention and treatment of psychiatric illnesses?

**7.** What steps would you take for the beginning plans for Mrs. J.'s eventual return to the family?

# 11 CASE SITUATION

# A Marijuana Smoker

The homeroom teacher at the junior high school looked across her desk at the nurse.

"I think," she said, "that is all I have this time—but, oh yes, there is a boy I wanted to ask you about. Do you know Henry J.?"

The nurse nodded slowly. "Yes, I've known him since he was in the fifth grade. Is he still here? I thought he was in senior high by this time."

"He should have gone in February, but he failed in two courses because he was absent so much. He's been absent a lot this term, too, and it seems to me he's losing weight. Do you suppose he gets enough to eat?"

"That family has lots of trouble," replied the nurse. "The mother is in and out of the state mental hospital, and the father misses work a lot because of illness."

"Are there any other children?"

"An older sister, Sadie. She's the one who shows the most emotional stability. She is married, with a family of her own, but she helps as she can. She goes to the house and cleans the place and takes them food. There were two younger brothers, but they were drowned last summer playing at the docks. What else do you notice about Henry?"

"Well, sometimes he seems as if he just wasn't here."

"Have other teachers mentioned anything about him?"

"His social studies teacher says that at times he seems dreamy and inattentive and sits and looks out the window. Another teacher told me yesterday there was a question whether or not he was involved in the robbery of that grocery store on the corner last week."

At this point, the class returned to their homeroom. The nurse watched Henry as he passed near her on his way to his seat. To the nurse, his appearance was not noticeably different from that of the other students, ex-

296

cept that he seemed pale and drowsy and shuffled a little as he walked.

As the nurse was returning to the district office, the thought occurred to her, could Henry be taking drugs or smoking marijuana? She recalled a statement she had read recently that problems presented by "present day narcotic addiction are essentially problems of social deviation and disorganization."[1] This boy's family situation included problems of social deviation and disorganization and the need for adjustment.

When she discussed the situation with her supervisor, it was agreed that the nurse should have a conference with the boys' counselor at the school regarding Henry as soon as possible. This was done, and a few weeks later, through the combined efforts of the school and the health department, psychiatric service was secured for Henry at the community mental health center, where it was determined that he had been smoking marijuana. A long-term program based on the cooperation of the school, the health department, the department of social welfare, and Mr. J. and Sadie was developed and followed.

## DISCUSSION

**1.** Assume the role of this nurse. What factors in Henry's background might alert you to the possibility of drug abuse?

**2.** What elements in his background might give strength to a rehabilitation program that could be worked out for Henry?

**3.** If Henry lived in your community, what specific resources would you be able to use to help him meet his drug problem?

**4.** What are some of the legal aspects to be considered when working with drug abuser patients?

**5.** What are some of the characteristics of the marijuana smoker that might alert the nurse in case finding?

[1]Alfred A. Freedman, Richard E. Brotman, and Alan S. Meyer, "A Model Continuum for a Community Based Program for the Prevention and Treatment of Narcotic Addiction," *American Journal of Public Health,* 54:791–802 (May) 1964.

# 1 CASE RECORD

## Stroke

**Mr. F., age sixty-six, a mechanic.**

Mr. F., a widower, lived alone in a small two-room house which he was buying. It was about two blocks from the garage where he worked. Since his wife's death, he had lived in various boarding houses and was happy to have his own home and to do his own cooking. His two married daughters, Mrs. A. and Mrs. B., and his married son, John F., lived in other sections of the city, and he saw them infrequently.

One evening he returned home from work, prepared and ate his dinner, and while washing the dishes, apparently suffered a stroke. Later that evening a neighbor found him lying on the floor. He was helped to bed but would not allow his family to be called. However, the next morning his children, Mrs. A., Mrs. B., and John, were notified, and they arranged for hospitalization.

Following his dismissal from the hospital, he went to the home of Mrs. A., where he remained a month. During this time, the community health nurse called once a week to teach the family to care for him. She demonstrated and supervised the passive exercises prescribed by the physician for his paralyzed left leg and arm. Mr. F. had some residual facial paralysis, which interfered with his speech, making it difficult for others to understand him. This made him impatient with those who were caring for him.

After a month, Mrs. A. said she could no longer care for her father in her home, and he was moved to the home of Mr. and Mrs. B. Mr. B. was employed by the gas and electric company. Another nurse visited Mr. F. weekly and, supervised the care and the exercises his daughter gave him.

About six weeks later, Mrs. B. told the nurse she could not continue to care for him because of the demands of her family and the overcrowding in the home. Mr. F. had to share a room with his two small grandsons. Furthermore, his personality changes made it difficult for Mrs. B. to handle him. He was tense and despondent about his condition, and he refused to cooperate. Mrs. B. said that she and her brother wanted help in having the patient hospitalized again or taken care of in his own home "in some way." Mrs. A. refused to do anything more for her father.

The nurse discussed the matter with the family physician, who said that if the family wanted this, they should go ahead with plans. The nurse referred them to the social welfare division of the health department for help in planning. At the same time the doctor referred Mr. F. for a medical evaluation and asked the nurse to increase the number of her visits to Mr. F. in order to give more passive exercises. Arrangements were made for the nurse to visit on a part-pay basis, three times a week, to help Mrs. B. with the passive exercises until other plans could be made.

At this time Mr. F. was still having pain in his left fingers, hand, and shoulder, and resisted whatever was being done for him. He found many reasons why he should not cooperate when the passive exercises were being carried out.

As the nurse was able to show him that the exercises were helping, and as he could see some improvement himself, his attitude slowly changed. However, the improvement in his arm was slow and the doctor doubted that there would be much more, so it seemed best to concentrate on improving his walking so that he could move around by himself. As he continued to improve and to be less dependent, Mrs. B. and her brother grew more interested in helping him, gave him support and encouragement, and were willing to work more closely with him. Mr. F. responded to this encouragement by trying to do more to help himself and by being more cooperative. He was able to get in and out of bed alone and to walk with a cane if someone was nearby. He could shave himself and began to feed himself if the food was cut up for him. Next he progressed to dressing himself but needed help in getting garments over his shoulders. This was frustrating to him and increased his impatience.

His progress continued to encourage the family to take more interest in him. John took him to his mountain cottage for weekends to relieve Mrs. B., but Mrs. A. refused to contribute to her father's care in any way.

On one visit, Mrs. B. talked to the nurse about her sister's attitude, which she said she could appreciate in a way but found very upsetting. She felt she had been forced to take their father into her home, that he was demanding, and that since she could not leave him alone, she was unable to leave the house or carry on her usual activities. She had thought and even dreamed of "getting rid of him." She had tried to be good to him and not let her feelings show; probably because of this she had done too much for him and that as he had become more dependent on her and demanding of her time and attention, she had grown more tense. She had always thought of her father as an independent person, and now his dependence on her was hard to accept. Because Mrs. B. was able to express openly her feelings regarding her father to the nurse, the nurse could discuss them with her and help her to understand her own reactions, the restrictions his illness placed on her father, and his reactions.

Nearly a month after a request was made, a medical evaluation conference for Mr. F. was held at the local hospital to determine if he would be a good candidate for the Rehabilitation Center. The team physician, a community health nurse, a social worker, and a physiotherapist reviewed his situation, and then he was presented to the staff. In evaluating the case, it was agreed that he would benefit from intensive therapy but that a letter was needed from his physician to confirm this. Following the receipt of the doctor's letter, he was declared eligible and was promised the next available bed at the Center.

Mr. F. and his family were greatly encouraged by his acceptance, and the patient worked harder than ever to regain his independence, with the hope that some day he would return to his job at the garage. The nurse took his affected arm through all possible ranges of motion, following the examples given in *Strike Back at Stroke.*[1] His shoulder was painful, but his arm could be elevated to about a 45° angle. It could be extended backward only a little way, but he could extend it forward and straighten it to about 125 °. Slowly Mr. F. developed the ability to maneuver his arm into various positions and, when standing, to raise his arm to waist level. He gained some voluntary movement in his fingers. His walking improved, he could take longer steps with less dragging of his foot; this gave him confidence.

About two weeks after the conference, Mrs. B. was requested to take her father to the Rehabilitation Center the next day. She notified the nurse but said she would not tell her father until the morning as it would excite him. The nurse visited Mr. F. the next morning to tell him some of the things he might expect at the Center, and promised to call on him there in a week or so.

Ten days later the nurse was able to visit the Center. Mr. F. was in the physiotherapy department, where he spent several hours each day having both passive and active exercises. He was pleased to see the nurse and appeared happy and contented in his new environment. He seemed to relate well to the staff and to other patients. The physiotherapist was not optimistic that further improvement could be made with Mr. F.'s arm, or that any additional motion would result. The social worker said that Mr. F. showed an ability for sketching, and the occupational therapist was working with him on it.

The nurse called on Mrs. B. a few days later to report on her visit with

[1]U.S. Department of Health, Education and Welfare, Public Health Service, Division of Chronic Diseases, *Strike Back at Stroke,* 1961.

Mr. F. Mrs. B. had just received a homesick letter from him, and he wanted to leave the Center. She hoped he would stay a little longer. The garage where Mr. F. had worked had gone out of business. Mr. and Mrs. B. had cleaned and painted his little house and hoped to rent it. Mrs. B. promised to let the nurse know when Mr. F. left the Center, and what plans they would make for him.

The next day the nurse summarized Mr. F.'s record. As she did so, she realized the importance of one's own attitudes toward a situation, the value of family-centered care, and the value of rehabilitation for both patient and family.

## DISCUSSION

1.  If Mr. F. lived in your area, what community facilities would you have available for his care?

2.  Assume the role of the nurse. How would you discuss with Mrs. B. her feelings regarding her father?

3.  As the nurse, how would you interpret Mr. F.'s personality changes to his daughter, Mrs. B.?

4.  Would it be possible to draw Mrs. A. into the family situation, so that she might participate in the care of her father? Give reasons for your answer.

# Rehabilitation

Frank L., age seventy.
Carmen L., age fifty-eight, patient.
Joe L., son, deceased.

Frank L. came from Italy as a young man and settled in a large Eastern city, where he worked for some years as a waiter in a well-known restaurant. He lived economically, saving as much money as possible in order to buy some land. Finally he was able to give up his job and with his savings buy a few acres on the outskirts of the city where he could raise fruit and vegetables for the city markets. At this time he met and married Carmen, a young woman who had arrived recently from her native Italy. Joe was their only child. Carmen was busy with her home and her little son, but she helped Frank when she could by waiting on customers at the little roadside stand he built not far from the house. Following high school graduation, Joe joined the Army, and was killed in action one year later.

Shortly after that, Carmen had a severe stroke that left her right side paralyzed, with an involvement of the left side of the brain and an almost complete aphasia. Her only means of communication was blinking her eyes, once for "No," twice for "Yes."

The family physician ordered complete bed rest and quiet. It was wartime, and hospitalization for civilians was difficult to secure. Furthermore, Frank did not want Carmen out of his sight, so Carmen remained at home. Frank took complete care of her, not allowing her to do anything for herself. He told her to lie still and get well. Occasionally, a next-door neighbor helped Frank to get Carmen up in a chair, but the neighbor moved away and Frank could not do it alone, so Carmen remained in bed for nearly twenty years.

There were relatively few resources for rehabilitation of stroke patients at that time. It was generally accepted that the best way to recover from a stroke was to lie quietly in bed.

Frank sold part of his property and invested the money with what he received from his son's war insurance. He was able to manage fairly well on this income and could give all his time to the care of Carmen. He continued to raise some flowers and produce, which he sold at his roadside stand, but most of his time was devoted to the care of Carmen, feeding, bathing, and nursing her with deep love and devotion. Carmen outlived two family physicians.

Finally, Frank could carry his nursing responsibilities alone no longer, and he asked the family physician for help. The physician requested the community health nurse from the health department to visit Carmen and evaluate the situation and report to him.

The nurse found the home neat and clean. Carmen, also neat and clean, lay in bed as she had for so many years, her neck, shoulders, spine, arms, wrists, fingers, legs, knees, ankles, and even toes contracted almost to immobility. As the nurse wrote in her report, "It is a classic picture of what should never happen." The doctor requested the nurse to visit twice a week in order to give Carmen a bed bath and other appropriate nursing care.

The nurse spent the initial visits giving the necessary nursing care and establishing a working relationship with Frank, who had rigid and set ideas regarding health matters. On the third visit, the nurse noted that, despite her physical incapacities, Carmen was more bright and alert than she had originally thought. She appeared to look forward to the nurse's visits. With Carmen's spirit and Frank's beginning interests and efforts to help her, the nurse saw possibilities of some rehabilitation. With this in mind she discussed the situation with the doctor, who gave her a blanket order to do whatever she thought would help Carmen to gain the maximum functioning of her apparently useless arms and legs. He suggested that if the nurse saw continued progress, it might be possible to send Carmen to the Blue Mountain Rehabilitation Center, a private rehabilitation center located in an adjacent township, for two or three days for a complete and thorough evaluation.

On her next visit, the nurse began passive exercises on Carmen's legs and arms, using a limited range of motion. She demonstrated the method of the exercises to Frank, suggesting that he do them every morning and evening for five minutes, gradually increasing the time. A few days later, while bathing Carmen, the nurse noticed numerous bruises. She asked Frank to demonstrate his passive exercises, and found him quick and rough. She cautioned him on the importance of gentleness. Frank learned to be more gentle, and soon Carmen showed some motion in one arm. At the nurse's suggestion, Frank purchased some small rubber balls for Carmen to squeeze; this helped Carmen also to develop some motion in her hands. It was small but perceptible and encouraging. The nurse taught Frank how to make doughnut rings for Carmen's heels, which showed the only evidence of skin breakdown after about twenty years of bed rest.

During all those years, Carmen had lain in any position she could, and Frank found it difficult at this time to understand the nurse's emphasis on the significance of body alignment. At each visit, the nurse discussed the value of bed boards and of a footboard, because Carmen had a marked degree of foot drop. For some time Frank appeared resistant to such ideas, but one morning the nurse arrived to find bed boards and the footboard in place. The nurse praised his accomplishments, hoping for further efforts on his part.

That morning while bathing Carmen, the nurse noted she had many insect bites on her body, and also that there were numerous blood specks on the sheets. She spoke to Frank about it, but he steadfastly denied there could be any fleas in his house, that Carmen had not complained, and that he had not seen fleas. On the next visit, the nurse succeeded in persuading him to buy flea powder, and for the next several visits she helped Frank to powder the mattress, the pillows, the bed frame, and the rugs. Finally the fleas disappeared.

During all this time, Frank faithfully and gently continued the passive exercises for Carmen, morning and evening, and at the nurse's urging, tried to get Carmen to talk. Carmen showed considerable progress, learning to raise her arms so that she could slip them into the sleeves of the gown when it was held for her. With proper use of pillows and the exercises, slowly her body grew straighter, and it was possible to get her up in a chair. On one occasion she attempted to stand, and it was obvious she wanted to take a step, but because of her foot drop, it was not possible. She learned to say three words, "Thank you" and "Bye."

In her three month's summary of progress which the nurse wrote for the doctor and the files, she said:

> Because of Frank's and Carmen's motivation, there is evidence that a great deal can be done for Carmen. The task is to convince Frank that further progress lies with an evaluation of Carmen's potential for further rehabilitation, and that she must go to Blue Mountain Rehabilitation Center for a few days. He is unwilling to have her go because they have not been separated for nearly forty years, so he continues to say 'No.' It appears that the place of the nurse is to continue the care and the exercises for Carmen, and to discuss with Frank the advantages of an evaluation by specialists at every opportune time.

## DISCUSSION

1. What are the goals of a rehabilitation program? How well did this nurse meet them?

2. What precepts of community health nursing did the nurse employ in this family situation?

**3.** What cultural values had to be considered in working with Carmen and Frank?

**4.** Was this nurse too permissive with Frank? What are the reasons for your answer?

**5.** If Carmen's stroke had happened today, what rehabilitation program could have been worked out for her if she lived in your community?

# 3  CASE RECORD

# Married Expectant Mother

**Mr. D., age twenty-one, truck driver.**
**Mrs. D., age seventeen, housewife.**

Mr. and Mrs. D. lived in a neat and clean little apartment. Mr. D. had recently secured employment after a four-month layoff. Mrs. D. was in about the eighth month of pregnancy. Her mother died several years ago, and her father was on welfare. Mr. D.'s mother, a widow in comfortable circumstances, refused to accept her son's marriage and would have nothing to do with the young couple.

Young Mrs. D. left high school at the time of her marriage. She appeared mature in her attitudes, accepting of her responsibilities, and was trying hard to make her marriage a success.

On the previous visit, the nurse's first one, Mrs. D. had told the nurse that her husband had frightening nightmares and had been advised by the city hospital clinic to seek psychiatric care, but as they were unable to afford it, they had done nothing about it. The nurse had promised to secure a list of possible resources in the community where Mr. D. might seek psychiatric help. Mrs. D. had just started to attend the prenatal clinic at the city hospital. She had expressed so many needs to learn and understand more about her pregnancy and her baby that the nurse had planned two visits with this in mind.

**Visit 1**  The nurse called in the middle of the morning and found Mrs. D. still in bed. She apologized for her laziness. The nurse thought it was probably because she had nothing definite to do except her household duties. She was eager to have the list of psychiatric resources for her husband. The nurse went over the list with her, and then Mrs. D. put the list away in a table drawer. She remarked that she had had "a terrible cold" for several days. However, her temperature was normal when taken. The nurse asked her about her eating and rest regimen. Following are excerpts from the remainder of the visit.

## Discussion                    ## Nurse's Thoughts

*Mrs. D.:* I try to sleep a lot.

*Nurse:* Rest is good. Taking lots of fluids, especially fruit juices, is also good.

*Mrs. D.:* I'll try that; anything to get rid of this cold. I'm worried about my bowel movements, they are dark and green.

*Nurse:* Are you taking pills?

*Mrs. D.:* Yes.

*Nurse:* Iron pills usually make the stool that color.

*Mrs. D.:* That's it then. I was worried.

*Nurse:* You should tell the doctor about it the next time you go to the clinic. I brought you a little book that shows you how to make formula. You may have your delivery and be home again before I see you and you will need to gather some equipment for this. I will try to be here the day you return from the hospital.

Mrs. D. examined the little book on formula making.

*Mrs. D.:* I think I understand, but will you come to show me how to do it?

The nurse promised. Mrs. D. told a rather long story about a neighbor who was not caring properly for her two-month-old baby.

*Mrs. D.:* She just doesn't give that baby any love. I want to do everything that's right for my baby. I don't want to feel it's my fault if anything goes wrong with it.

*Nurse:* I am sure you will do everything you can for your baby. Babies are wonderful, but there may be times, especially during the first few

Nurse realized that this was an opportunity for anticipatory guidance.

weeks, when things get a bit difficult. It may seem that all you do the whole day long is to feed him and change diapers. Some babies want to eat every three hours for the first few weeks, others may eat oftener. Since feeding takes about half an hour, you may think you'll never get any rest.

*Mrs. D.:* How about at night?

*Nurse:* At first, every baby wants to eat at night as well as in the day.

*Mrs. D.:* Do you believe in putting them on a schedule?

*Nurse:* Babies are the best judges. After a little while they will sort of set their own schedules and you will be able to tell when they are hungry. Having a rigid schedule usually upsets both mother and baby. He may want to eat when it's still an hour until feeding time, or not be hungry at all when he is supposed to be taking his bottle. It's a bit difficult to let the baby set up his own schedule the first few days, but they usually do it quite early. Then he may sleep through one of his nighttime feedings.

*Mrs. D.:* That's wonderful. I like the idea of feeding him when he is really hungry, rather than on schedule. I wish he'd come, I'm getting so fat! I used to weight 125 pounds, but now I'm 160. It's too much, isn't it?

*Nurse:* Yes, 35 pounds is rather a lot to gain. When did you gain most of it?

*Mrs. D.:* During the first few months. The first time I went to the clinic they told me not to gain any more, and that actually I should lose some.

That's why they gave me this low-salt diet and told me to watch for sodium. By the way, what is sodium?

*Nurse:* It's one of the chemicals in ordinary salt. It keeps fluids in the body, especially during pregnancy. That is why your hands are swollen. Many prepared foods have salt, such as bacon, breads, and some canned foods. It makes it a bit difficult to shop, doesn't it?

*Mrs. D.:* It sure does. If I was going to go by that, I couldn't eat much. I don't like things with no salt. They told me I should be careful because of some kind of poison. I can't remember the word.

*Nurse:* Toxemia, perhaps?

*Mrs. D.:* Yes, that's it. They told me to watch for headaches, spots before my eyes, and blurry vision.

*Nurse:* Have you had any of these?

*Mrs. D.:* No, I'm trying to follow the diet they gave me, but you see, I think I'll go to the hospital any day now, and my husband doesn't know how to cook, so we've been buying canned and frozen foods; otherwise he wouldn't eat anything while I'm gone.

*Nurse:* Couldn't you buy a few things on your diet list for yourself?

*Mrs. D.:* It's just too difficult. We shop once a week, and, well, we can't afford too much right now. I buy things like ham and bologna for my husband, and bananas, apples, and grapefruit, too.

*Nurse:* Cold cuts have a lot of salt in them. What else do you have besides fresh fruits?

Nurse wonders how much Mrs. D. is interested in following her diet.

*Mrs. D.:* Nothing, I really don't know how many calories I'm getting, I never can keep track of what I eat.

*Nurse:* Try keeping a list of every thing you eat during the day and the amounts. I'll bring you a pamphlet that gives the calories in different foods. That will help.

*Mrs. D.:* I'd like to have it.

*Nurse:* I'll bring the birth atlas, too. It has some good pictures showing the growth of the baby, and of the delivery.

*Mrs. D.:* Oh! I want to see it. When are you coming again?

Nurse wonders how much can be accomplished so late in pregnancy.

The nurse closed the visit and made an appointment for the next one the following week.

**Visit 2**   Mrs. D. was up and dressed, sitting by the window watching for the nurse. At first, Mrs. D. dominated the interview with small talk. This was understandable to the nurse, as the patient was young, somewhat lonely, and had no mother figure. Finally the nurse could open her visit.

*Nurse:* Did you talk to your husband about the list of mental health resources I gave you?

*Mrs. D.:* Yes. We decided to let it go until after the baby comes. He's much better now, but he will go after a while, because he needs help. He's going to get more money pretty soon on his new job, maybe as much as a hundred a week. This is the budget I made. If we can follow this, in two more months we won't have any more debts and we can start to save money.

The nurse was impressed with Mrs. D.'s concern for their debts, and complimented her on her planning.

*Nurse:* I brought you the calorie book, but don't follow the diets here as long as you are pregnant. Stay on the one the clinic gave you.

*Mrs. D.:* Oh, I threw that one away a long time ago, but I drink milk, eat meat, fruits, and vegetables.

*Nurse:* Did you keep a list of what you have been eating for the doctor at the clinic?

*Mrs. D.:* No, but I will now.

*Nurse:* Good, we'll talk about it next time.

*Mrs. D.:* I don't know when I'm going to have this baby.

*Nurse:* When was your last period?

*Mrs. D.:* I can't remember, April or May.

*Nurse:* Perhaps you gave the doctor the wrong month, and you're not as far along as you thought. It seems to me, though, that the baby has dropped. You'll see what I mean when I show you the birth atlas.

*Mrs. D.:* The doctor said the baby had dropped. Perhaps it won't be too long now. Let's look at your book, I'm real curious about it.

The nurse went through the atlas, slowly explaining the anatomy and physiology. Mrs. D. was very much interested, but her knowledge was limited, and the nurse found the visit was growing too long.

*Mrs. D.:* Please leave the book with me. I want to show it to my husband. He would love to see it.

*Nurse:* I'm sorry, but I can't. It's the only one I have, and I use it all the time, but I will bring it again.

*Mrs. D.:* Please do. When will you come?

The nurse summarized the visit, and arranged for a visit the following week, suggesting that they review diets at that time.

Before it was time for the next visit, Mr. D. called the nurse to say that Mrs. D. had had a cesarian section and the baby had lived only a few hours. The nurse expressed her sympathy; she asked him to let her know when Mrs. D. would be home again and said that she would visit her. Several days later Mr. D. called again and asked the nurse if she would call the following day, and she arranged to do so.

**Visit 3**  Mrs. D. was lying down when the nurse arrived at midmorning, but the small apartment was in order. Mrs. D. insisted on sitting up in a chair while the nurse was there. The nurse said she was sorry about the baby, and Mrs. D. began to cry. The nurse waited quietly for a little while and then asked Mrs. D. if she would like to talk about it. Mrs. D. nodded.

"Did you see the baby?" asked the nurse. Again Mrs. D. nodded.

"Was it a boy or girl?" At this point Mrs. D. stopped crying and began to talk about the baby, a girl. She said that even though she had died so soon, they wanted her to have a name, and had called her Hazel, after Mrs. D.'s mother. Mrs. D. described the baby, her dark hair, and her tiny fingernails. "She even held my finger—I think," and the nurse agreed that this was possible.

The nurse asked how she felt when she knew the baby had died. Mrs. D., between her sobs, expressed at length her feelings of loss and disappointment. Then she apologized for talking this way as she tried to stop crying, but the nurse explained that it was good to cry and that it helped to accept the loss. The nurse asked if she and her husband had talked about it together, and Mrs. D. said they had not, as she didn't want to keep reminding him of it. The nurse suggested that perhaps he was feeling the same way. This seemed a new idea to Mrs. D.

The nurse talked a little about Mrs. D.'s health, her diet, the need for rest and exercise, and about her next clinic appointment. She asked if Mr. D. was working; Mrs. D. replied that he had been laid off for a few days but would return to work the next day, and that at the moment he was doing the shopping. The nurse inquired about his nightmares; his wife said they seemed to have stopped but that she was keeping the list of resources in case they needed them. The nurse promised to return in a few days.

As she was leaving the apartment house, the nurse met a young man with a bag of groceries. She asked if he were Mr. D., and introduced herself. She expressed her sympathy at the loss of the baby and asked him if he and his wife talked about the baby. He said they had not, as he was afraid it would make her cry. The nurse explained the value of facing their loss together and told him that it would help in overcoming their grief.

When the nurse called a week later, Mrs. D. was packing the baby clothes. She had been to the clinic, and the doctor had told her it would be possible for her to have another baby.

"I thought I would never have another one, and I was going to give these away, but now I'll keep them." She told the nurse she wanted to finish high school now before she had another baby. Her husband had agreed to this. The nurse saw that Mrs. D. had accepted the loss of her baby and would adapt to it. Mrs. D. had a few questions regarding nutrition which the nurse answered. She gave Mrs. D. the agency's card, asked her to call if she needed help at any time, and told her to be sure to call early in her next pregnancy, and that a nurse would come to see her. The case was closed.

## DISCUSSION

**1.** What were Mr. and Mrs. D.'s most important problems? What do you think were the bases for these problems?

**2.** How effective was the nurse in meeting these problems?

**3.** How do you evaluate the nurse's teaching?

**4.** How important do you consider Mr. D.'s nightmares in this situation?

**5.** The nurse planned to teach Mrs. D. formula making. Should she have done this without first determining whether Mrs. D. could or would breast-feed her baby?

# 4 CASE RECORD

## Single Expectant Mother

**Helen O., age sixteen, schoolgirl, pregnant.**

A single expectant mother, Helen O. lived with her mother and two younger sisters in a small upstairs apartment in a rapidly changing part of the city. Helen finished junior high school and attended a nearby vocational school for a little more than a year, but dropped out at Thanksgiving time. Her mother did housework three days a week, and also received an aid-to-dependent-children grant. Helen had visited the prenatal clinic at the city hospital at the nurse's suggestion. Afterwards, the clinic requested a follow-up home visit by the community health nurse, as the patient was listed as being preeclamptic. The baby was due in February.

The nurse made her second call one morning early in January. Helen, in her bathrobe, answered the nurse's knock and invited her to come in, saying that her mother had just left to go to the store and to visit a neighbor. After an exchange of pleasantries, the nurse felt that Helen was glad to see her and was accepting of the visit. Following are excerpts from the patient-nurse discussion, and the nurse's thoughts as the discussion proceeded.

| Discussion | Nurse's Thoughts |
|---|---|
| *Nurse:* Did you get your pills from the pharmacy when you were at the clinic last week? | The nurse was concerned about Helen following clinic orders, and felt she didn't realize fully the significance of her physical condition. |
| *Helen:* No, but I'll get them tomorrow. I go back then. | |
| *Nurse:* Do you understand how important they are for you? Be sure to get them tomorrow. | The nurse made a mental note to return to this point in her visit summary. |
| *Helen:* Yes, I will, but I lost weight without them. | The nurse questioned this, but realized that Helen probably weighed herself at different times of the day. |
| *Nurse:* How much do you weigh today? | |

*Helen:* Two hundred pounds.

*Nurse:* You have lost 5 pounds then since you were at the clinic.

*Helen:* I guess so.

*Nurse:* What have you been eating?

*Helen:* Not much. I have a weak stomach.

*Nurse:* What did you eat yesterday?

*Helen:* I had an apple.

Nurse saw she must ask specific questions, since Helen was so vague.

*Nurse:* Was that all you had all day long?

*Helen:* No, I had a hamburger for breakfast.

*Nurse:* How did you cook it?

*Helen:* I broiled it, like you said last time.

*Nurse:* Good for you, that helps to cut down on calories.

*Helen:* But I still drink lots of water, I get so thirsty. I told them that at the clinic.

Nurse wonders if Helen could be eating salty foods.

*Nurse:* What did they say?

*Helen:* Nothing, except it's probably all the salt that's in me. I guess it's what makes my hands and feet so big.

Nurse wonders if this showed Helen was beginning to recognize her problem.

*Nurse:* Have you thought of any more questions since last time?

*Helen:* No, I'm just plain scared. Every week I hope the baby will come next week. Oh! I hope I never have the baby. No, I don't really mean that.

Nurse saw that Helen was showing how unsure and frightened she really was.

*Nurse:* I understand how you must feel. It's normal to be afraid of something you have not experienced and can't really know what it's like until

you go through it. You remember
last time you said you would like to
know more about the birth process?
I brought some pictures that I think
will help you to understand. Would
you like to see them?

*Helen:* Yes, perhaps it will help
some.

    The nurse explained the birth process with the use of pictures from the
birth atlas, and Helen listened attentively:

*Nurse:* Are you glad I showed them
to you or not?

*Helen* (shuddering): I don't know. In
a way I'm glad; yet it brings it awful
close to when I'll have mine. Will
they give me shots?

*Nurse:* I'm sure they will. If you try to
relax and take things as they come
and breathe the way they tell you, it
will be much easier for you. It will be
hard, but don't you think it will be
worth it for the baby?

*Helen* (laughing uneasily): If the
baby is cute. Say, can I have a mis-
carriage this late? Some folks say
it's even worse than having a baby.
Don't get me wrong, I don't want to
lose my baby.

*Nurse:* You won't have a miscar-
riage this late. That occurs before
the sixth month. Why do you ask?

*Helen:* I know a girl. She took pills,
she was two months along and she
lost her baby.

*Nurse* (sharply): That's a very serious
thing to do. Often pills won't do
any good and the girl doesn't lose
her baby, but she can bring definite

Nurse saw this as a sign of im-
maturity. Nurse thinks Helen may
have asked this question for one of
three reasons: (1) she may be just
curious; (2) she might attempt an
abortion now in order to avoid labor;
(3) she may have tried abortion early
in pregnancy and may be afraid now
of the consequences because it did
not work. Nurse thought question
was asked for the second reason.

If Helen's reason was the third
above, nurse realized she was too
harsh in her reply.

harm to herself and the baby. [Pause] Can you think of other questions you'd like to ask?

*Helen:* No, I just get scared thinking about it, that's all.

*Nurse:* Does it help for you and me to talk about it?

*Helen:* Yes, you help while you're here, but when I'm alone in a few hours I'll start thinking about it, and I'll get scared.

Nurse wonders how supportive and helpful the mother is.

*Nurse:* Have you talked with the caseworker yet?

*Helen:* No, I told my mother to, but I don't know whether she did or not.

*Nurse:* Do you have some things for the baby yet?

Nurse wonders if family is afraid caseworker will want to take baby away.

*Helen:* Don't have a thing. My mother is going to town soon, and she'll pick up something I guess.

The nurse summarized and closed the visit, reminding Helen to go the next day to the clinic for her pills and to take them regularly. She arranged for the next visit, and suggested that Helen write down any questions she might have.

## DISCUSSION

1. What particular needs did this patient have?

2. In her teaching, was the nurse sensitive to the cues the patient gave her? Illustrate by examples.

3. What barriers to communication existed in this visit?

4. Was there evidence that the nurse imposed her standards of social behavior on Helen? If so, in what way?

5. How much empathy did the nurse have for Helen's problems?

# 5 CASE RECORD

# Communicable Disease— Typhoid Fever

Mr. A., age thirty-four, insurance adjuster, at 2000 Elm Avenue.

Mrs. A., thirty-three, housewife.

Jane, thirteen, junior high school pupil.

Bob, twelve, junior high school pupil.

Bill, ten, fifth grade pupil.

One Tuesday morning in early October, the nursing division of the community health department was requested to call on the A. family by the division of communicable disease control. Mr. A. had been hospitalized for a week at the West Side General Hospital. A positive diagnosis of typhoid fever had been established, confirming the physician's tentative diagnosis. Mr. A.'s condition was satisfactory. The nurse was asked to determine if the home situation would permit the patient's return there early in his convalescence. If so, the nurse was asked to teach the family communicable disease care and control, and to assist in the epidemiologic study.

In planning for the visit, the nurse reviewed the office manual relating to the health department's rules and regulations regarding care and control of communicable disease, especially as it related to typhoid fever. She telephoned Mrs. A. for an appointment for the visit, and was asked to call that morning.

**Visit 1. Tuesday morning** The nurse found 2000 Elm Avenue to be an attractive home, similar to others on the street and set back in a well-kept garden. Mrs. A., a trim, competent-looking person, invited the nurse into the dining room, where she was ironing. Mrs. A. said she had been disturbed at her husband's diagnosis, but was happy with his continued progress. The nurse explained the reasons for her call, and Mrs. A. was most cooperative. The family had a three-bedroom, two-bathroom house. One bathroom opened off the master bedroom. There was adequate kitchen, dining, and living room space, and automatic laundry facilities in the utility room. The house was supplied with city water and was connected with the city sewer system.

None of the family had ever had typhoid immunization. "We just didn't think it was necessary," Mrs. A. said. The nurse urged Mrs. A. and the children to secure their typhoid immunization. She gave the mother literature relating to immunization and to the home care of the communicable disease patient. She arranged to return the next afternoon so that she could see the children.

**Visit 2. Wednesday afternoon**   Mrs. A. had visited her husband that morning and was further encouraged by his progress. The nurse asked Mrs. A. to help her to complete the forms that the health department needed regarding possible sources of Mr. A.'s illness. Mrs. A. said the family had gone to the ocean on a camping trip early in September, using the camp facilities of a state park. One afternoon they dug for oysters on the beach near Pine Point in Ocean County. Mr. A. had cleaned the oysters, eating a few raw ones as he worked. The rest of the family did not eat any until after they were cooked.

Two days after their return from the beach, Mr. A. made a quick trip to a neighboring state to attend the funeral of a younger brother who had died following an appendectomy. The brother lived with his parents on their farm, and Mr. A. spent two nights at the farm, which was on River Road, Dale City. At the farm they had their own well, grew their own vegetables, and used unpasteurized milk. There was a septic tank some distance from the well. The family had lived on this farm for forty years, and Mrs. A. could not recall hearing of any illnesses similar to typhoid. Except for their camping trip and Mr. A.'s trip to his old home, the family had not been away from home; they had had no overnight guests.

Mrs. A. said that the family physician had suggested that they go to the city health department for typhoid immunization. The nurse made appointments for them for the following afternoon. She left stool containers for each member of the family, and asked Mrs. A. to bring in a specimen for each of them. She also emphasized the need for good hygiene on the part of every member, stressing that immunization was no substitute for cleanliness and sanitation. She pointed out that because of the manner of the spread of the disease, and the possibility that anyone of them could have, at this time, a nonclinical case, the use of caution and proper hygiene, especially with food handling, were essential for the safety of them all. She supported the doctor's recommendation that, for the time being, the children's friends be discouraged from visiting in the home and that the A. children not eat or sleep away from home. She explained that this was not a restriction of the health department, but was a wise precaution for the present.

At this point the children returned from school. They appeared to be healthy, active children, with no obvious physical or emotional health problems. The nurse explained to them the need for good personal hygiene and asked them to demonstrate safe handwashing procedures for her. They had questions about their father's illness which she answered to their apparent satisfaction.

The nurse asked Mrs. A. if she could recall places outside the home where Mr. A. could have eaten. She replied that he always came home for lunch and that they seldom had dinner away from home. However, two evenings before the onset of his illness they went to dinner at the home of neighbors, Mr. and Mrs. J. at 2100 Elm Street. The evening that Mr. A. returned from attending his brother's funeral the family had had dinner at Joe's Hamburger Stand, and the following evening Mr. A. had had dinner with a business associate at the Steak House, a popular restaurant in the financial district. She could not remember that he had been away from home for any other meals.

The next morning (Thursday) Mrs. A. telephoned the nurse to say that she had forgotten that Mr. and Mrs. J. had come to play cards with them the evening before Mr. A. had become ill. Mrs. A. had prepared the sandwiches, cake, and coffee for the group. Mr. A. did not assist her and did not eat any of the food. She wished to bring these neighbors with her when she and the children came for immunization. The nurse encouraged her to do so. At that time, the nurse arranged for a home visit for the following Monday afternoon.

Before making visit 3, the nurse telephoned the doctor regarding Mr. A.'s return to the home. The doctor felt that a discharge date was tentative but that if the patient continued to progress, he might return home in six or seven days. He wished the isolation precautions to be continued and directed that the patient's low-residue diet and present medications also be continued.

The nurse selected some suggestions for low-residue menus that were high in calories, nonirritating, and non-gas-forming. She secured a pamphlet of instructions prepared by the health department on the care of patients with communicable diseases. It described isolation procedures, such as safe care of patient's linens, dishes, and body wastes, and general isolation techniques.

**Visit 3. Monday** The nurse discussed with Mrs. A. the preparation of the master bedroom as an isolation unit, emphasizing that a basic principle in isolation of a communicable disease patient was the protection of the contacts and the community. She suggested that all unnecessary furniture and bric-a-brac be removed from the room, and that a small portable television set, a comfortable plastic-covered chair, and a metal wastebasket be placed in the room. The nurse urged Mrs. A. to have a generous supply of paper towels, large paper bags, and large coverall aprons. Mrs. A. thought she would have time to make the aprons before Mr. A. came home. The screening of the doors and windows of the room was discussed. The nurse demonstrated the use of paper towels in turning water faucets on and off and opening and closing doors. She stressed the importance of frequent cleansing of toilet seat, flush handle, television knobs, the plastic chair, and anything else the patient might touch. She asked Mrs. A. to demonstrate how she would prepare to leave the patient's room after caring for the patient, e.g., washing hands and removing apron and hanging it up without contaminating it. The washing of bed linens, pajamas, and aprons was discussed. The nurse demonstrated the care of the patient's dishes, advising that the tray remain in his room, and that the dishes be scraped there and brought in a container to the kitchen after the family's dishes had been washed, boiled for twenty minutes, and then washed in the usual manner. The nurse suggested that Mrs. A. use sturdy dishes for the patient, and that she keep them separate. Uneaten food scraps should be placed in a paper bag and burned, together with newspapers and other materials discarded from the patient's room. The nurse told Mrs. A. that she would need to keep a thermometer and a jar of clean cotton in the room. She demonstrated the cleansing of the thermometer with soap, water, and friction. The next visit was arranged for the day of Mr. A.'s return.

**Visit 4. Monday**  The nurse visited the home one week later. Mrs. A. reported that she and the children and Mr. and Mrs. J. had had their second immunizations, and that the A. family had taken their second stool specimens to the laboratory. Mrs. A. had everything in readiness for her husband's return home that afternoon. The nurse praised her for the thoroughness of the preparations she had made. There was some discussion on how the children might help their mother and participate in their father's convalescence. The nurse promised to visit the following morning.

**Visit 5. Tuesday**  Mrs. A. and the children seemed equal to the problems involved in Mr. A.'s care, and the nurse arranged to call once a week to make sure proper precautions were being taken and to assist Mrs. A. in any problems that might arise. She assured Mrs. A. that she could call her at any time she needed help.

   The sanitarian checked out the personnel at the Steak House; all help had been on the staff for the past two years, all had current health cards, and none had had any apparent illnesses. The same general findings obtained at Joe's Hamburger Stand. The state department of health had been notified of the case and of Mr. A.'s trip to his old home in the neighboring state, and the state health department of that state was notified of the trip and the dates. The Ocean County Health Department was notified of the facts of the case, since the A. family's camping trip had taken place in their health jurisdiction.

The nurse closed the case when Mr. A.'s laboratory reports were negative and Mrs. A. did not need further help. All stool specimens for the family were negative, and all immunizations were completed. No other case was traced to Mr. A.'s illness or to the raw oysters, and no cases materialized in the neighboring state. However, the epidemiology of a typhoid case remains an open question in communicable disease control files until positive proof of source is established.

One by-product of this case was that the nurse discovered she had let her typhoid immunization lapse, and she promptly brought it up to date.

## DISCUSSION

**1.** In this situation, what steps were taken by the local health department to protect the community? the family? the patient?

**2.** Was this nurse's teaching regarding communicable disease care and control up to date? What might have been omitted with safety?

**3.** What *specific* knowledge did this nurse need in order to function satisfactorily in this situation?

**4.** This family apparently had a fairly high social and economic background. Plan a sample day's menu for Mrs. A. and the children. Adapt your menu as far as possible to the doctor's orders for a low-residue, nonirritating, and non-gas-forming diet for Mr. A., a patient convalescing from fever.

**5.** While caring for a patient with an elevated temperature in a home, what symptoms or group of symptoms that the patient exhibited might make you suspicious of typhoid fever? What would be your next steps?

**6.** List at least six methods of typhoid prevention carried on by a health department.

# Tuberculosis

John G., age twenty-seven, college instructor.

Mary G., age twenty-three, housewife and patient.

Mary G. and her husband, John, had grown up in the same neighborhood in a large Eastern city. They had been married about four years prior to Mary's diagnosis. Mary had worked as a secretary to help John finish his university studies and obtain his doctorate. That autumn John accepted a position to teach biology in a small liberal arts college in a Western state.

John and Mary came from large families of Irish descent, and in their new home they missed these close family ties. Prior to moving to the West, while visiting her family, Mary had a chest x-ray in a mass tuberculosis survey in her home neighborhood but thought nothing of it.

Six weeks after their arrival in their new home, the local health department received an interstate reciprocal notification to the effect that Mary had a suspicious x-ray that needed a follow-up. The community health nurse was asked to make a home call. The nurse found Mary working in her garden. She was a small, wiry young woman, quick and alert. She told the nurse she had had marked fatigue lately and had visited a physician a few days ago, when an x-ray was taken. She had an appointment to see the physician again the following day. The nurse urged her to keep her appointment.

The nurse reported on her visit to the director of the tuberculosis division of the health department. He arranged a conference with the private physician. Later a definite diagnosis of moderately advanced tuberculosis was established. It was believed that the disease had been present for over a year.

Mary was hospitalized on a part-pay basis in the county tuberculosis sanatorium. She was placed in isolation, and antituberculosis therapy and bed rest were instituted. She responded satisfactorily to treatment. While Mary was hospitalized, John, temporarily a bachelor, was being invited to many college-centered and faculty social activities. It was disturbing to Mary that John was having these activities without her, and she begged to go home. After seven weeks she was sent home to continue her regimen under the care of a practical nurse and with the supervision of her physician and the community health nurse.

Tuberculosis creates many home problems relating to family health, and the nurse tried to include John in her home contacts, as she found that he had some emotional problems in relation to his wife's illness. Both Mary and John resented the tuberculosis, for it meant delaying parenthood to which they had been looking forward.

The nurse arranged to visit Mary on a weekly basis. The first few visits were used to establish rapport with the patient and her husband, to determine how much they knew about tuberculosis, and to give them an opportunity to bring up other health problems (none were raised). The nurse spent time in determining and appraising the health needs of the family on the basis of their health situation, their ages, patterns of behavior, socioeconomic background, and the family environment. What was to be the impact of a long-term disease on this young couple who found it almost impossible to accept the diagnosis? She realized the importance of being objective and nonjudgmental in her appraisal of the family's needs.

Mary's needs appeared to be:

**1.** Help in accepting physical and mental rest as a way of life and in directing her energies into less strenuous activities than gardening and skiing

**2.** Understanding in facing the fact that she must delay motherhood

**3.** Appreciation of her loneliness in her new home far from her immediate family and friends

**4.** Education about symptoms of tuberculosis, transmission, isolation techniques, complications, contact finding, conscientious drug administration, drug toxicity, good body alignment, nutrition, and the ill effects of smoking and sunbathing

**5.** Someone to whom she could verbalize about her problems, for her husband refused to listen to her fears. He was afraid, too

The nurse saw John as a confused and somewhat frightened young man. Although he had a sound scientific background, he knew little about tuberculosis and could see it only as a social disgrace, something to keep hidden. His needs appeared to be more intangible than Mary's but just as important.

The nurse saw John's needs to be:

**1.** Help in understanding and accepting the modern concepts of tuberculosis and its therapy

**2.** Help in accepting his wife's illness in relation to his position in the college and in the community

**3.** Understanding as he tried to face the fact that they would not be able to have children for a long time

**4.** Understanding of his fears that he would be rejected by the college community because of tuberculosis in his family

**5.** Understanding of his rejection of outside help in the care of his wife

**6.** For someone with whom he could discuss his problems, as he had no close friends or relatives in the community

The nurse wondered if some of his rejection of her and his refusal to accept Mary's illness might be based on guilt feelings because Mary had worked to help him gain his education.

When she had defined the needs of Mary and John, the nurse began to consider the immediate and long-term nursing goals she wished to accomplish—those goals which might be met within a few weeks, and those which might take much longer. The immediate goals appeared to be:

**1.** To help the family recognize and accept tuberculosis

**2.** To educate the family regarding the disease

**3.** To interpret the therapy, e.g., the nutrition, the drugs, and the bedrest

**4.** To improve the family's general health practices

The long-term goals appeared to be:

**1.** The eradication of the disease by care, prevention, and control

**2.** The rechanneling of the family's energies into hobbies and light recreation

**3.** Providing information regarding community agencies and their services

**4.** Providing information on all aspects of tuberculosis care

**5.** A recognition that no tuberculosis case once discovered can be forgotten, but that each case should be followed on a periodic basis to ensure that the disease remained "inactive"

**6.** Helping the family to become independent of the health agency but assuring them of further health services and health supervision as needed

Teamwork was the basis for the nursing care plan. The nurse worked closely with the director of the tuberculosis division in the health department, with the family physician, with the practical nurse, and with the patient and her husband. Based on the objectives of family health care, the plan included help to the family for their personal and social development, securing other nursing services as needed, the reinforcement of the physician's teaching, and the discovery and appraisal of other health problems. In some family situations, the plan might have included helping the family toward independence of the health service, but with this family, the problem was to get them to accept even temporary necessary help.

After about two years, Mary recovered sufficiently to resume many of the activities of normal living. The health supervision and teaching program that had been carried on by the health department was discontinued. It was possible for the agency to close the case except for periodic checkups.

## DISCUSSION

**1.** What precepts of community health nursing were observed by this nurse?

**2.** Discuss in detail the information regarding tuberculosis that this nurse needed in order to help this family.

**3.** What implications for her new community did Mary G.'s illness have? For her former community?

**4.** How practical were the nurse's goals for this family?

**5.** How would you have helped Mary in her concern for her husband's social life in which she could not participate? This problem was serious for Mary and caused her great concern.

**6.** How would you have helped John and Mary in accepting the delay in parenthood? Consider their cultural and socioeconomic background.

Mr. U., age fifty-two, farmer.
Mrs. U., age forty-eight, patient.
Fred U., age twenty-five, married, with
Army, overseas.
Ruby B., age twenty-two, with her service
husband, overseas.
Pearl U., age fourteen, high school
student.
Mr. K., 74, retired.
Mrs. K., 71, housewife (parents of Mrs. U.).
The county health department received a re-
ferral from the local Cancer Society, stating
that Mrs. U., who had advanced carcinoma of
the colon, needed nursing assistance. She and
her daughter, Pearl, were staying with Mr. and
Mrs. K. in a small town about 20 miles from
the county seat. Dr. A. was her physician.

The nurse for that district called Dr. A.'s
office for any orders that he might have for
Mrs. U., but learned that he was out of town for
a week. The office nurse said that Mrs. U.'s
standing orders were:

1.  General bedside care and a light diet

2.  Morphine by hypodermic injection every
four hours as necessary

The office nurse added, "Mrs. U. knows
her diagnosis and her prognosis." With this
limited information, the community health
nurse planned her first visit for the next morning. Her objectives were to:

1.  Establish rapport with Mrs. U. and her
family

2.  Secure necessary information in order to
determine and assess the patient's needs

3.  Secure necessary information in order to
determine and assess the family's needs

**Visit 1**   The nurse found the family living in a
small frame house, badly in need of paint, on
a side road on the outskirts of the little town.

# Terminal Cancer

Mr. and Mrs. K. were watching for her at the gate, as they had been told that she would visit them that morning, and they greeted her eagerly. Mr. K. said, "We didn't know the Cancer Society had a service like this. It's wonderful to have a nurse take care of our daughter for two or three hours every day."

It was necessary for the nurse to begin her visit by explaining the relationship of the Cancer Society, a private agency, to the county health department, and the duties, responsibilities, and limitations of the community health nurse. Mr. and Mrs. K. accepted the explanation and asked the nurse to teach them how to care for Mrs. U. They led the nurse into a crowded living room, containing an oil-circulating heater, a davenport, a buffet, two chairs, a hospital bed, and a bedside table. Through the door, the nurse could see a small kitchen with an electric stove and a refrigerator, and a table and chairs. Through the kitchen window, she saw a chicken house and a rabbit hutch and, on the back porch, an old washing machine. There were two bedrooms and a small bathroom. One bedroom was used by Mr. and Mrs. K. and the other by Pearl, their granddaughter.

Mrs. U., the patient, appearing weak and emaciated, lay supine on the hospital bed near a large window that gave a broad view of the valley beyond. She was receptive to the nurse but, because of dyspnea, experienced difficulty in talking. Her abdomen was extended, and the nurse noted pitting edema of ankles and legs. The patient complained of diarrhea and of sternal and axillary pain. Her fluid intake was 2 to 3 qt daily. She was able to explain her medications on the bedside table to the nurse—pills for nerves, pills for diarrhea, and the morphine. From time to time she called fretfully to her mother to give her a drink of water, shift her position, or remove the blanket. Mrs. K. said she followed the doctor's orders of light diet, such as milk, soups, puddings, and custards.

Mr. and Mrs. U. owned a farm on the other side of the state. Mrs. U. left her home five months ago when she became too ill to continue working on the farm, where she had cared for the livestock, driven a tractor, plowed the fields, and done the cooking and the housework. A year previous, she had had a laparotomy, which was followed by x-ray treatment. Then, friends on neighboring farms had raised money, which, with family savings, had been spent for a trip for Mrs. U. to another state for treatments and medications by a "cancer specialist," who, they learned later, was a quack doctor. Mrs. U. returned to the farm, where she continued to work until she had to give up; she had then come to stay with her parents.

"My husband worked us all. When we were sick, we still worked. I brought Pearl over here because I knew her father would take her out of school to work on the farm," she told the nurse.

Mr. U. came from a southeastern European country and belonged to the Catholic faith. Mrs. U.'s family had been American for several generations. She belonged to the Pentecostal faith, as did her parents.

Mr. U. sent money for medications when he could, but he had had poor crops for the past two years. Mrs. U.'s married sister sent money as she could, and visited frequently to relieve her mother in the care of Mrs. U.

The nurse noted that most of the nursing was done, however, by Mrs. K., a quiet and friendly person. She was fearful of hurting her daughter and was timid in approaching her nursing duties. Mr. K. was a tall old gentleman with twinkling blue eyes and a sense of humor. He was devoted to his church, and spent much of his time reading the Bible to his daughter. He was a known diabetic and administered his own insulin. Two weeks prior to the nurse's visit, he had discontinued the insulin without consulting his physician. Mr. and Mrs. K. had a pension that under ordinary circumstances was sufficient to meet their needs; he also did carpentry jobs in the neighborhood. The nurse was keenly aware of the emotional support and devotion given to one another by members of the family.

After listening to the family for some time, the nurse recognized that the immediate nursing need was to teach Mrs. K. the following:

**1.** How to change the patient's position from time to time, to add to her comfort

**2.** How to help the patient to use a pan on a bedside chair

**3.** The need to continue the medications on schedule

**4.** The importance of recording the amount of narcotic given and the time

These points were demonstrated and discussed with Mrs. K., and the nurse arranged to return the next day to demonstrate a bed bath. She explained to Mrs. K. the equipment needed. She thought the patient and family recognized and understood her role as a community health nurse.

As she drove away, the nurse had a warm sense of accomplishment and of being wanted; then suddenly she began to wonder whether she was meeting her own needs, or those of the patient and family? She realized how easy it would be to let this family become dependent on her, and that then she would not be able to accomplish her objective of helping them to help themselves. She saw the need of a plan involving both short- and long-term objectives. Later that day she set up objectives and developed her plan.

For Mrs. U.:

**1.** To use those nursing skills that could be taught readily to the family so that Mrs. U.'s remaining days would be as comfortable as possible, including:

    *a.* Bed bath
    *b.* Turning and changing position

    *c.* Use of bedpan
    *d.* Preparing and giving medication by hypodermic syringe
    *e.* Mouth care
    *f.* Skin care
    *g.* Perineal care

**2.** To give emotional support to Mrs. U. and her parents

**3.** To teach the family to give nursing care independently of the nurse

**4.** To call the physician for further orders regarding specific care

**5.** To request sickroom supplies, such as bedding and gowns, from the Cancer Society

She saw, too, that specific objectives should be considered for Mr. K., the diabetic. These included:

**1.** To help him to understand the need for continued medical supervision of his diabetes

**2.** To help him to understand the importance of taking his insulin regularly

**3.** To help him to understand the need to do fractional tests

**4.** To teach him and Mrs. K. the use of sugar substitutes

**Visit 2** When the nurse called the next morning, she found Mrs. U. restless and apprehensive, and complaining of generalized lower abdominal pain. The nurse used this as an opportunity to demonstrate to Mrs. K. again how to assist the patient to use the bedpan on the chair by the bedside. The patient protested, saying she wished to be helped to the bathroom. The nurse explained that use of the pan would save her strength and that of her elderly parents, trying to be understanding but firm in her approach, for it was evident that soon the patient would not be able even to use the pan on the chair, but until that time it would help Mr. and Mrs. K.

Mr. and Mrs. K. had not given Mrs. U. an injection for six hours, as they were waiting for the nurse. Because of her restlessness and pain, the nurse prepared the hypodermic syringe, using it as another opportunity to demonstrate to Mr. and Mrs. K. She discovered that the parents experienced difficulty in removing air from the syringe and in maintaining sterilization. After the medication, the patient grew quiet and relaxed, and the nurse demonstrated the bath procedure to Mrs. K., emphasizing skin care, ways of turning and positioning the patient, and the care of fingernails and toenails.

In evaluating her visit later, the nurse realized that she had been pushed by a sense of time, and probably had tried to teach too much. She planned on subsequent visits to see how much the family had learned and how well they could put it into practice.

**Visit 3**   The nurse was unable to return for three days. On her arrival, Mr. and Mrs. K. were preparing to give the morphine. The nurse was encouraged on observing how well they were doing this, and complimented them. They were shyly pleased by her approval.

Mrs. U. had reddened areas over the sacrum and right shoulder. She was too tired to have a bath, so the return demonstration was deferred until the next day. In its place, massage was demonstrated, and skin care and positioning were reemphasized. The nurse noted a shortage of bed linen and gowns. Later that day, she secured four sheets, four gowns, a rubber drawsheet, and a fracture bedpan from the Cancer Society.

**Visit 4**   The nurse returned two days later, which was the day before Thanksgiving, with the equipment from the Cancer Society. Mrs. K. satisfactorily demonstrated the bed bath and the changing of the bed, and the nurse praised her skills. She still showed a fear of moving her daughter and of cleansing the painful areas. The nurse recognized that these were the feelings one had in caring for a beloved member of one's family and that since the fear of hurting may be so intense, nursing care may not always be completed. Mrs. U. needed to be handled slowly and firmly, with explanations of what was being done. She disliked using the bedpan because of the odor, and again wanted to be helped to the bathroom. In order to conserve her strength and that of her parents, the nurse explained once more the importance of using the bedpan. Mrs. U. accepted this direct approach. On this visit, perineal care, use of the pan, and nursing skills to encourage the patient to void were demonstrated.

**Visit 5**   The following Monday, the nurse arrived to find Mrs. U. emotionally upset. Mr. U. had visited her over the weekend, and while there had asked the local Catholic priest to visit Mrs. U. and administer the last rites of the Church to her, which she refused. Mr. U. wanted Pearl to return to the farm with him, but Mrs. U. insisted that Pearl must stay with her until she died and then she wanted the girl to go to live with Fred and his wife, as they would soon return to the States and had asked that Pearl live with them. Mrs. U. begged that under no circumstances was Pearl to return to the farm. The nurse realized she had been so busy teaching Mrs. K. the care of the patient that she had not arranged to see Pearl. She decided to go to the high school the next day and talk with the girl and learn her feelings about her mother's serious illness, about her father, and about going to live with her brother and his wife.

The nurse discussed eye hygiene for Mrs. U. with Mrs. K., and the importance of closing the eyes when Mrs. U. was asleep. The reddened areas over the sacrum and the shoulder had disappeared. The nurse complimented Mrs. K. on her excellent nursing care. The nurse was concerned that Mrs. U.'s respirations appeared to have Cheyne-Stokes characteristics.

As the nurse was leaving, Mr. and Mrs. K. followed her to the car to tell her they felt they would not be able to carry the strain of caring for their daughter much longer, but they could not bear to think of sending her to the county hospital where she might die alone, and what were they to do? The doctor was coming that afternoon, so the nurse suggested they ask him if he would request the Cancer Society to employ a private duty nurse to assist them temporarily.

The request was made and accepted by the Cancer Society. A private duty nurse was sent by the Cancer Society the next morning. That afternoon, Mrs. U. died at home with her family.

During her visits to Mrs. U., the nurse had talked to Mr. K. about his diabetic condition. He was not receptive at first to talking about it but finally agreed to see his doctor, which he did. He resumed his insulin and obtained the necessary tablets to do his fractional tests. The nurse secured a book of sugar-free recipes for Mrs. K. to use, and she suggested some of the sugar-free soft drinks on the market because he was so fond of them. The nurse thought that Mr. K.'s attitude toward medical supervision for himself should be explored.

In summarizing and closing Mrs. U.'s record, the nurse was aware of the relative unimportance of the nursing care she had given, except that it was a valuable tool to help her meet the tensions and emotions that this family were experiencing. Nursing care for Mrs. U. was only a small segment of the total family care, for her illness and death had an impact on every member of the family, directly or indirectly.

In summary, the family problems appeared to the nurse to be economic problems, Mr. K.'s diabetes, the health of Mrs. K., the future of Pearl, religious differences, the impact of a death of a family member, and the attitudes of each member to the death of Mrs. U., e.g., what had Mrs. U.'s illness and death meant to Mr. U.? to Fred, Ruby, and Pearl? and to Mr. and Mrs. K. and their other daughter?

The nurse regretted that she had not been able to talk with Mr. U., or Pearl, or Mrs. U.'s sister. She planned to visit Mr. K. as necessary because of his diabetic condition.

## DISCUSSION

**1.** How well did the nurse meet the objectives for this family?

**2.** In appraising this total family situation, do you feel you need additional information? If so, what further information would help you?

**3.** What evidences of family solidarity are revealed in this total family?

**4.** How do you see Mr. U.? Assume the role of the nurse, and interview Mr. U. as of that Thanksgiving weekend.

**5.** What cultural conflicts do you see in this total family?

**6.** Following the death of Mrs. U., what assistance do you think the nurse should continue to offer this family?

# 8  CASE RECORD

## Venereal Disease

**Margery X., age twenty-one, typist.**

The communicable disease division of the state department of health reported Miss Margery X. to the Ocean County Health Department as having a gonorrheal infection and as being a possible contact. It requested a visit to her and a follow-up of her contacts. Margery's address was given on the report with the specific request that she not be contacted at her home. The report also stated that Margery was under the care of her private physician, Dr. R., who had reported the case.

The community health nurse telephoned Margery at her place of employment and arranged to meet her for a conference that afternoon after work. The young woman arrived promptly as prearranged. The nurse carefully explained that she was not connected with the court in any way and that she was on the staff of the county health department, which was interested in preventing further spread of the infection that Margery had acquired. The nurse told Margery she wanted to help her and, furthermore, that she wanted Margery to help her.

When Margery was over the initial fright of the idea of the interview and understood what she could do to help the nurse in controlling the spread of the infection, she responded to the nurse's interest and friendliness. Her parents had died during her childhood, and she lived with an aunt who was very strict.

Margery told the nurse that she had been dating a young serviceman, Andy, for about two years, and that they had been intimate on several occasions. About a month ago they had had a quarrel. She did not see him for two weeks, but heard he had been dating Grace Y., a civilian employee at the base where Andy was stationed. Grace had recently returned from a three-week trip to Italy.

One Saturday evening, Andy called Margery and made up their quarrel, and later that evening they went out on a date. They were intimate during the evening. The next morning, Sunday, Andy flew to his home in another state, 2,000 miles away, to spend a thirty-day furlough. On Wednesday morning, Margery had severe urethral pain and vaginal discharge, which frightened her. That afternoon, after work, she went to her physician who diagnosed the condition as acute gonorrheal infection and started treatment immediately.

"Have you had any other sex contacts in the past thirty days?" the nurse asked. (This is a routine question in a venereal disease investigation interview.)

"No," Margery replied. "Andy is the only one I've ever dated, and since I've never had an infection before, I know there must be a third party, and I think it was that girl Andy was dating, Grace."

The nurse told Margery to write to Andy immediately and tell him to consult a doctor at home promptly, and that if he did not see a doctor, the health department would have to report him to his commanding officer at the Base, and he would be examined on returning from furlough. Margery promised to write that evening and let the nurse know as soon as she heard from him. The nurse stressed the importance of Margery's keeping up her treatments.

Three days later, Margery telephoned the nurse that Andy had called her long distance to say he had had her letter and that he had stopped off in a city en route home and had received treatment. He had telephoned Grace and told her to have an examination and secure treatment as soon as possible. He said that Grace told him that she might have contracted the infection on her recent trip to Italy.

The nurse closed Margery's case.

## DISCUSSION

**1.** What objectives did the nurse have in her work with Margery?

**2.** Do you think the nurse should have closed the case when she did? Why?

**3.** What particular skills and abilities are needed by the nurse in a venereal disease control program?

**4.** Considering the sexual behavior of the three young people exposed in this case, could you predict the possible number of contacts?

**5.** What has been the history of gonorrhea in our civilization? On a world basis, how widespread is it today?

# Alcoholism

Fred W., age twenty-nine, construction worker.

Marie W., age thirty, housewife.

Bobby W., age six, first grade pupil.

Billy W., age four, in nursery school.

The community health nursing agency's first contact with the W. family was through a school referral for Bobby by the teacher, who told the nurse that she was concerned about him as he seemed such a nervous and tense child and appeared considerably underweight. The teacher asked the nurse if she would make a home visit. The nurse observed Bobby in the classroom and agreed that a home visit would help in planning for the child. She found the family living in a small house in an average neighborhood in a new section of the city.

**Visit 1** During the visit, the mother told the nurse that Bobby slept poorly, was restless and talked in his sleep, and had frequent colds. He was not interested in food, and it was difficult to get him to eat. The family had moved many times because of the father's work. The children had not been immunized, so the nurse explained the importance of immunizations. The mother promised to take both children to the child health conference as soon as she could arrange it. The nurse discussed the children's eating habits and encouraged the mother to provide more fruits and vegetables in their diet, though the mother said, "They will never eat them." The mother was not receptive to the nurse's visit, her attitude was negative, and she gave the impression that she did not need help.

**Visit 2** Six weeks later, a case of diphtheria developed in Bobby's classroom. The nurse made another home call to determine if the children had been immunized. The mother explained that she had been too busy to attend to it, but was planning to take the children to have it done as soon as she could arrange it.

At this point, Mrs. W. started to cry. She told the nurse she was having a great deal of trouble because Mr. W. was drinking very heavily. He had been drunk most of the past week, and only that morning had been able to return to work. Finally Mrs. W. stopped crying and began to talk freely about her husband's problem and about their family background. Mrs. W. was a college graduate and had taught school for one year. The following summer, she had worked as a receptionist at a hotel in one of the national parks. While there, she met her husband at a dance and fell in love with him. They were married at the end of that summer, seven years ago, with considerable opposition from her family, who had had little to do with her since the marriage except to send the children toys and clothing at Christmas and for birthdays.

Mr. W. was raised by his maternal grandmother, who came from Prague. He had not learned to speak English until he went to school and still spoke with a marked accent. He did not complete high school, leaving to go to work when he was seventeen. He had had a good work record until he started drinking heavily about three years ago. Shortly after Billy's birth he had told his wife that she should never have married him. He said that he was sorry he had not told her before that he was an "illegitimate child" and did not know who his father was, that his mother had always refused to have anything to do with him, and therefore he did not think he was the kind of person who had any right to have children. He was bitter, also, because some of the men at work made fun of his foreign accent. "At times," Mrs. W. continued, "he comes home from work, silent, irritable, bitter, and withdrawn."

The nurse asked her how she met the situation. Mrs. W. replied that she hugged and kissed him and tried to get him to tell her what had happened, but that he became more withdrawn and usually left the house, returning at midnight—drunk.

At this point, Billy, home from nursery school, came in crying because of a slightly scratched knee. Mrs. W. hugged and kissed him vigorously and told him it was a naughty old sidewalk that scratched her baby that way. The nurse watched this interaction, wondering if Mr. W. received the same sort of treatment.

When Billy left, Mrs. W. said that a year ago she had started suit for a divorce but had withdrawn it when Mr. W. promised to stop drinking. He kept his promise for several months, but now he had begun again, she was considering divorce, and this time she would carry it through and return to teaching.

The nurse explained that it was possible that help for Mr. W. was available, and asked Mrs. W. if she had thought of seeking it for Mr. W. and for herself and the children. Mrs. W. hesitated a minute and then said she had no idea where to go. The nurse suggested their clergyman; Mrs. W. said they had no church connection because they had moved so often, but that the little boys went to a Sunday school in the next block, and perhaps she could go and talk to the minister there.

"This has been going on now for three years, and something has to be done." She paused and then said slowly, "I think now he is a real alcoholic, or soon will be."

"Could you and your husband go together to see the minister about your problems, not only the drinking, but his sense of insecurity and inadequacy?" the nurse asked. "Or perhaps he would like to go alone," she added.

The nurse then mentioned other community resources, such as the local Alcoholics Anonymous or AA group and the local Council on Alcoholism, a branch of the National Council. She inquired if these problems had been discussed with the family physician; Mrs. W.'s reply was that they did not have a family physician, and that she did not think her husband would go to see the company doctor about it. The nurse thought that was understandable, as it might jeopardize his job.

In summarizing her visit, the nurse again emphasized the need for having the children immunized. She suggested that, if possible, Mr. and Mrs. W. try to face their problems together and consider also the community clinic for alcoholics as a resource. She gave Mrs. W. the address and telephone number of each of the agencies she had mentioned, pointing out that Mr. W. would have to want to seek help and take some initiative in seeking it. The nurse said that in some instances it was helpful if man and wife went together, but that there were times also when it worked out better if they went separately. She suggested that Mrs. W. give her husband the list of resources and let him decide, as after all he was an adult and should make the decisions.

On returning to the office, the nurse talked to her supervisor about the family.

"I go to see them about a simple matter of immunization and wind up with a big problem like alcoholism, and all kinds of social problems," she said ruefully.

"That is the challenge of community health nursing," replied the supervisor. After some discussion of the family situation, the supervisor and the staff nurse agreed that perhaps a great deal could be done to help this family face their problems. The supervisor suggested that the nurse talk with the social worker at the clinic for alcoholics. The nurse made an appointment for the next day.

At the meeting with the social worker in his office, the nurse described her two visits to the W. home. The social worker pointed out that families try to hide their drinking problems from the community, and that frequently the community health nurse is the first person with whom they can face their problems. He explained that then the nurse becomes a channel between the family and the community resources. At no time, he pointed out, should the nurse feel responsible for the patient's successes or failures in meeting his problem. Her function is to take or to meet the patient where he is and give him and/or the family information relating to community resources, as well as facts regarding the dangers of alcoholism and suggestions for meeting the problems, but that the final responsibility for utilizing the available help lies with the patient and family, that they are the ones who must work at it. He explained that the alcoholic patient is frequently an egocentric person, often because of severe emotional deprivation in his early years. He has little interest in anything but himself and his own problems, and frequently is maladjusted before he ever begins to drink compulsively. Usually his personality since childhood has not developed normally because of a gradual realization of his own inadequacy and anxiety. For such a patient, the use of alcohol provides an escape from his emotional life and from his tensions, tensions which he himself does not understand.

The social worker agreed with the nurse that Mrs. W.'s "momism" and her sense of superiority because of her education and background, even though she might not be conscious of it, might be a factor in Mr. W.'s drinking, and that if they sought help at the community clinic, she would need consideration and help also. He thought that a change in her attitudes might well be a part of a constructive treatment program. It was agreed that the nurse would not visit the family, unless a crisis involving the children arose, for a couple of weeks at least, in order to give the family time to take some action on their own initiative.

Two weeks later, the social worker at the clinic notified the nurse that Mr. and Mrs. W. had made an appointment and kept it. About a month later, the teacher reported to the nurse that Bobby seemed much better and was showing progress in his school work. Occasionally, the nurse met Mrs. W. on the street or in the shopping center. She told the nurse that the children had completed their immunizations and that Mr. W. was fine and working steadily.

Nearly three months later, the community clinic for alcoholism called the nurse to say the W. family had missed their last two appointments, and to ask if there was some sort of crisis in the family. The nurse telephoned Mrs. W. to make an appointment for a home visit for the following day, but Mrs. W. asked her if she could come that morning.

**Visit 3**  Mrs. W. said that things had been going well with them until about three weeks ago when Mr. W. had some difficulty at work with a fellow employee. That evening he came home morose and withdrawn and refused to play with the children as he had been in the habit of doing lately; he had even knocked little Billy down when the child persisted in wanting to play with him. A little later, without waiting for dinner, Mr. W. went out, returning about midnight, and it was evident that he had been drinking. On the next day, Friday, on his way home from nursery school, Billy was run over by a car, receiving serious head injuries. The child was improving but was still hospitalized. On that evening, following the accident, Mr. W. left the house and was gone for two days. He apparently drank very heavily, for when he came home he was so remorseful and self-incriminating that his wife felt she could not take it; she was thinking of a divorce again. The nurse pointed out that perhaps Mr. W. had had more tensions than he could take. She told Mrs. W. that she had strengths and had learned to recognize the problem, and that a supportive attitude on her part could probably help Mr. W. at this time. Mrs. W. thought for a few minutes; then she said that she believed she and her husband could work out their problems more satisfactorily now, and that they would ask for another clinic appointment.

The nurse asked for a conference with her supervisor shortly after this visit, as she was somewhat disturbed by Mrs. W.'s talk of divorce and considered this a punitive action on her part.

In their discussion, the supervisor raised the point that quite possibly Mrs. W. was being punitive but that this might be a normal human reaction in relation to all she had gone through, that it might be something that could be expected. Would it be wise to accept the fact that the wife cannot be nonjudgmental at this point and recognize her frustration? On the other hand, the nurse might ask her to delay thinking of the divorce a little longer, as sometimes a family crisis like Billy's accident can help to resolve a situation such as the W. family was facing. Mr. W. should really want to go to the clinic for help, not to please his wife or to avoid the divorce but because he recognized his need for help. The staff nurse agreed and realized that this would be a helpful course of action.

Soon after this episode, the nurse resigned from the staff, but the agency maintained a contact with the W. family for several years; during this period Mr. W. had a few lapses, but as time went by they were less frequent. He learned and accepted the fact that it was not illegal to be born, and that the illegality rested on the parents, not on the child. He came to look more tolerantly on his Eastern European heritage, and slowly grew more mature emotionally. He joined Alcoholics Anonymous, became friends with those who had similar problems, and read widely on the nature and causes of alcoholism.

Mrs. W. learned to be more tolerant also, less judgmental and aggressive. She became less maternal and possessive toward her husband, and assumed more of the role of a wife. She joined the Alonon group in her community, which she found helpful. She, too, read widely on the nature and causes of alcoholism. She came to realize, to a degree, that perhaps her attitudes toward her husband had heightened his emotional problems and tensions, and the demands of these tensions contributed to his alcoholism as a means of escape.

## DISCUSSION

1. What evidences of family solidarity did you note in the W. family?

2. Do you think it might have been better for Mrs. W. and the boys if she had been encouraged to go ahead with her divorce? Why?

3. What does the nurse contribute to the alcoholic patient and his family by having a nonjudgmental attitude?

4. What knowledge and philosophy does a community health nurse need in order to work effectively with an alcoholic patient and the family?

5. If the W. family lived in your district, what community organizations could you suggest to them for help?

# 10  CASE RECORD

## Cuban Refugee Family

Mr. F., age forty, laborer.
Mrs. F., age thirty-five, mother.
Manuel, age fifteen.
Tito, age fourteen.
Rosita, age twelve.
Carlos, age seven, patient (cerebral palsy).
Maria, age five.
Juan, age three.
Panchita, new baby.

The F. family, Cuban refugees, was referred by their social worker to the nursing service of the city-county health department. She reported that Mrs. F., about seven months pregnant, had been in the county hospital for a week because of high blood pressure, and was being discharged that day. The social worker said the parents spoke little English. They were living in a three-bedroom apartment in a large public housing complex. The family was Protestant.

**Visit 1**  The nurse made a home visit the next day. Talking in broken Spanish and English with Mr. and Mrs. F., the nurse learned that the family had been in the United States less than a year. In Cuba, Mr. F. had made a fairly comfortable living as a fisherman and had had additional employment in a factory. The family escaped from Cuba in Mr. F.'s small fishing boat, which was wrecked off the Florida coast. Two of their children were lost in the accident. After a short stay in Miami, the family moved to the West Coast. At the time of the nurse's visit, Mr. F. did not have steady employment and the family had been on welfare for three months. The three elder children attended a nearby grade school but were not doing well because of language difficulties.

During the visit, the nurse became aware of strange gutteral sounds and an unusual crying. Mrs. F. finally left the room and returned with Carlos in her arms. The child was undersized, emaciated, unable to walk, and had uncontrolled head movements. The nurse thought he had a cerebral palsy condition. Throughout the visit, Maria and Juan clung, whimpering, to their mother and watched the nurse fearfully.

The nurse reviewed the doctor's orders for Mrs. F. regarding diet and rest with Mr. and Mrs. F. and felt there was little more she could do at the time because of language difficulties. She promised to return in a week. As she was leaving, the Protestant minister arrived. The nurse explained to him that her knowledge of Spanish was insufficient for her to help the family as she wished to do, and asked if there were someone who might act as interpreter. He suggested Mrs. L., a neighbor who spoke English and Spanish fluently and would be acceptable to the family.

*Later*  The nurse called on Mrs. L., a friendly young woman of Spanish-American descent. She said she and her husband felt sorry for the F. family. Her husband had tried to help Mr. F. find work, but his lack of knowledge of English made it difficult. Mrs. L. worked part-time in a neighborhood grocery store. She said if the nurse could arrange her visits to the family when she was free, she would do all she could to help. She gave the nurse her telephone number.

*Later*  The nurse reported to the social worker, who had not known of Carlos' condition. She offered to work with the nurse in getting him to the children's clinic for a diagnosis.

*Later*  The nurse telephoned the school nurse, who reported the children were absent a great deal and were seriously handicapped in their school work by their lack of English. The teachers were concerned and wished the children could have extra help in learning English.

**Visit 2**  With Mrs. L.'s help, the nurse had arranged for another visit to the family a week later. With an interpreter, the nurse found it easier to build interpersonal relationships. She discovered Mrs. F. had been eating some foods not on her prescribed diet, but thought this resulted from a misunderstanding. With Mrs. L.'s help, she was able to explain the importance of following the doctor's orders. The nurse told the parents that the social worker had made a tentative appointment for Carlos at the children's clinic the latter part of the next week if they could take him at that time. The parents quickly agreed, and Mrs. L. said she would either take them herself or find someone who could provide transportation.

*Later*  The nurse confirmed the appointment with the social worker and notified Mrs. L.

Because of unusual pressure of work in the agency, the nurse was unable to visit the family for two weeks. However, she telephoned Mrs. L., who said the family had taken Carlos to the clinic and that institutional care had been recommended for him. The family was given an application to River Falls, a state school for handicapped children about 20 miles away. A neighbor had taken them to visit the school and they were satisfied that Carlos would have good care there, and they were eager to file an application and wanted the nurse's help in filling it out. Several days later, Mrs. L. phoned to say that Mrs. F. had been taken to the hospital by ambulance, and had had a baby girl by cesarian section. Mrs. F.'s condition was good and she was expected home in a few days.

*Later*   The school nurse telephoned that the F. children had been absent for several days and wanted to know if they were ill. The nurse explained that Mrs. F. was in the hospital for delivery and thought it was possible Mr. F. had kept them at home. She planned a visit soon and would let the school nurse know if the children were ill.

The nurse learned that a summer "head start" program would begin soon at the school and that Maria would be eligible and also that there were plans to offer English classes for the foreign-born at the school building in the evenings during the summer.

**Visit 3**   When the nurse and Mrs. L. called they found the children had returned to school. Mr. F. had kept them at home during Mrs. F.'s hospitalization because he was lonely and afraid. With the help of their minister, they had filled out Carlos' application for River Falls, had mailed it and were waiting to hear from the institution. The nurse explained the "head start" program for Maria and the English classes for the parents and older children. Mrs. F.'s condition appeared good. She was obviously trying hard to follow the doctor's orders and the prescribed diet. Panchita appeared to be a normal, healthy baby.

**Visit 4**   A few days later, as the nurse was in the neighborhood, she stopped to see Mrs. F. and check on her clinic appointments. When Maria saw the nurse, she ran out the door and soon returned with Mrs. L. Mrs. F. showed the nurse a letter from River Falls to the effect that Carlos was on the waiting list, and that there would be a place for him in about a month. Mrs. L. and Mrs. F. had a conversation in rapid Spanish. Then Mrs. L. explained that Mr. and Mrs. F. felt that they should not have any more children, and could the nurse tell them of a clinic where they could go for help. The nurse explained about the Planned Parenthood clinic and gave Mrs. F. a card to the clinic. The nurse arranged for a call about a month later.

**Visit 5**   Mr. and Mrs. F. were home when the nurse called. Mr. F. had found work as a fisherman and thought it would be permanent. He had arranged for time off so that he could be home when the nurse called. Manuel and Jose had summer jobs, thanks to Mrs. L.'s help and that of their minister. Carlos had been admitted to River Falls. A neighbor had taken them to visit him, and they were happy with the care he was receiving. They and the older children were attending the evening classes and Maria was enrolled in the "head start" program. The parents had attended the Planned Parenthood clinic. Mr. F. hoped they would be able to go off welfare the following month. The nurse urged Mrs. F. to take the preschool children to the children's clinic for immunizations. It appeared to the nurse that this family had achieved a certain amount of independence and could probably handle future health problems. She left her card and asked the family to call the nursing service if a need arose.

*Later* The nurse reported to the social worker and the school nurse that she had closed the case, as Mr. and Mrs. F. now seemed able to manage their own situation. Case closed.

## DISCUSSION

**1.** What resources did this family appear to have within itself?

**2.** What emotional problems might you expect this family to have as a result of their experiences since leaving Cuba?

**3.** Should the nurse have closed the case when she did? Why?

# 11    CASE RECORD

# Rediscovery of a Tuberculous Patient

Mr. D., age fifty-two, bartender.
Mrs. D., age thirty-three, waitress, former tuberculous patient.
Perry H., age fifteen, tuberculous patient.

Perry H. had lived with his maternal grandfather and stepgrandmother since babyhood. The grandparents had a fairly adequate pension to live on, but not enough to provide for emergencies.

At the urging of the school nurse, who was concerned with Perry's weight loss and persistent cough, the grandparents took him to the city tuberculosis clinic. It was known that his mother had had tuberculosis. A few days later, a diagnosis of moderately advanced active tuberculosis with positive sputum was made and Perry was admitted to the tuberculosis unit of the county hospital.

Perry's own parents were divorced, and the grandfather had not heard from his daughter for five years but believed she was living at a certain address in A., a city about a hundred miles away. Nothing was known of the whereabouts of his father.

The chief of the tuberculosis clinic notified the health officer in A. of Perry's diagnosis and requested a visit to his mother, if possible, to inform her of Perry's condition. The request was referred to the nursing bureau. A staff nurse made a home visit to the last known address of Perry's mother, an old apartment building. The landlord said she had remarried and that the last address he had for her was a small hotel on the waterfront. A check of old files in the A. city health department revealed that Perry's mother had been a patient in the county tuberculosis hospital for ten months, six years previously. She had been given a weekend pass, but had not returned; her status was AWOL. There was some question as to whether she was an alcoholic.

After several attempts, the nurse located Mrs. D. living with her second husband on the third floor of an old waterfront hotel. They occupied a single room with housekeeping facilities. The room was exceptionally clean and neat and had good light and ventilation. Both Mr. and Mrs. D. were home when the nurse called about three in the afternoon. Mr. D. said he was just leaving, but would return in half an hour.

Mrs. D. had just arrived home from work. She was a tall, slender woman, neat in appearance, and friendly, although the nurse noted that her eyes constantly roamed about the room and that at times she seemed out of contact, yet she answered questions easily and frankly. When she heard of Perry's diagnosis, she was shocked and remarked that her own mother had died from tuberculosis and that her family had "weak lungs."

Mrs. D. was startled when the nurse told her she was considered AWOL from the tuberculosis hospital. She said it was her understanding that she left with permission and that her sputum was negative. She added that she had had no symptoms of tuberculosis since leaving and that recently she had begun to gain weight and that her appetite was excellent. She had had no follow-up since leaving the sanatorium. She commented that she learned two things while in the sanatorium: (1) to get plenty of rest; and (2) to eat an adequate diet at regular intervals. The nurse thought she must have lived by these two rules and that could be the reason the disease had not been reactivated.

When Mr. D. returned, Mrs. D. told him of Perry's hospitalization, that she, too, had been a tuberculous patient at one time, and that she was sorry now she had not told him. He said it was all right and that he had not told her of his medical problems either. Mr. D. was neat and clean in appearance, with a shy but kindly manner.

The nurse discussed the general nature and communicability of tuberculosis with Mr. and Mrs. D., making the following points:

1. That it is caused by an organism too small to see

2. That the disease itself is not inherited

3. That it can become inactive

4. That it is a chronic disease in the sense that it takes a long time to recover from it, and then may reactivate after a period of inactivity

5. That it is communicable and anyone can contract it

The nurse thought that Mrs. D. had had a severe emotional shock on learning of Perry's illness and of her own health situation. The nurse made an appointment for another visit a few days later. In the meantime, Mrs. D. would telephone her father.

On her return to the office, the nurse discussed the case with her supervisor and the chief of the tuberculosis clinic. Since Mrs. D. had been

known to the tuberculosis clinic as an active case six years before, arrangements were made for her to attend the chest diagnosis clinic at the health
department. Mrs. D. belonged to a group health plan and she was entitled
to have work done at their clinics on a part-pay basis. It was suggested that
she have follow-up medical care there also when her diagnosis had been
established. Mrs. D. was anxious to clear her status with the health department, where she had had a food handler's examination under her current
name. That examination had been negative. She had told no one of her
previous hospitalization.

Mr. D. was not home when the nurse called a few days later. The
nurse's objective was to give Mrs. D. support in following through with her
examinations. Mrs. D. had attended the group health clinic and had completed most of the diagnostic work there, except for a gastric analysis,
which would be finished the following day.

In succeeding visits, the nurse worked closely with Mrs. D. and gave
her needed encouragement. Mrs. D. was able to verbalize her feelings regarding tuberculosis. She had many fears and qualms over her status with
the health department, thinking that they might cause her to lose her waitress work. On some visits, she appeared to the nurse to repress her feelings
as though trying to deny any knowledge of tuberculosis and her relation to
it.

Mrs. D. showed a growing interest in Perry. At first the nurse wondered
if this was in order to secure her approval, but then she saw that Mrs. D. was
genuinely interested in her son and sorry for her years of neglect. Several
times she grew emotional over this. When present, Mr. D. supported the
nurse's suggestions and encouraged Mrs. D. in many little ways.

Mrs. D. had lost custody of Perry "because I was considered an unfit
mother." On the nurse's final visit, both Mr. D. and Mrs. D. wanted to know
if it would be possible for them to gain Perry's custody, although they were
currently unable, financially, to take legal action. The nurse referred them
to the legal aid society for advice. At this visit, Mrs. D. said that she had
received a friendly letter from her father, and he reported Perry was making
satisfactory progress.

The problems relating to tuberculosis that Mr. and Mrs. D. had encountered seemed to the nurse to have brought them closer together. Mrs. D. was
asked to keep in touch with the health department for future checkups, and
the nurse felt she would cooperate. The case was closed.

## DISCUSSION

1. What positive factors did the nurse have to work with in this case?
2. What dangers did she have to watch for?
3. Do you consider Mrs. D. a liability in her community?

Mr. H., age twenty-six, laundry driver.
Mrs. H., age twenty-three, housewife.
Tommie, age four months.
A student nurse made the visit described here.
She wished to do a self-evaluation of her call,
and wrote it up on a process recording basis.

**Purpose of visit**   On my previous visit I had
suggested that Mrs. H. attend the well-baby
clinic with Tommie, which she did. On this visit
I planned to discuss the clinic experience and
any problems that Mrs. H. might have in caring
for her baby.

**Introduction**   Mr. and Mrs. H. are high school
graduates and have been married for two
years. They are buying their home, which is in
an old part of the city, in a middle-class neighborhood and close to a college where Mr. H.
attends night school. He hopes to be a certified public accountant some day. Prior to her
marriage, Mrs. H. worked for the telephone
company. She is an intelligent young woman,
eager to learn to care for her first child.

**The visit**   Mrs. H. greeted me warmly at the
door, but then her facial expression became
one of grave concern. After we were seated,
Mrs. H. opened the conversation.

# 12 CASE RECORD

# Infant
# Health
# Supervision

| Mother-Nurse Verbal and Nonverbal Exchange and Interaction | Nurse Comments and Analysis |
|---|---|
| *Mrs. H.:* Last week at the well-child clinic, the doctor took my baby's diaper and handed it to the nurse. He told her to do a PKU test. At the time I didn't think to ask him what that meant, but I have been wondering: does this mean he thinks something is wrong with my baby? | Mrs. H. was obviously quite anxious about this test and the baby's health. I wondered if the test were the real cause of her anxiety or if she had some other reason for inquiring. I needed more information before answering her question. |
| *Nurse:* You're concerned about your baby's health? | This reinterpretation would allow Mrs. H. to expand upon the problem further, and allow me to evaluate it. |

349

*Mrs. H.:* Yes, I am. [Silence, but she seemed to want to say more.]

I nodded, telling her nonverbally to go on.

*Mrs. H.:* You see I've been leaving the window open in the bedroom at night because the baby's been perspiring so much. My husband keeps telling me the baby is going to get sick sleeping in that draft, and I knew deep down he was right. When I went to the clinic I was afraid the doctor would find something wrong with him.

It seems Mrs. H. may feel guilty that she might have caused an illness in her baby. Before clarifying her first question I wanted information about the general condition of her baby in order to relieve her fears.

*Nurse:* I see.

This was said in an understanding tone to let her know that I understood her explanation.

*Nurse:* What did the doctor say about Tommie's health?

I wanted to ascertain if the baby had a cold or other symptoms that could be related to the draft.

*Mrs. H.:* Oh, he said the baby was in absolutely perfect health and gaining weight.

The mother smiled for the first time —she seemed very pleased.

*Nurse:* That's fine, Mrs. H.

I shared in her delight and showed my approval.

*Mrs. H.* (her face clouded): I was so happy until I came home and remembered that PKU test. What does it mean?

She still may have connected the test with the draft in the bedroom, and now was the time to clarify this misunderstanding of her initial question.

*Nurse:* Do you remember, Mrs. H., when you had your chest x-ray at the health department?

I knew she had had an x-ray for tuberculosis.

*Mrs. H.* (puzzled): Yes, but that was a routine check for TB. My baby doesn't have TB, does he?

I was going to use this to correlate it with her baby's test, and I accepted her momentary puzzlement.

*Nurse:* No, but you see, just as you had a routine x-ray to check for tuberculosis, so the PKU test is a routine check for a disease in children called phenylketonuria.

I was going from the known (her own x-ray) to the unknown, the PKU test, so that she could understand better.

*Mrs. H.:* What does that mean?

Mother wants more explanation.

*Nurse:* Well, remember when we talked about the importance of protein, fats, and sugar foods in the diet?

*Mrs. H.:* Yes, I understand that.

*Nurse:* This disease is concerned with proteins. Before they can be used to build strong bodies they have to be broken down to smaller parts, and to do this there is a substance called an enzyme. Do you understand so far?

*Mrs. H.:* Yes, I think I do. What you're saying is that a substance breaks proteins down in order to give my baby a strong body.

*Nurse* (smiling): That's right. In the disease phenylketonuria this substance, or enzyme, that breaks down a particular part of the protein isn't there and can't be used by the body. Therefore this part of the protein keeps building up in the body and can cause brain damage. Some of it comes out in the baby's urine, too, and that's one way to know if the baby has the disease. Do you understand so far?

*Mrs. H.:* I see, then this is what the nurse was testing for?

*Nurse:* That's right.

*Mrs. H.:* Can the nurse do the test there, or did she take something off the diaper and send it somewhere?

*Nurse:* No, they do the test right away at the clinic. Do you remember when your mother stayed with you after she was told she had diabetes and you did her urinalysis for her—

Again, I attempted to enable the mother to recall what she knew in order to help her understand this condition.

She was eager for me to go on and I now knew she was following and understanding my explanation so far.

This feedback from Mrs. H. was evidence that she understood and was able to relate her learning to incident concerning the baby.

I wanted to show my approval.

I was explaining it in lay terms, but before proceeding I asked for indication of her understanding.

Again, feedback from Mrs. H. showed she understood.

I smiled to show my approval.

It seemed she was worried that she might be informed later about the test, and was concerned about whether her baby had the condition.

Again going from the known to the unknown and using my knowledge of family history.

and how the urine changed color after you dropped the tablet into the tube?

*Mrs. H.* (with interest): Yes.

*Nurse:* They tested the baby's urine like that. They drop a testing solution on a small spot on a wet diaper, and if the spot turns green, they know the baby has the disease. That is, they are pretty sure of it.

Using correlation in explanation.

*Mrs. H.:* Then my baby doesn't have it, because the nurse brought the diaper back, smiled at me, and didn't say anything. Come to think of it, it was after the nurse talked to the doctor that he came back and said Tommie was in perfect health. Oh! I feel so much better now that I understand it wasn't the draft that had anything to do with this.

Evidence she understood the test; she seemed happy—perhaps in knowing that the draft had caused no harm.

There was marked relief in her voice. I nodded.

My suspicions were confirmed, and this was the opportunity to deal with the draft problem, which I did.

**Summary** Although Mrs. H. was concerned about the test for PKU, her concern stemmed from her guilt feelings about the draft. By allowing the mother to talk further about her feelings and not answering the question directly at the beginning of the visit, I found a problem that could be dealt with. After answering Mrs. H.'s questions about the test, I focused on the draft problem. It was discovered that Mrs. H. had kept the four wool blankets she had used during the winter months on Tommie's bed. She had not removed any of the blankets with the approaching spring weather, and this was the reason for the baby's perspiration. Hence the open window, which was creating a draft, would not be necessary if some of the blankets were removed. This action served two purposes: first, alleviating the draft on the baby, and second, alleviating the guilt feeling of Mrs. H. that she might cause the baby illness. Mrs. H. was pleased and happy at the end of the visit and appeared relieved. From the course of the discussion, Mrs. H. now also understood something about PKU. I planned to discuss it further with her next time so that she would be a well-informed mother regarding this current problem.

## DISCUSSION

**1.** What purposes did this visit serve?

**2.** What principles of learning did this nurse utilize?

**3.** What concomitant learning is it reasonable to hope took place?

**4.** How does the process recording method help in self-evaluation?

**5.** Should or should not the nurse have completed the discussion of PKU (e.g., incidence, symptoms, treatment, and problems) on this visit? Why?

Alcoholism, 217–219
  case record, 336–341
  case situation, 290–291
American Red Cross, 264–265

Cancer, case record, 327–333
Case records:
  alcoholism, 336–341
  cancer, 327–333
  heart disease and stroke, 298–301
  process recording in home visit, 349–353
  rehabilitation, 298–301, 302–305
  tuberculosis, 323–326, 346–348
  typhoid, 318–322
  venereal disease, 334–335
Case situations:
  alcoholism, 290–291
  diabetes, 282–283
  drug abuse, 296–297
  mental illness, 294–295
  venereal disease, 289
Children's Bureau:
  division of HEW, 265
  founded, 263
Chronic degenerative diseases and death,
    223–225
  diet in disease, 207–212
Communicable diseases:
  tuberculosis, case records, 323–326,
    346–348
  typhoid, case record, 318–322
Communication (*see* Groups; Interview;
    Learning; Teaching)
Community, the:
  characteristics and health practices of,
    74–87
  defined, 75
  organization process, 83–85
  social classes in, 80–82
Community health, 3
  six basic functions of, 3–4, 10
  trends in, 272–273
  United States Constitution and, 8–9

Community health nurse:
  functions of, 118–123
  services of, 22
  selected concerns of, 214–234
Community health nursing:
  agencies:
    combination, 20–21, 266
    health department nursing
      service, 19–20
    specialized nursing services,
      20
    support, responsibilities, and
      programs, 14–17
    visiting nurse agencies, 17–19
  concepts of practice, 5
  defined, 4–5
  functions and setting, 6–8
  history of, 258–267
  philosophy of, 273–274
  precepts of, 23–36
  trends, 267–272
Concomitant learning, 177–178
Consultation, use of, 71–72

Department of Health, Education
  and Welfare (HEW):
  Children's Bureau, 265
  Public Health Service, 9
Departments of health:
  local, 10–12
  state, 10
Diabetes, 207–210
  case situation, 282–283
Diet in disease, 207–212
Drug abuse, 219–221
  case situation, 296–297

Ecologic health problems,
  225–226
Elderly, the:
  consumer groups, 227–229
  diet problems, 205–207

Family, the, 89–116
  defined, 89
  factors in assessing, 128–130
  function of, 95–99
  representing cultural groups,
    106–109
    cultural gap, 108–109
    cultural shock, 107–108
    families:
      black, 109–113
      Indian, 113–115
      other cultural groups,
        115–116
    meaning of culture, 106–107
  representing socioeconomic
    groups, 99–108
    low income, 99–104
    middle and high income,
      104–108
  systems approach, 90–93
Fee schedules, 131–133

Goodrich, Annie W., 264, 265,
  274
Groups, working with, 59–65
  criteria for growth, 65
  group discussion, 183–184
  group process, 62–63
  techniques in leading, 63–65

Health officer, responsibilities, 16
Health team, 66
Heart disease and stroke:
  case record, 298–301
  diet in, 210–211
Hill, Octavia, 260
  philosophy of, 273–274
Home visit, 118–167
  case finding and referral,
    154–156
  closing and recording visit,
    156–159

Home visit (*cont'd*):
  components of, 123
  contract with family, 125–126
  nurse's introduction to family,
    124–125
  nursing process, 126–165
    assessment, 126–130
      nursing diagnosis, 130–131
    evaluating, 159–165
    implementing, 148–159
    planning, 134–148
    preparation for, 123–124
    process recording, 162–163
    case record, 349–353
Howard, John, prison reform, 260
Human sexuality, 215–217

Interdisciplinary personnel, 66–70
International health organizations:

  Food and Agricultural
    Organization (FAO), 14
  International Council of Nurses,
    272

  International Red Cross, 260

  World Health Organization
    (WHO), 13, 272
Interview, 184–189
  concerns of interviewer, 188
  defined, 185
  evaluation of, 187–188
  teaching techniques in, 184–189
  with venereal disease patient,
    187

Koch, Robert, 261

Learning, 173–178
  barriers to, 189–191
  concomitant, 177–178
  principles of, 173–177
Local departments of health,
    10–12

Mead, Margaret, 196
Medicare and Medicaid, 133–134,
    166, 264
Mental health, 221–222
Mental illness, case situation,
    294–295
Milio, Nancy, 37, 79, 113

National League for Nursing, 264
National Organization for Public
    Health Nursing, 264
Nightingale, Florence, 18–19, 23
Nursing, defined, 4
*Nursing Outlook,* founded, 264
*Nursing Research,* founded, 266
Nursing studies, 266
Nutrition, 194–213
  diet in disease, 207–212
  needs:
    of elderly, 205–207
    of infants, preschool, and
      school children, 202–203
    of middle aged, 205
    of pregnant and lactating
      mothers, 198–201
    special health problems,
      201
    superstitions, 201
    of teen-agers, 203–205
  purposes of adequate diet,
    195–196

Phenylketonuria (PKU), 211–212
Public health (*see* Community
    health)
Public health nursing (*see*
    Community health nursing)
Public Health Service, 9

Rathbone, William, 260
  early precepts of community
    health nursing, 23

Rehabilitation, 270–271
  case records, 298–301,
    302–305
Relationship skills in community
    health nursing, 38–45
  coordination of interdisciplinary
    personnel, 66–70
  interpersonal approaches, 45–54
  therapeutic relationship skills,
    54–56
  use of consultation, 71–72
  working with families and
    groups, 56–65
Rogers, Carl, 41–42, 193

Sheahan, Marion, philosophy of
    community health nursing,
    274
Social legislation:
  Children's Bureau, 263
  Medicare and Medicaid,
    133–134, 166, 264
  Sheppard-Towner Act, 263
  Social Security Act, 22, 263
State departments of health, 10
Statistics, 235–257
  concepts and techniques,
    237–238
  data, 236–237
    analysis of, 243–251
    collection of, 239–241
    graphical presentation of,
      241–243
    measurement, 251–256
    sources of, 236–237
    tabulation of, 241
    types of, 238–239
  defined, 236
Suicide, 222–223

Teaching:
  components for success,
    172–173
  philosophy of, 192
  plan for, 178–179
  techniques, 178–192
    demonstration, 180–182
    group discussion, 183–184
    interview, 184–189
    lecture, 180
    problem solving (or inquiry),
      49–54, 182–183
Tuberculosis, case records,
    323–326, 346–348
Typhoid, case record, 318–322

Vincent de Paul, St.:
  basic precepts of community
    health nursing, 23
  philosophy of service, 259–260
Venereal diseases:
  interview, 187
  case record, 334–335
  case situation, 289

Wald, Lillian, 20, 262, 263, 264,
    275
Working with individuals, 45–54
  approach:
    goal-oriented, 52–54
    interpersonal, 45–46
    mutual, 46–47
    problem-solving, 49–54
    strengthening, 47–49

Youth groups,
  diet needs, 203–205
  special concerns for, 229–233